CW01066479

current
nursing
practice

Applied Nutrition and Dietetics

Current Nursing Practice titles

Already published

Accident and Emergency Nursing
Ear, Nose and Throat Nursing
Neuromedical and Neurosurgical Nursing
Plastic Surgical and Burns Nursing

In preparation

Anaesthesia and Recovery Room Techniques
Ophthalmic Nursing
Orthopaedic Nursing

Applied Nutrition and Dietetics

Joan Huskisson BSc (Hons) Dietetics

Part-time Lecturer in Nutrition
Medical School
University of Cape Town, Cape Town
and Lecturer in Nutrition and Dietetics
Cape Technikon, Cape Town

Second edition

Baillière Tindall London Philadelphia Toronto
Mexico City Rio de Janeiro Sydney Tokyo Hong Kong

Baillière Tindall   1 St Anne's Road
W.B. Saunders   Eastbourne, East Sussex BN21 3UN, England

West Washington Square
Philadelphia, PA 19105, USA

1 Goldthorne Avenue
Toronto, Ontario M8Z 5T9, Canada

Apartado 26370—Cedro 512
Mexico 4, DF, Mexico

Rua Evaristo da Veiga, 55, 20° andar
Rio de Janeiro—RJ, Brazil

ABP Australia Ltd, 44–50 Waterloo Road
North Ryde, NSW 2064, Australia

Ichibancho Central Building, 22–1 Ichibancho
Chiyoda-ku, Tokyo 102, Japan

10/fl, Inter-Continental Plaza, 94 Granville Road
Tsim Sha Tsui East, Kowloon, Hong Kong

First edition published as a Nurses' Aids Series Special Interest Text under the title *Nutrition and Dietetics in Health and Disease* 1981
Second edition 1985

Typeset by M.C. Typeset, Chatham, Kent
Printed in Great Britain by Biddles Ltd of Guildford

British Library Cataloguing in Publication Data

Huskisson, Joan, M.
  Applied nutrition and dietetics.—(Current
  nursing practice)
  1. Nursing   2. Diet in disease
  I. Title   II. Huskisson, Joan M. Nutrition
  and dietetics in health and disease   III. Series
  613.2′024613   RT87.N87

ISBN 0–7020–1101–0

Contents

Every careful observer of the sick will agree in this that thousands of patients are annually starved in the midst of plenty, from want of attention to the ways which alone make it possible for them to take food.

Florence Nightingale in *Notes on Nursing*, first published by Harrison and Sons, 1859, reprinted by Gerald Duckworth and Company Ltd., 1970.

Preface to the second edition

Nutrition, like many other sciences, has made major strides forward in recent years.

Vitamins as a class of nutrients were unknown before this century and insulin was only isolated in 1922.

The Space Age has brought with it remarkable advances in unrelated fields of knowledge and technology, and inventiveness and achievement are also reflected in the products on supermarket shelves.

Hence it is essential to question and update facts and information of even a few years ago — the objective of this edition. New details have been included and a change of emphasis is applied where necessary. For example, the current trend of referring to a variety of convenience foods as 'junk foods' emphasizes the need to look at this subject in some depth, and to recognize both the disadvantages and the merits of this widespread practice of eating. Furthermore, the role of diet in the causation of migraine headaches (a condition suffered by nearly one in ten people in Britain) and cancer has become more prominent. Recent references have been added at the end of each chapter.

Two extremely relevant chapters have been added. In the first place, the subject of anaemia is comprehensively discussed in the new chapter on haematological disorders. Anaemia is widespread in the Third World, as a result of nutritional deficiencies and parasitic infestation, as well as in the most sophisticated and developed areas. In the latter countries, causes include the increasing tendency to vegetarianism as well as the escalating cost of meat and other sources of significant nutrients. It is thus appropriate to devote attention to the causes, problems and treatment of this condition.

The second additional chapter is devoted to the practical nursing problems associated with the provision of optimal nutrition to hospital patients. The day-to-day feeding of patients both with and without physical or mental handicaps and the efficient administration of special diets is fully discussed. This chapter has been contributed by Vivien Coates, a practising nurse with a special interest in nutrition.

In keeping with the new format, a summary of nursing considerations has been listed at the end of several chapters.

Wherefore I say that such constitutions as suffer quickly and strongly from errors in diet are weaker than others that do not, and that a weak person is in a state very nearly approaching to one in disease . . . And this I know, moreover, that to the human body it makes a great difference whether the bread be fine or coarse, of wheat with or without the hull . . . whoever pays no attention to these things, or paying attention does not comprehend them, how can he understand the diseases which befall man. For every one of these things, whether in health, convalescence or disease, nothing else can be more important or more necessary than to know these things.

HIPPOCRATES

Acknowledgements

I wish to acknowledge the help of the following specialists and express my appreciation to them for reading and commenting on the sections related to their subjects. I am indebted to them for their constructive criticism and helpful guidance. They are: Professor M. Berger, F. Bonnici, J. Dommisse, W. Gevers, R. Kirsch, Dr. S. O'Keefe and Professor R. van Zyl-Smit.

My grateful thanks are extended to Mrs Nan Oosthuizen for secretarial help and to Mrs Phyl Greenwood for painstakingly reading the manuscript and her attention to linguistic details.

Finally, my family: I wish to record my appreciation to my husband, Ian, who has, as always, given me his unfailing support and help. Our daughters, Sally, Janet and Nikki, have encouraged me with their enthusiasm and interest in this project, and for this I thank them. I also thank my father, Professor G.M. Dreosti, for his guidance and helpful advice.

JOAN M. HUSKISSON

I Normal nutrition

1 The components of food

Ever since Adam and Eve ate the apple from the tree of life in the Garden of Eden, food has been endowed by Man with attributes far beyond the known nutritional properties. Throughout history, Man's relationship to food has been emotional and mystical. Grain and pottery food-holders have been found in old Egyptian tombs, and we read that in early times specific foods were blamed for the passions and deeds of men. To a large extent food has shaped the history of the world. Ships sank and men drowned attempting to find spices to enhance the flavour of their meals, and colonies — such as the Cape of Good Hope — were started to combat scurvy. The science and practice of nutrition and dietetics has come a long way since those early days, and, although quackery and misconceptions still abound, the many known basic principles of the subject form the background for a scientific approach to foods and feeding.

With regard to the individual it is not an overstatement to suggest that both body and mind reflect one's level of nutrition. In the absence of adequate intakes of essential nutrients, body tissue, bones and metabolic processes will be affected, impairing one's feeling of well-being, one's attitudes, and one's physical and mental development.

Nutrition is the study of food (and the properties of its constituents, including digestion, metabolism and utilization), and the conversion of food to living tissues by the body.

Dietetics refers to the modification of the intake of food according to the pathological requirements of the individual who is ill.

The normal diet has certain basic constituents. Energy and tissue materials are derived from fats, carbohydrates and protein, whereas vitamins and minerals — the two other essential classes of nutrients — are generally body process regulators or microcomponents, not energy providers. Water is also an essential dietary component. Alcohol (ethanol) is an energy source but cannot be classed as a nutrient.

ENERGY

Energy is required for

1. basal metabolism (maintaining life),
2. voluntary exercise and activity,
3. additional needs such as growth.

Energy is derived from the oxidation of carbohydrates, fats, proteins and alcohol in the diet. The bodily reserves of these substances are present in the liver and muscle as glycogen, but the vast majority occur in adipose tissue. Energy production is defined in terms of kilojoules (kJ). (This unit has replaced the Calorie.) One gram (g) of protein or carbohydrate yields 16.5 kJ, 1 g of fat yields 37.5 kJ, and 1 g of alcohol yields 29 kJ. The kilojoule is the preferred term today, although many food tables in international use still give the energy content of food in terms of Calories.

The *Calorie* (Cal) is a unit of heat measurement and is the amount of heat needed to raise the temperature of 1 kg of water by 1 °C. This is the large Calorie, or kilocalorie. It is 1000 times the size of the small calorie, the unit used in physics. However, through common usage (and partly due to the unenlightened journalists in the lay literature) the capital letter has largely been replaced by a small 'c' (i.e. use of the word *calorie* not the correct *Calorie*) in popular magazines. Although this is confusing, it is generally accepted today and, when addressing the subject of food and diets, the words *calorie* and *Calorie* indicate the same size of unit.

The *kilojoule* is a unit which can be used to indicate heat, electricity or muscular energy. In comparison with the Calorie, it can be defined as the amount of heat needed to raise the temperature of about 240 g of water by 1 °C. Use of the kilojoule can involve reference to very large numbers, so the megajoule (MJ), which is equal to 1000 kJ, is sometimes used instead. To summarize:

1 cal = 4.2 J
1 Cal = 1000 cal = 4.2 kJ
1 kJ = 240 cal = 0.24 Cal
1 MJ = 10^6 J = 10^3 kJ

To calculate the energy production of a person, either direct or indirect calorimetry is used. *Direct calorimetry* is a difficult and expensive technique. The individual is placed in a specially constructed room in which all heat produced can be accurately determined. Energy expended in controlled physical activity is measured and added up to obtain total energy production. *Indirect calorimetry* is the measurement of oxygen consumption and carbon dioxide production arising from the combustion of specific nutrients. The method is based on the fact that the amount of energy expended is always in direct relationship to the amount of oxygen utilized in the combustion of the various food components.

Basal metabolic rate (BMR)

This is the energy requirement of the body when totally at rest. It is the sum of the needs of the processes of life such as peristalsis, respiration, cardiac function, etc. This amount of energy is influenced by various factors, such as sex (women have a lower BMR than men) and age. The BMR is highest in childhood and decreases with age. Hormonal control influences the energy used at rest — the thyroid plays a major role in regulating the BMR. Emotional stress and tension increase BMR. Climate, too, influences energy requirements, in that a drop in temperature results in increased body heat. However, the use of central heating and protective clothing, as well as reduced exposure to cold in most societies, minimizes the need for increased energy intake under day-to-day conditions. Nevertheless, calculations of requirements for expeditions in cold climates should include cognizance of increased needs. Davidson and Passmore suggest an increase in energy intake of 3% per 10 °C drop in temperature below 10 °C. Growth and pregnancy markedly increase the BMR and this should be born in mind when calculating the requirements of individuals. Energy needs also increase considerably during lactation — up to 4000 additional kJ may be required daily.

Specific dynamic action (SDA) is the term previously used to define the additional energy utilization arising from the metabolism of food. Today, this is referred to as the *thermogenic effect*, a term which covers many aspects of heat and energy production in the body and as a result is thought to play a role in weight maintenance. This thermogenesis is most evident in a high-protein diet, which has led some individuals to the fallacious belief that if certain foods are eaten they will use up more energy than they produce and so result in weight loss! In practice, little emphasis is placed on this type of thermogenesis and it is considered to be of little importance in the calculation of daily dietary requirements.

Physical activity increases energy requirements considerably, and when calculating a person's energy needs the BMR may have to be doubled for a very active person. Under most conditions it is adequate to determine whether the individual is one whose normal life includes mainly light exercise (e.g. office workers and teachers), moderate exercise (those in light industry, nurses, etc.), or heavy exercise (e.g. manual labourers). Useful tables based on the age and ideal body weight of an appropriate group of people are available to help one determine quickly the needs of individuals (Tables 1 and 2, pp. 8–10).

PROTEIN

Proteins are unique organic compounds containing not only carbon, hydrogen and oxygen (as do the other major dietary constituents) but also nitrogen. Some proteins also contain sulphur, and other essential mineral elements may also be present. Protein is needed by the body for:

1. the production and repair of tissues,
2. the manufacture of various hormones,
3. helping to maintain fluid balance — low serum protein levels result in oedema.

Protein-malnourished people are also less resistant to disease.

The constituent units of proteins are known as amino acids and each protein is made up of a particular number of some 20–22 possible amino acids. This situation is often compared to the alphabet where selection and rearrangement of the 26 letters makes possible a variety of words. Certain amino acids are known as *essential* amino acids as human tissue cannot be made without them and they cannot be synthesized by the body. The nine essential amino acids required by the human adult are leucine, isoleucine, lysine, methionine, phenylalanine, threonine, tryptophan, valine and histidine. Histidine was previously thought to be required only by infants. However, current opinion is that it is also essential for adults. Arginine is probably also an essential amino acid for babies.

Dietary proteins which contain all the essential amino acids have been characterized by a variety of terms, but are usually called *complete proteins*, whereas those lacking in one or two essential amino acids are called *partially complete*. Those that are totally inadequate for tissue manufacture and repair are called *incomplete proteins*.

The term '*biological value*' is also used to denote the degree of adequacy of a protein food. It reflects the percentage of absorbed nitrogen, derived from the protein, that is retained by the body and can be utilized for tissue production. Complete proteins are also those with a high biological value whereas the more inadequate proteins are lower in biological value. It is obvious, therefore, that protein quality is determined largely by the type and quantity of the individual amino acids present. If two partially complete protein foods are eaten at the same meal, and each provides the essential amino acids absent in the other, they result together in a nutritionally balanced or complete protein food.

With the exception of gelatin, which is a protein of extremely poor quality, animal and fish proteins are complete, thus a high proportion is utilized by the body. Wheatgerm and yeast are also complete protein foods. Vegetable sources such as nuts, peas, beans, lentils and soya, and certain cereals such as oats, are extremely satisfactory but cannot be termed complete because of the limited number of amino acids. Because of the high cost of meat and fish it is sound nutritional practice to include 'meat replacement' meals in the form of legume dishes, emphasizing those foods mentioned above. Texturized vegetable proteins and other soya products are widely used in this way, particularly in institutional meals (school lunches, etc.). Such combination meals are readily given a variety of flavours, are relatively inexpensive, and provide less fat in the meal than does meat.

Incomplete proteins include cereals such as maize and wheat products, and gelatin. Adults should receive at least one third of their daily requirement of protein as complete protein to ensure an optimum intake of essential amino acids.

It is important that the nurse fully understands the importance of such grading of protein foods according to their biological value, for two reasons. Firstly, when calculating the adequacy of

Table 1. Recommended daily amounts of food energy and some nutrients for population groups in the United Kingdom.

Age range[a] (years)	Occupational category	Energy[b] MJ	kcal	Protein (g)	Thiamine (mg)	Riboflavin (mg)
Boys						
under 1					0.3	0.4
1		5.0	1200	30	0.5	0.6
2		5.75	1400	35	0.6	0.7
3–4		6.5	1560	39	0.6	0.8
5–6		7.25	1740	43	0.7	0.9
7–8		8.25	1980	49	0.8	1.0
9–11		9.5	2280	57	0.9	1.2
12–14		11.0	2640	66	1.1	1.4
15–17		12.0	2880	72	1.2	1.7
Girls						
under 1					0.3	0.4
1		4.5	1100	27	0.4	0.6
2		5.5	1300	32	0.5	0.7
3–4		6.25	1500	37	0.6	0.8
5–6		7.0	1680	42	0.7	0.9
7–8		8.0	1900	47	0.8	1.0
9–11		8.5	2050	51	0.8	1.2
12–14		9.0	2150	53	0.9	1.4
15–17		9.0	2150	53	0.9	1.7
Men						
18–34	Sedentary	10.5	2510	63	1.0	1.6
	Moderately active	12.0	2900	72	1.2	1.6
	Very active	14.0	3350	84	1.3	1.6
35–64	Sedentary	10.0	2400	60	1.0	1.6
	Moderately active	11.5	2750	69	1.1	1.6
	Very active	14.0	3350	84	1.3	1.6
65–74	Assuming a	10.0	2400	60	1.0	1.6
75+	sedentary life	9.0	2150	54	0.9	1.6
Women						
18–54	Most occupations	9.0	2150	54	0.9	1.3
	Very active	10.5	2500	62	1.0	1.3
55–74	Assuming a	8.0	1900	47	0.8	1.3
75+	sedentary life	7.0	1680	42	0.7	1.3
Pregnant		10.0	2400	60	1.0	1.6
Lactating		11.5	2750	69	1.1	1.8

[a] Each figure represents the amount recommended at the middle of the age range. Within each age range younger children will generally need less and older children more than the amount recommended.

[b] 1 MJ = 10^6 J = 1000 kJ = 240 Cal.   1 Cal = 4.2 kJ

[c] 1 nicotinic acid equivalent = 1 mg available nicotinic acid or 60 mg tryptophan.

[d] No information is available on children's folate requirements. The figures shown are merely graded between the figure for children under one, which is based on the folate content of mature human milk, and the figure of 300 μg daily which is recommended for adults.

[e] 1 retinol equivalent = 1 μg of retinol, 6 μg of carotene or 12 μg of other biologically active carotenoids.

Nicotinic acid equvalents (mg)[c]	Total folate[d] (μg)	Ascorbic acid (mg)	Vitamin A retinol equivalents (μg)[e]	Vitamin D[f] cholecalciferol (μg)	Calcium (mg)	Iron (mg)
5	50	20	450	7.5	600	6
7	100	20	300	10	600	7
8	100	20	300	10	600	7
9	100	20	300	10	600	8
10	200	20	300	—	600	10
11	200	20	400	—	600	10
14	200	25	575	—	700	12
16	300	25	725	—	700	12
19	300	30	750	—	600	12
5	50	20	450	7.5	600	6
7	100	20	300	10	600	7
8	100	20	300	10	600	7
9	100	20	300	10	600	8
10	200	20	300	—	600	10
11	200	20	400	—	600	10
14	300	25	575	—	700	12[h]
16	300	25	725	—	700	12[h]
19	300	30	750	—	600	12[h]
18	300	30	750	—	500	10
18	300	30	750	—	500	10
18	300	30	750	—	500	10
18	300	30	750	—	500	10
18	300	30	750	—	500	10
18	300	30	750	—	500	10
18	300	30	750	—	500	10
18	300	30	750	—	500	10
15	300	30	750	—	500	12[h]
15	300	30	750	—	500	12[h]
15	300	30	750	—	500	10
15	300	30	750	—	500	10
18	500	60	750	10	1200[i]	13
21	400	60	1200	10	1200	15

[f] Dietary sources may be unnecessary for children and adults sufficiently exposed to sunlight, but during the winter children and adolescents should receive 10 μg (400 IU) daily by supplementation. Adults with inadequate exposure to sunlight, e.g. those who are housebound, may also need a supplement of 10 μg daily.

[h] This intake may not be sufficient for women with large menstrual losses.

[i] For the third trimester only.

This table is reproduced, by kind permission of Her Majesty's Stationery Office, from *Report on Health and Social Security Subjects: 15*. It is Crown copyright.

Table 2. Energy expenditure over 24 hours*.

Distribution of activity	Light activity		Moderately active		Very active		Exceptionally active	
	Cal	MJ	Cal	MJ	Cal	MJ	Cal	MJ
65 kg man								
In bed (8 h)	500	2.1	500	2.1	500	2.1	500	2.1
At work (8 h)	1100	4.6	1400	5.8	1900	8.0	2400	10.0
Non-occupational activities (8 h)	700 to 1500	3.0 to 6.3	700 to 1500	3.0 to 6.3	700 to 1500	3.0 to 6.3	700 to 1500	3.0 to 6.3
Range of energy expenditure (24 h)	2300 to 3100	9.7 to 13.0	2600 to 3400	10.9 to 14.2	3100 to 3900	13.0 to 16.3	3600 to 4400	15.1 to 18.4
Mean (24 h)	2700	11.3	3000	12.5	3500	14.6	4000	16.7
Mean (per kg of body weight)	42	0.17	46	0.19	54	0.23	62	0.26
55 kg woman								
In bed (8 h)	420	1.8	420	1.8	420	1.8	420	1.8
At work (8 h)	800	3.3	1000	4.2	1400	5.9	1800	7.5
Non-occupational activities (8 h)	580 to 980	2.4 to 4.1	580 to 980	2.4 to 4.1	580 to 980	2.4 to 4.1	580 to 980	2.4 to 4.1
Range of energy expenditure (24 h)	1800 to 2200	7.5 to 9.2	2000 to 2400	8.4 to 10.1	2400 to 2700	10.1 to 11.8	2800 to 3200	11.7 to 13.4
Mean (24 h)	2000	8.4	2200	9.2	2600	10.9	3000	12.5
Mean (per kg of body weight)	36	0.15	40	0.17	47	0.20	55	0.23

*Passmore *et al* (1974).

diets of individual patients, it is imperative to avoid a false impression. By merely adding the amounts of protein present in individual foods one may reach a completely misleading total, as the food tables used may indicate the quantity but not the quality of protein present. For example, a patient consuming a large loaf of white bread per day will be taking in 70 g of protein in bread alone. It is obvious that, although this theoretically meets his requirement of protein, his diet cannot be regarded as adequate.

Secondly, the combination of a variety of plant foods including legumes and nuts can result in a totally adequate diet and the nurse need not fear that the adult vegetarian who selects his food intelligently will be consuming a deficient diet. Furthermore, eating both animal and vegetable foods at the same meal results in far greater efficiency in terms of protein utilization than dependence on animal proteins as the sole source of protein.

Protein requirements

Understandably, in situations where there is additional need of tissue production, greater quantities of protein are required. As can be seen from Table 1, infancy, childhood, pregnancy and lactation all cause increased demand for protein. Surgery, trauma and burns, associated with tissue destruction, increase individual requirements; up to two and a half times the normal requirement may be needed, as all cells need protein for growth or repair. Growth is also impaired.

As discussed above, the biological value of a protein is very important. For purposes of simplicity, egg or milk protein, which is complete protein, is often used as a measure of requirement in food tables, but sometimes total protein (i.e. including the approximate proportions of various proteins in the normal diet) is given. When making use of these tables the nurse should first determine the yardstick of measurement.

Protein deficiency

Mild protein deficiency, although unusual in the UK, is widely encountered among underprivileged people who rely on a cheaper high-carbohydrate diet for their nutritional needs. Infants and children are particularly affected. Reduced resistance to infections and slow wound healing are the most general symptoms of the condition. Lethargy, malaise and fatigue also occur and there is an increase in the incidence of tuberculosis due to a disturbed immune response. Growth is also impaired.

There is also a strong correlation between protein deprivation and mental development. During the first five years of life the overt growth of childhood is accompanied by the final stages of development of the brain. Protein deprivation will retard the physical growth of the brain and permanently affect mental performance if left untreated for some months. Added to this, the concomitant lethargy will limit a child's reaction to the stimuli in his environment at a very crucial stage in his life.

In adults, low serum protein levels are often the first indication of protein deficiency. Although the condition is uncommon in Western societies where a plentiful supply of food and strong supportive social services are available, careless vegetarians who voluntarily restrict their animal protein intake without substitution of sound plant sources occasionally have low serum protein levels. This is discussed in detail in Chapter 2 (pp. 58–62).

In various Eastern countries and in Africa, severe long-term protein-calorie (energy) malnutrition is a common and far-reaching problem. Because mental and physical growth can be inhibited, whole nations may be affected. An interesting example of the effect of diet on physical growth may be observed in some Eastern peoples. Japanese born and bred in the USA are comparable in weight and stature to their American compatriots, and thus diet, not genetics, is now considered responsible for the slight build previously associated with this race.

There are two classical forms of protein deficiency — marasmus and kwashiorkor. However, there is a wide range of conditions within these two extremes of protein malnutrition.

Marasmus

The name 'marasmus' is derived from the Greek word meaning 'to waste'. The condition occurs mainly in the first five years of life and results from a chronic deficiency of both protein and energy in the diet. It is often caused by premature weaning and replacement of breast milk with dilute artificial formulas or black tea. Lowered resistance to infection and unhygienic living conditions result in repeated bouts of gastroenteritis and debilitation. The situation is often aggravated by the long-term withholding of food from the child with diarrhoea, when further wasting occurs. The child becomes wizened, underweight, stunted and weak (Fig. 1). Temperamentally, he may be apathetic or highly irritable. Severe watery diarrhoea is usually present.

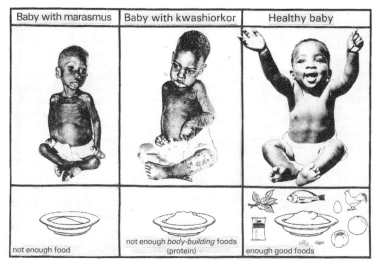

Baby with marasmus	Baby with kwashiorkor	Healthy baby
not enough food	not enough *body-building* foods (protein)	enough good foods

Fig. 1. *Nutritional deficiency diseases.* (Reproduced by kind permission of the National Food and Nutrition Commission, Zambia.)

Kwashiorkor

Kwashiorkor is a Ghanaian word given to the condition when it was first described in that country. It means 'deprived child' (meaning displaced from the breast when the new infant arrives). The child is fed a very starchy diet and the energy intake is often adequate. As with marasmus, lowered resistance results in repeated infection and diarrhoea. However, because of nutritional oedema, caused in part by the low level of serum protein, the child looks less ill. At first impression the child may appear to be plump, but when he is compared to height–weight charts the growth failure is obvious (Fig. 2). Skin changes are usually apparent and areas of increased and decreased pigmentation may occur. The hair, too, may be affected. In fact the word kwashiorkor was originally thought to refer to the red tinge on the hair as the word is similar to this term in one of the African languages. Today this is not regarded as a specific symptom of the condition and the name of the disease has been verified.

In summary, marasmus refers to the severe emaciation and tissue catabolism resulting from severe deprivation of food, protein deficiency being particularly evident in the wasted, wizened child. The child with kwashiorkor, on the other hand, has

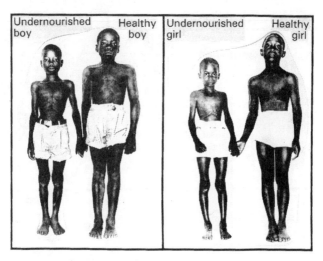

Fig. 2. *The effects of undernourishment.* (Reproduced by kind permission of the National Food and Nutrition Commission, Zambia.)

been fed an unbalanced diet with grossly insufficient protein to meet his needs; he may look more healthy but is stunted and undersized for his age. Marasmic kwashiorkor is a combination of the two conditions to a lesser or greater extent.

However, even within this range of symptoms, there is not uniformity of expert opinion. In a recent article on the subject, Keller and Fillmore suggest that classification systems that specify kwashiorkor, marasmic kwashiorkor and marasmus are more suitable for clinical purposes than field surveys. For the latter, many nutritional experts suggest the terms nutritional stunting or dwarfing (past or chronic malnutrition) and nutritional wasting and emaciation (acute malnutrition).

Table 3 summarizes the major sources of protein and their main functions and characteristics.

FATS

Fats are composed essentially of carbon and hydrogen, with little oxygen. They are the most concentrated source of energy in the diet, providing 37 kJ/g — more than twice as much as proteins and carbohydrates.

Table 3. Summary of major sources and characteristics of proteins, fats and carbohydrates.

Major sources	Functions	Effect of deficiency	Chemical and physiological characteristics	Daily adult allowance
Protein				
Complete proteins: meat, fish, eggs, milk Incomplete proteins: legumes, grains, nuts	1. Building and repair of body tissue 2. Maintenance of water and acid–base balance 3. Necessary for enzyme and hormone action	1. Kwashiorkor and marasmus 2. Increased susceptibility to infection 3. Physical and mental development adversely affected	1. Generally unaffected by cooking procedures and temperatures 2. Body proteins made from combinations of selected ingested amino acids	54–75 g (0.8 g/kg body wt.)
Fats				
Butter, oil	1. Carrier of fat-soluble vitamins 2. Combined with other constituents as essential metabolic compounds (e.g. phospholipids)	Inadequate intake of fat-soluble vitamins, dermatitis	1. Available as saturated (solid) polyunsaturated (liquid) 2. Addition of hydrogen to liquid oils causes hydrogenation or solidification 3. Bile emulsifies fats and assists digestion	30–35% of total energy intake
Carbohydrates				
Sugars: jams, honey, fruit Starches: bread, potatoes, cereals	1. Essential energy source 2. Protein-sparing	Ketosis	Sugars broken down by specific enzymes; stored as glycogen — immediate source of energy	Minimum 15% of total energy

Most dietary fats are *triglycerides*, which are combinations of one molecule of glycerol with three molecules of fatty acid. Depending on the number of carbon atoms in each of the three chains in the fat molecule, the fat is regarded as *short-, medium-* or *long-chained*.

The fats we eat are the glycerides of *even-numbered fatty acids*, usually predominantly with a long chain length. Each food fat has a mixture of various fat types. For example, palmitic (C_{16}), stearic (C_{18}) and arachidonic (C_{20}) acids are found mainly in animal fats. In dairy fats a small amount of short-chain *n*-butyric (C_4) and caproic (C_6) acids are present with the longer chain fats, thus allowing slightly easier digestion where mild pancreatic enzyme, or bile, deficiency is present.

A group of fats encountered more sparsely in the diet comprises the *phospholipids*, which mostly contain phosphate and nitrogen in the composition of the molecule. The most commonly occurring phospholipid is *lecithin*, which is found in egg yolk, brain, liver and kidney. *Sterols*, which are polycyclic lipid alcohols of animal or vegetable origin, have properties like fats. *Cholesterol* — the only sterol which occurs in animals or man — is today widely researched on account of its relationship with coronary artery disease (see Chapter 9).

Medium-chain triglycerides (MCT)

Triglycerides (often termed neutral fats) are compounds of glycerol combined with three fatty acids, linked together by ester bonds. As stated above, the fatty acids may vary in length: long-chain triglycerides are those with twelve or more carbon atoms, medium-chain triglycerides have eight to eleven carbon atoms, and those fats which have fewer than eight carbon atoms are known as short-chain triglycerides.

Medium-chain triglycerides are found predominantly in coconut oil, the commercial source of MCT. Most commonly eaten fats contain predominantly long-chain triglycerides, which are hydrolysed to their constituent fatty acids by pancreatic lipase. Digestion is assisted by bile salts. In the mucosal cells of the gut, these fatty acids are then incorporated into chylomicrons and transported via the lymph to the systemic circulation. In contrast, MCT does not require hydrolysis and inclusion in chylomicrons, but enters the portal vein directly from the gut, thus going directly to the liver.

Although medium-chain triglycerides have no therapeutic properties, they are used to advantage in several disease states, particularly where minimal fat intake is required. MCT is occasionally included in the diets of patients with hyperlipidaemia types I and V (see Chapter 9) as it has little effect on the serum lipid levels. Similarly, MCT may be used to replace other fats in disorders of the biliary system, pancreatic insufficiency and intestinal resection. MCT is also used in diseases accompanied by severe malabsorption and has recently been included in ketogenic diets prescribed for epilepsy (see Chapter 15).

MCT can be used as a fat replacement in baking, in desserts and for roasting. Fried foods (fish, chips, etc.) can be prepared most successfully in MCT but foods should be cooked for a slightly longer time and at a lower temperature than with ordinary oils which have a higher smoking temperature. MCT can be incorporated in feeds for infants and may be combined with ice-cream or fruit juice if required by children.

An important disadvantage of these fats is the associated side-effects which may occur with administration of MCT, particularly at the start of the regimen. Hyperosmolar diarrhoea may occur, accompanied by abdominal pain and vomiting, and it is thus imperative to introduce MCT into the diet slowly. Initially only 20–25% of the required daily intake is given, distributed over the three meals and buffered by other food items. The next day this may be increased to 50% of the required amount, and this quantity can be doubled over the following two days.

Another important disadvantage of MCT is that it is an extremely expensive commodity.

Saturated and unsaturated fats

Of particular relevance in the field of nutrition is the *degree of saturation* of fats. This term refers to the number of double bonds between the carbon atoms in the fatty acid chain. The presence of these bonds allows for the addition of hydrogen atoms, which in turn results in an increase in the firmness or solidity of the fats. Fats may be either saturated, i.e. unable to accept hydrogen ions, or unsatured. Monounsaturated fats have one double bond; oleic acid (found particularly in peanuts and olive oils) is the most common fatty acid.in this group. Monounsaturated fats appear to have no effect on serum cholesterol, whereas the presence of two or more double bonds promotes a cholesterol-lowering effect.

Natural fats contain a combination of various fatty acids. In those types where polyunsaturated fats predominate, the oil is liquid at room temperature. Solid fats contain mainly saturated fats. Thus, depending on their composition, fats are classified as saturated or unsaturated and are appropriately hard or liquid at room temperature. In general, fish and plant oils (except coconut fat) are unsaturated and animal fats are saturated.

The current use of hydrogenation to convert oils into the solid state, producing margarine which is more versatile in cookery, is a process in which hydrogen is added to the fat to saturate it either partially or fully. Those fats which remain relatively unsaturated and thus softer in texture are packed in plastic cartons and the degree of polyunsaturation may be indicated on the carton (e.g. 'contains more than 40% polyunsaturated fat') for the information of people on a diet modified for coronary heart disease.

Functions of fats

Although the role of dietary fats appears to be less important than that of proteins, fats none the less play a major physiological role. As mentioned earlier, they are the most concentrated source of energy in the diet..Thus they are invaluable for a person with a high energy requirement, who can markedly increase his energy intake with a relatively small amount of food. Fats also act as vehicles for the fat-soluble vitamins and greatly enhance the palatability of foods. Fats delay gastric emptying and consequently have a high satiety value, prolonging the period before the recurrence of hunger. They act as lubricants in the bowel, assisting in regular bowel actions. Within the body, fat around the organs forms a buffer for their protection, and subcutaneous fat provides insulation for the body. However, much anatomical fat can be produced from energy sources in the diet other than fats — in particular carbohydrate — and the consumption of fat is not essential for its production.

Fat deficiency

Animal studies show that certain fatty acids are vital for animals but to date there is only one fatty acid known to be essential for Man. *Linoleic acid* must be taken in the diet; all other fatty acids can be synthesized in the body, either from other fats consumed or from surpluses of other foods. Linoleic acid is invariably included in the diet of healthy people but deficiency of this fatty acid has recently been observed following long-term hyperalimentation with a fat-deficient diet. Dermatitis is the first and most obvious symptom to occur.

Table 3 summarizes the major sources of fats and their main functions and characteristics.

CARBOHYDRATES

Carbohydrates are made up of carbon, hydrogen and oxygen, the latter two elements being in the same proportion as in water. Carbohydrates are used preferentially to fats for immediate energy needs. They include sugars, starches, cellulose (the fibre forming the framework of plants) and glycogen. One gram of carbohydrate provides 17 kJ of energy.

Carbohydrates represent the cheapest and most commonly encountered class of food in the diet, accounting for approximately 40–60% of the energy in the normal balanced Western diet. The more inexpensive the diet the higher the proportion of carbohydrates, and among grossly underprivileged people the carbohydrate intake can account for up to 90% of the energy intake. Apart from lactose (the carbohydrate in milk) and glycogen, carbohydrates are derived from plant sources.

Sugars

Sugars are the simpler carbohydrates. The most basic forms of sugar are the *monosaccharides* — glucose, galactose and fructose. These simple sugars can be directly absorbed from the digestive tract independently of digestive enzymes. Glucose and fructose are found particularly in sweet fruits, fructose also being present in large amounts in honey. Galactose does not occur in natural sources but is produced in the gut by hydrolysis of lactose (milk sugar). The monosaccharide with which the nurse will be most familiar is glucose, the form to which all other sugars are broken down in the body. It is from this basic compound that glycogen — the carbohydrate storage product in the liver and muscle — is produced. Glucose is also a very important direct source of energy in the blood.

Disaccharides are sugars which occur widely in the diet. They are broken down to simple sugars or monosaccharides by hydrolysis or specific digestive enzymes in the gut. *Sucrose* is obtained from cane sugar or sugar beet and is the sugar most commonly used for culinary purposes. Used mainly in its refined form, it is prevalent in the diet in confectionery, sweets and cakes. Sucrose is a non-essential food and studies show that a high sugar content in the diet is harmful. Communities with a high sucrose intake suffer from a greater incidence of overweight and diabetes. It is also thought that tooth decay is promoted by a high sucrose intake. Furthermore, the consumption of quantities of a concentrated source of energy such as sugar often precludes the inclusion of more important nutrients. The nurse should thus discourage her patients from taking excessive quantities of sugar. The ingestion of 10% of energy in the form of sucrose is thought by many to be the very maximum desirable. *Maltose* is a disaccharide encountered in malted cereals and beer. It is also formed during the breakdown of starch in the body prior to the production of glucose. *Lactose* is a disaccharide found exclusively in milk and milk products.

Sucrase, maltase and lactase are digestive enzymes which split the above sugars as follows:

1. *sucrase* converts one molecule of sucrose into one molecule of fructose plus one molecule of glucose;
2. *maltase* converts one molecule of maltose into two molecules of glucose;
3. *lactase* converts one molecule of lactose into one molecule of galactose and one molecule of glucose.

The absence of any one of these specific enzymes will result in malabsorption and its associated symptoms, which are discussed in Chapter 8.

Polysaccharides

Starches are more complex sources of carbohydrates and are known as polysaccharides. They are found predominantly in cereals and certain vegetables such as potatoes and legumes, and provide a major source of energy in the diet. During digestion starch is broken down to glucose and is either used directly as energy or stored as glycogen for later use.

Cellulose is another polysaccharide in the diet. It is minimally broken down in the human gut and is therefore not available to be used as energy, but it is of major importance as a source of bulk in the digestive tract. Wheat bran can absorb up to 200 times its weight in water and is thus invaluable in preventing constipation. *Glycogen* is encountered in animal muscle and liver. While it is theoretically a source of carbohydrates, it does not in practice contribute materially to one's diet. This is because the cell changes that occur after slaughter result in rapid breakdown of glycogen.

Carbohydrate requirements

No empirically derived quantity for carbohydrate requirement is to be found in food tables nor is it common to find someone taking a long-term carbohydrate-deficient diet. Carbohydrate is used as the most efficient energy source but in its absence both protein and fat can be utilized for this purpose. Carbohydrate is therefore 'protein-sparing', i.e. it allows protein to be retained for its prime functions in the body instead of being utilized for producing energy. Carbohydrate is required to produce glycogen, the first-call energy reserve product, which is stored mainly in the liver but also in lower concentration in the large mass of muscles throughout the body. In total, this reserve supply of energy does not exceed the approximate requirement of 12–13 h, and for optimum efficiency ingestion of carbohydrate is essential to maintain optimum storage levels. If necessary, Man is able to obtain energy from other sources in the body, particularly adipose tissues, but only in the longer term, i.e. for sustained energy demand. Excessive oxidation of fats is associated with an accumulation of acidic ketones (intermediary products of fat oxidation), which can cause acidosis of the blood. This situation can also occur in uncontrolled diabetes where carbohydrate utilization is impaired and abnormal demands are made on the fat resources.

Carbohydrate deficiency

Carbohydrate deficiency is not often encountered; in Western society the opposite condition, resulting in obesity, is prevalent. However, strict adherence to an unbalanced weight reduction regimen, with severely restricted carbohydrate intake, may result in acidosis. Recent research has shown that these diets may have long-term side-effects including calcium depletion, dehydration and hyperlipidaemia, thus accelerating atherosclerosis. They also promote gout and renal stones in patients with a tendency to these disorders. Interestingly, a study of two men fed an exclusively meat diet providing 8400–12 600 kJ a day for a year showed that their usual weight could be maintained in spite of the absence of carbohydrates. Although reduction of carbohydrate is advisable in a weight reduction regimen, its absence from the diet is not a prerequisite for weight loss nor is the consumption of a moderate amount inadvisable. In a study of Canadian troops during World War II, the ingestion of an emergency diet of pemmican (beef with added suet) and tea resulted in severe symptoms within three days. There was a reduction in performance, and nausea, vomiting, dehydration and fatigue were evident in these soldiers.

In conclusion, while excessive amounts of *refined* carbohydrates probably play a major role in the diseases prevalent in Western society, such as diabetes, coronary artery disease and cancer of the colon, the inclusion in the diet of a small to moderate amount of carbohydrates, with emphasis on those sources with a high fibre content, is to be encouraged. Ironically, in underprivileged communities where these diseases are hardly encountered, up to 80% of the diet may be derived from carbohydrates, but these are natural unrefined foods. The presence of fibre — a dietary constituent being widely researched today — may well play a major role.

Table 3 summarizes the major sources of carbohydrates and their main functions and characteristics.

VITAMINS

Vitamins are nutrients essential for the normal functioning of the body. Present in minute quantities in natural food sources, they participate in specific metabolic activities and must be taken regularly to ensure continuous adequacy. The sources and characteristics of the principal vitamins are given in Table 4.

Certain vitamins can be manufactured by the body, but not in amounts sufficient to meet requirements. It would seem that the need for consumption of the others is a disadvantageous result of increasing genetic 'refinement' of the human body. This has ultimately become an inborn error of metabolism which is harmless in the vast majority of people because they have an adequate intake from outside sources.

Vitamins produce enzymic action at a multitude of body sites, but their precise role is still being studied. They are either fat- or water-soluble and are named according either to their original alphabetical classification or, more recently, to their chemical composition. Deficiency diseases occur widely in developing countries among impoverished people eating inadequate diets and living in conditions which promote infections and undermine well-being. The reasons for the appearance of specific selective symptoms with dietary deficiency of particular vitamins are not fully understood as these symptoms sometimes do not appear to have any bearing on the physiological role of the vitamin concerned.

Fat-soluble vitamins

Vitamin A (retinol)

This is present in the diet either in the form of the vitamin (retinol) or as its precursor, carotene, which is partially water-soluble. The latter is found particularly in plants that are yellow, bright green or orange — colours characteristic of the carotenoid pigments. Man can convert the provitamin in these pigments to vitamin A.

Vitamin A is required for the formation of rhodopsin (visual purple) in the retina, thus ensuring visual acuity in poor light. This vitamin is necessary for the integrity of the epithelium of the eyes and the membranes of the nose, throat and gastrointestinal tract. It is an essential dietary component for reproduction and lactation and is necessary for normal growth. Deficiency causes night blindness and keratinization of the mucous membranes. With severe deficiency, xerophthalmia (conjunctivitis and atrophy of the cornea) and eventual blindness can occur, and the skin becomes progressively more dry and scaly. Deficiency had been seen to occur in infants fed solely on skimmed milk and was

Table 4. Sources and characteristics of major vitamins.

Vitamin	Major sources	Functions	Effect of deficiency	Chemical and physiological characteristics	Recommended daily adult allowance (see also Table 1)
Vitamin A (retinol)	Dairy fats, fish oil, egg yolk, liver	Formation of rhodopsin — required for visual acuity in poor light Essential for normal growth and reproduction	Night blindness; keratinization of mucous membranes	Insoluble in water; fat-soluble; stable in cooking	750 μg retinol equivalent
Carotene	Carrots, pumpkin, spinach, broccoli, apricots, yellow peaches	As vitamin A	As vitamin A	Water-soluble; converted to vitamin A in the body; stable in cooking	5000 IU
Thiamine (vitamin B₁)	Milk, meats, particularly organ meat, wholegrain products, green leafy vegetables	Coenzyme in carbohydrate metabolism	Beri-beri in severe cases; in moderate deficiency cases loss of appetite and weight, emotional and psychological symptoms	Water-soluble; destroyed by heat in alkaline medium, heat-stable in acid medium	1.3 mg (approx. 0.5 mg per 4200 kJ)
Riboflavin	Milk, meats, particularly organ meat, wholegrain cereals, green leafy vegetables	Essential for normal cell growth and development	Cheilosis (cracks at the corners of the mouth), burning eyes and affected vision	Slightly soluble in water, unstable in light	1.6 mg (approx. 0.6 mg per 4200 kJ)
Niacin	Wholegrain cereals, lean meat, poultry, fish and organ meats, green vegetables	Active compound of enzyme systems involved with energy production	Pellagra. Early symptoms: loss of appetite and weight, weakness	Slightly soluble in water; unaffected by external factors such as light, alkali, acid, etc.	18 mg nicotinic acid equivalent

Vitamin	Function	Deficiency	Source	Properties	Requirement
Vitamin B$_{12}$	Participates in production of nucleic acid, necessary for haemopoiesis	Pernicious anaemia; long-term deficiency results in subacute degeneration of the spinal cord	Liver and kidneys, meat, milk	Absorption dependent on Castle's intrinsic factor. Heat-stable; adversely affected by light, alkalis and strongly acid media	3 µg
Folic acid	As vitamin B$_{12}$	Megaloblastic anaemia	Dark green vegetables, liver and kidneys, yeast	Fairly stable in; water; unstable in light and strongly acid media	300 µg
Ascorbic acid (vitamin C)	Maintains intercellular substances; assists in iron absorption	Scurvy, evidenced by bleeding gums, subcutaneous bleeding, corkscrew hair follicles	Citrus fruits, tomatoes, potatoes, strawberries	Water-soluble; adversely affected by light, heat, air, alkalis; minimal reserves retained in body	30 mg
Vitamin D	Necessary for efficient calcium metabolism and deposition, thus essential for development of bones and teeth	Rickets: soft, fragile bones, skeletal deformities, retarded growth. Osteomalacia in adults; dental caries; tetany	Sunlight, fish-liver oil, fortified milk, margarine	Ultraviolet light synthesizes the vitamin in the skin; fat-soluble; stable in air and heat	0–10 µg 400 IU
Vitamin E (tocopherols)	Counteracts oxidation of certain essential components (e.g. vitamin A) in the body, needed for cell respiration	Not seen in humans under normal conditions	Oils of vegetable origin (e.g. sunflower seed oil, nut oils), peas, beans, leafy vegetables, wheatgerm	Fat-soluble; antioxidant of oil; protects red blood cells against haemolysis	15 IU
Vitamin K	Essential for blood clotting	Haemorrhagic disease of the newborn; increased tendency to bleed	Green leafy vegetables	Fat and water-soluble; can be synthesized in gut; heat-stable	Dietary deficiency unlikely

reported from Brazil following the distribution of skimmed milk by UNICEF (United Nations International Children's Emergency Fund). This was attributed to the fact that the vitamin A capsules which accompanied the milk distribution were not, for one reason or another, taken by the children.

The recommended intake of vitamin A is 750 μg (i.e. 5000 International Units, IU) per day.

FOOD SOURCES. As mentioned previously, carotene is found mainly in green, yellow and red fruit and vegetables. Carrots, pumpkin, spinach, broccoli, apricots and peaches are rich sources of this provitamin. Vitamin A is found in fish oils and dairy fats, such as butter and full cream milk, although there is a seasonal variation in its amount in dairy products. An excellent constant source of vitamin A is margarine, which in the UK is vitaminized. Approximately 50% of the ingested vitamin A in a Western-type diet is of animal origin, whereas the other 50% is in the form of carotene.

HYPERVITAMINOSIS. Excessive intake of the fat-soluble vitamins will result in accumulation in the body and symptoms of toxicity. Patients should be cautioned to take both vitamins A and D in carefully controlled amounts. Hypervitaminosis can occur as an acute or chronic condition. The former situation is more likely and was recently seen in the family of a woman whose occupation was fish filleting in a small fishing harbour. Having collected the day's fish livers, she then fed them to the family for supper. Symptoms are transient hydrocephalus and severe vomiting. Chronic hypervitaminosis A can occur following long-term over-administration of vitamin A supplements. The symptoms are fatigue, abdominal discomfort, headache, joint pain and loss of hair. The symptoms disappear upon withdrawal of vitamin A.

Carotenaemia occurs occasionally when overenthusiastic mothers feed excessive quantities of green and yellow vegetables to their infants. It can also occur among food faddists and people on a weight reduction regimen endeavouring to 'fill up on vegetables'. The skin, in particular the soles of the feet and palms of the hands, is tinged with yellow. This has no adverse effect and disappears when smaller quantities of these foods are consumed.

Vitamin D

Vitamin D is present in food fats and is absorbed with fat from the gut. Man is able to produce it from a precursor present in the skin in the presence of ultraviolet light. This means that when we are exposed to regular sunlight vitamin D in the diet is unnecessary. In the absence of sunlight, dietary vitamin D is essential, and the fortification of many foods (including margarine) with this vitamin emphasizes this need.

Although vitamin D has various functions in the body (including adaptation to low calcium intakes and maintenance of plasma calcium levels) its main function is associated with the action of parathyroid hormone which affects calcium metabolism. Adequate vitamin D intake does not reduce the body's calcium requirement but assists in its most efficient utilization. Deficiency of the vitamin will thus be particularly apparent in infants and growing children and during puberty, due to the high rate of bone formation at this stage. For this reason many infant formulas are supplemented, and breast-fed babies should be given an oral supplement in areas of limited sunshine. *Rickets* is the classical deficiency disease encountered. It is a disease characterized by crooked and deformed bones, delayed closure of the fontanelle and pain in the muscles. Tetany and increased dental caries also occur in children. *Osteomalacia* is the adult equivalent of the disease. It occurs especially in pregnant and lactating women on a low-calcium and low-vitamin D diet and is manifested by increased softness and fragility of bones. The above conditions can also result from disorders where fat absorption is reduced, such as biliary obstruction and coeliac disease. The nurse should be alert to the possibility of rickets in babies who are left in the care of an inactive or elderly adult unable to supervise the infant out of doors and to expose it to sunlight very often.

The main sources of vitamin D are fish-liver oils, exposure to sunlight, fortified milk and margarine. Small amounts are present in egg yolk and butter. Supplementation to infants should be accurately administered as there is a relatively small margin between adequate and toxic doses. Hypervitaminosis D is characterized initially by diarrhoea, loss of weight and nausea. Long-term overdosage can result in irreversible renal damage and calcification of the soft tissue. The recommended intake for infants and young children is 10 μg (400 IU) per day, but by the age of seven the requirement drops to a quarter of this and remains constant thereafter, except during periods of stress, such as reduced absorption, or increased need during puberty, pregnancy and lactation and in old age. Melanin pigment interferes with the manufacture of vitamin D through radiation and thus dark-skinned people may require more in their diet than those with light skins.

Vitamin E

This is the name given to a group of compounds known as tocopherols (from the Greek *tocos*, meaning childbirth, *phero*, meaning to bring forth, and *ol*, alcohol). The role of this vitamin is not clearly understood in Man, although it has an important function in preventing both fetal resorption and muscular degeneration in the rat. Deficiency states induced in experimental animals have wide-ranging effects on the muscular, nervous, circulatory and reproductive systems. In Man, the main effect of vitamin E is its potent antioxidant properties in the metabolism of fats. There is to date no scientific evidence to support the contention — made particularly by health food faddists — that vitamin E deficiency is related to ageing and conversely that increased amounts will retard it.

The daily requirement is small and related to the amount of polyunsaturated oil in the diet. The higher the oil content, the greater the need for vitamin E as an antioxidant. Vitamin E is found in vegetable oils, in particular wheatgerm oil, the vitamin E content depending on the refinement the oil undergoes before consumption. The estimated intake in a normal diet is approximately 15 IU and deficiency is unlikely. Secondary deficiency may occur as a result of malabsorption of fats or the consumption of rancid fats.

The therapeutic use of vitamin E in cardiovascular disease and menstrual disorders is controversial, although some vascular surgeons consider that it has a specific role in peripheral vascular disease.

Vitamin K

Vitamin K is the coagulation vitamin. It stimulates the synthesis of prothrombin and plays a major role in blood clotting. About 50% of the dietary requirement is probably synthesized in the ileum and the rest is derived from a wide range of dietary sources. This ingested vitamin K is absorbed relatively inefficiently, with only approximately 50% of this source being absorbed. Green vegetables and cheese are particularly good sources and dietary deficiency is seldom seen. Failure of synthesis or failure of absorption due to reduced bile output will result in an increased tendency to bleed. This is particularly relevant in newborn infants who in the first few days of life may be unable to synthesize the vitamin due to the sterility of the gut. Haemorrhagic disease of the newborn may occur and thus as a precautionary measure many doctors now routinely administer vitamin K at birth. This is particularly necessary where the infant shows a tendency to bleed.

Note: The absorption of fat-soluble vitamins is inhibited by the use of mineral oils, which are often used to increase lubrication of the gut by constipated individuals. Such oils will dissolve a proportion of these vitamins from ingested foods which make contact with them, and retain them in solution. The nurse should strongly discourage the regular use of mineral oils as a laxative.

Water-soluble vitamins

Vitamin B

'Vitamin B' was the name originally given to a single substance isolated from rice polishings and found to cure beri-beri. Later this was found to have a number of constituents which were essential for a variety of functions.

THIAMINE (VITAMIN B_1). Thiamine forms part of an essential coenzyme system required for the metabolism of carbohydrates. The daily requirement is directly related to the intake of energy. Vitamin B_1 is of historical interest in that beri-beri — the classical deficiency disease — was formerly endemic in the East where polished rice was the staple diet. In the period since the isolation of the missing factor (which is now just less than 100 years) the situation has improved dramatically owing to education and the wider variety of foods available. In the Western world, beri-beri is mainly encountered today in alcoholics on a deficient diet. Mild deficiency results in loss of appetite and weight, depression, fatigue and irritability — relatively mild emotional and psychological symptoms which are reversible with administration of thiamine. In the areas of low intake, feeding mothers produce milk with a low thiamine content, causing a high death rate from deficiency in breast-fed infants.

Clinically, two types of frank beri-beri are seen. They were formerly called wet beri-beri and dry beri-beri. The wet type is mainly exhibited by cardiovascular abnormalities such as tachycardia, rapid pulse and enlarged heart, oedema and an abnormal EEG. Epigastric pain can also occur. The symptoms of the dry type are mainly neurological — peripheral neuritis, tender and later atrophied muscles, fatigue, decreased attention span and confusion. Cardiac failure and sudden death, either with or without exertion, are features of the disorder. In severe acute deficiency due to alcoholism, Wernicke's encephalopathy can occur. Symptoms of the syndrome are vomiting, ataxia and severe mental symptoms leading to dementia.

The most important source of thiamine is wholegrain products, but it is also found in pork, beef, organ meats, peas and beans. Because it is soluble in water, much of the vitamin may be lost if cooking liquids are discarded, but in practice most foods rich in thiamine, apart from peas and beans, are not prepared in this way. Of much greater relevance is the use of bicarbonate of soda to preserve the green colour in peas and beans. Like ascorbic acid, thiamine is rapidly broken down in the presence of alkali.

RIBOFLAVIN. This is a component of coenzymes involved in a range of metabolic activities. In particular, riboflavin plays a major role in cell growth and development. Wound healing is impossible without it, and at times of major cell production, such as growth, pregnancy, lactation and following surgery, the body's need for riboflavin is increased. If it is not taken by mouth the body can to a small extent utilize its own reserves by catabolism.

The daily requirement bears a direct relationship to protein intake. Inadequate amounts of either riboflavin or protein will result in less efficient utilization of the other.

Riboflavin is slightly soluble in water and is most unstable in the presence of light. A major source of riboflavin is milk, and long exposure of delivered milk to sunlight outside kitchen doors results in vast losses of riboflavin in summer. Other major sources are eggs, organ meats and green leafy vegetables.

NIACIN. This is the active compound of a group of enzymes. As with thiamine, the amount required is related to the energy intake. Tryptophan is converted to niacin in the body, approximately 60 mg of tryptophan being required for 1 mg of niacin. Deficiency results in pellagra, the symptoms of which are known as the three D's — dermatitis, dementia and diarrhoea. Pellagra is particularly encountered in populations eating a predominantly maize diet. Early symptoms are anorexia, weight loss, weakness and lassitude, but with continued deficiency, itching skin lesions with characteristic distribution occur and occasionally the mouth becomes painful. Diarrhoea is a prominent feature, and mental disturbance — confusion, nervousness and depression — is also a symptom of this deficiency. The main sources of niacin are wholegrain cereals, lean meat, fish and poultry, green vegetables, liver and kidneys. Niacin is extremely stable in the presence of external factors such as sunlight and alkali, and is only slightly soluble in water. Losses during food preparation are negligible.

VITAMIN B$_6$. Vitamin B$_6$ is more commonly known as pyridoxine, which is one of its active forms. It occurs in a wide range of foods. It can also be produced by the intestinal flora, but this is unlikely to be necessary in Man. It is involved in a multitude of enzymatic reactions and plays a major role in the metabolism of the amino acid tryptophan. The daily requirement increases with protein intake. The USA Food and Nutrition Board recommends an intake of 2 mg/day for a daily intake of 100 g of protein or more. Less protein will require less pyridoxine. Vitamin B$_6$ occurs in practically all foods, good sources being wholemeal cereals, yeast and liver.

Dietary deficiency is rare, although it has been seen in infants receiving a commercial milk product manufactured by a process which destroys the vitamin. Symptoms are nervousness and epileptic-type convulsions. The use of an antivitamin experimentally can also cause deficiency.

Massive doses of pyridoxine are sometimes used as therapy for nausea and vomiting in pregnancy and in the treatment of hyperoxaluria and recurrent kidney stones.

PANTOTHENIC ACID. Like vitamin B_6, pantothenic acid can be made in the gut but as it is universally available in foods it is unlikely that this mechanism is normally required. Pantothenic acid is part of a variety of enzymic systems and is found in almost all plant foods, so that deficiency is virtually unknown. Like vitamin B_6, an experimental deficiency can be produced by administering an antivitamin.

BIOTIN. This is also found widely in food. A deficiency is unlikely. Biotin is of special interest to the nurse because of the antagonistic effect of avidin, a protein present in egg white which prevents the absorption of biotin. Avidin becomes ineffective with heating, so mothers are frequently told not to feed their infants raw egg white until the baby is several months old.

FOLIC ACID (FOLATE) AND VITAMIN B_{12} (CYANOCOBALAMIN). These vitamins are discussed under one heading as they both have the same physiological function in that they are both haemopoietically active and deficiency of either causes megaloblastic anaemia. They were originally thought to be the same compound and it was only in the 1940s that it became clear that two different substances were under investigation. The major difference between them is that vitamin B_{12} occurs almost exclusively in sources of animal origin, whereas folic acid is found widely in dark green vegetables. The significance of this for vegetarians is obvious. In the short term, megaloblastic anaemia can occur: after 12–15 years subacute degeneration of the spinal cord may result from a diet excluding all foods of animal origin. On the other hand, a folate deficiency is the more likely cause of nutritional anaemia in alcoholics who replace a major part of their necessary nutrient intake with alcohol. Pregnant women on deficient diets and others living in certain areas of low intake also readily develop folate deficiency. In some places this deficiency is common and folate is routinely administered at antenatal clinics. Folate deficiency is widely encountered in the tropics, and in premature babies where it is due to malabsorption. Folate is found in liver, kidney, wholegrain cereals and milk, apart from leafy green vegetables.

The absorption of vitamin B_{12} is dependent on the so-called intrinsic factor of Castle, a glycoprotein normally produced by the cells in the stomach wall. Vitamin B_{12} plays a major role in the production of nucleic acids and haemopoiesis. Liver is the major source of this vitamin; indeed it was the early therapy used for pernicious anaemia long before the disease entity was defined. Vitamin B_{12} is also found in kidneys, meat and milk.

Vitamin C (ascorbic acid)

The story of vitamin C is fascinating and Hodge and Baker's account in *Modern Nutrition in Health and Disease* (edited by Goodhart and Shils) briefly traces the repeated discovery of the value of certain foods in combating scurvy and the impact of the human need for this nutrient on the course of civilization. Scurvy was recognized by the ancient Egyptians, was the reason for the establishment of the Cape of Good Hope as a refreshment station, and was a cause of the tragic end to Scott's expedition to the South Pole, yet it was identified less than 50 years ago. Vitamin C plays a role in a limited number of coenzyme systems, where its reducing (antioxidant) ability may be of vital importance. Its presence is critical for the production of extracellular materials, and the amount required is increased when there is extensive tissue production such as occurs during growth, following surgery, etc. Vitamin C also plays a role in erythropoiesis but it is as yet uncertain whether this is due to its effect on folic acid, vitamin B_{12} or iron conversion.

Recommended intakes vary enormously. This is because whilst only 10 mg are required per day to prevent scurvy, complete saturation of the tissues requires 60–100 mg. The usual recommendation is thus somewhere between these two figures. Vitamin C is highly unstable and is rapidly denatured in the presence of light, oxygen and heat. Extensive losses occur both during the preparation of food and from allowing it to stand exposed at room temperature. To minimize the loss of vitamin C from source foods the following points should be observed:

1. limit the time lapse between preparation and consumption to the minimum;
2. heat foods rich in vitamin C only when necessary and for the minimum length of time;

   3. serve salads in large pieces to reduce the amount of surface
      area exposed.

Rich sources of vitamin C are tomatoes, citrus fruits, blackcurrants, potatoes and green leafy vegetables. Deficiency results in a
tendency to bleeding of the gums and delayed healing of wounds.
A unique symptom of hardened hair follicles surrounded by a
haemorrhagic halo also occurs in this condition. Of importance to
the nurse is the fragility of the capillaries under pressure (e.g.
when a tourniquet is applied for blood sampling) and the
spontaneous haemorrhages which are evident in these patients.
Prolonged deficiency causes scurvy, a disease in which these
symptoms are aggravated.

   A complicating factor is the importance of the medium in which
the vitamin is consumed. Acid foods promote absorption. Differences in the food types may be of major importance in causing the
conflicting results obtained with trials using massive doses of this
vitamin to prevent colds. Although dismissed by many, there is
considerable well documented evidence to support the theory that
huge doses of vitamin C have a protective effect with regard to
colds.

Excessive intakes of water-soluble vitamins

Further to the above statement regarding the use of vitamin C for
the prevention of colds, a word of caution is appropriate regarding
the intake of massive doses of any of the water-soluble vitamins.

   Vitamins were unknown before the twentieth century and
undoubtedly great advances in knowledge have occurred over the
years. However, the recent trend of faddists of taking megadoses
(massive doses) of specific individual vitamins merely in the hope
of ensuring continued good health is not only wasteful, extrava-
gant and unwise, it may in fact have the opposite effect. A recent
study by Schaumberg et al showed that vitamin B_6 toxicity could
result in neuropathy of the arms and legs. Furthermore, instances
of 'withdrawal scurvy' have been reported when megadoses of
vitamin C are discontinued. There have even been reports of
scurvy in infants of mothers taking massive doses of vitamin C
during pregnancy. Patients should be firmly cautioned about the
common fallacy that 'if a little is good, more must be better'.
Recommended allowances should be used as a guide, wherever

possible consuming the vitamins in fresh food rather than as isolated compounds in tablet form.

MINERAL ELEMENTS

Mineral elements make up a small (3–4%) but vital part of the human body. This is the 'ash' substance which remains when tissue is burnt — carbon, oxygen, nitrogen and hyrdrogen are converted to gases and driven off. Minerals form an integral part of tissue and bone. Many of them must be regularly ingested to ensure adequacy. The major minerals, or macro-elements, are calcium, phosphorus, iron, magnesium, sodium, potassium, sulphur and fluorine. (The sources and characteristics of these elements are given in Table 5.) A large number of other elements exist in the body in such small amounts that until recently their exact function and concentration could not be measured. These became known as 'trace elements' and at present there are 14 of these micro-elements believed to be essential for animal life. Their study is fraught with problems and since much of the evidence related to single elements has been found during this decade, the subject is not well defined or totally understood. Complicating factors are:

1. the possibility that with future scientific advancement and more precise techniques, other, as yet unknown, essential elements may be discovered;
2. the doubtful extent to which conclusions drawn from experiments on laboratory animals are relevant to man;
3. the toxicity levels of both essential and non-essential elements;
4. the effects of urbanization, including methods of food preservation and a sophisticated diet;
5. the atmosphere effects of industrialization and the impact of various manufacturing processes;
6. the effect of known and unknown elements found in a mixed diet on the functions and properties of a specific single trace element.

Calcium

This is the element occurring most abundantly in the body. It forms an essential part of bones and teeth, where it is present with phosphorus in a ratio of 2:1. It is also vital for blood clotting and

Table 5. Sources and characteristics of major minerals.

Mineral	Major sources	Functions	Effect of deficiency	Chemical and physiological characteristics	Reccomended daily adult allowance
Calcium	Milk and milk products, canned fish eaten with bones, fortified flour	Essential part of bones, teeth; major role in blood clotting, cell permeability and enzyme systems	Rickets, including skeletal deformities, soft, fragile bones and retarded growth; osteomalacia in adults; dental caries; tetany	Uptake and utilization adversely affected by phytate, oxalate; vitamin D essential for efficient utilization; absorption enhanced by lactose and ascorbic acid	500 mg
Iron	Liver, red meat, egg yolk, dried apricots, raisins	Essential component of haemoglobin	Hypochromic anaemia. Moderate deficiency causes lethargy; in severe cases, palpitations and oedema	Poorly absorbed; uptake further reduced by certain food components (e.g. phytate, oxalate); absorption enhanced by acid (ascorbic acid, gastric acidity)	10–12 mg
Magnesium	Milk, legumes, nuts, wholegrain cereals	Essential component of several enzyme systems, (in particular carbohydrate metabolism) and neuromuscular transmission	Irritability, muscle weakness, arrhythmias, depression	Normal component of sweat, therefore major losses in extremely hot climates and intense exercise	300–350 mg Deficiency unlikely but may occur in malabsorption state
Iodine	Sea foods, iodized salt	Constituent of thyroxine which has profound overall effect on metabolism	Goitre. In areas of extreme deficiency cretinism can occur endemically	Radioactive form widely used as a diagnostic measure of thyroid activity	100–140 μg

cell permeability and plays a major role in certain enzyme systems. Yet in spite of this knowledge, D.M. Hegsted, a world authority on the subject, has commented that 'calcium is a nutrient in search of a disease'.

There is still much argument about the precise metabolic pathways of calcium utilization. This may in part be due to the fact that Man can adapt to a wide range of calcium intake. For instance, although calcium needs are higher during pregnancy and lactation, osteomalacia (a disease characterized by painful softening of the bones) is not common in women who have had multiple pregnancies and lactations. Although it was formerly thought that the body calcium reserves were mobilized during pregnancy if an inadequate diet was eaten (i.e. 'a tooth lost for every baby'), it now appears that there is, in fact, *increased* deposition of bone during pregnancy. This surprising situation appears to be an aspect of enhanced utilization, which is hormonally induced. It appears that during lactation inadequate dietary intake of calcium will prompt depletion of body stores. However, this depletion is temporary and reserves will be replaced when the need for milk production drops.

The role of a calcium-deficient diet as the cause of osteoporosis has in the past been disregarded but is now being reconsidered. Osteoporosis, a condition in which there is reduced bone density resulting in increased susceptibility to fractures, is widely seen in elderly people. Postmenopausal women are particularly prone to the disease and oestrogen deficiency and calcium deficiency are the major causes of the condition. Long-term use of steroids and prolonged bed-rest have also been strongly implicated. As the daily intake of calcium of many individuals falls well below the recommended daily allowance (RDA) and as a high calcium intake reduces the age-related loss of bone density, it is important to encourage patients (particularly women) to take a high-calcium diet in an attempt to reduce the incidence of osteoporosis.

Apart from individual adaptive response to intake, calcium absorption is also dependent on various other dietary factors. The absence of adequate vitamin D, hypermobility of the gut or chronic renal insufficiency will all inhibit its absorption, as may certain unabsorbed fatty acids. The presence of phytic acid, present in wholegrain cereals, and oxalic acid, found particularly in spinach, rhubarb and beetroot tops, will also impair absorption:

both phytic and oxalic acids form insoluble salts with calcium. However, the adaptive ability of the human body in obtaining calcium appears to be very effective and it is unlikely that these organic acids in the diet are of day-to-day relevance for people on normal diets. Although it may theoretically be better for people on diets containing minimum amounts of calcium to avoid whole-wheat bread due to the phytate content, the presence in such bread of other essential nutrients (especially vitamin B complex) negates this as a practical suggestion.

Absorption of calcium in the gut is enhanced by the presence of other nutrients such as ascorbic acid and lactose.

Requirements of calcium

Although dependent on various factors, including the vitamin D content of the diet, the recommended allowance is generally given as approximately 600 mg/day. However, as stated previously, the body can adapt to a low calcium intake and as little as 300 mg/day is probably not harmful. Indeed the levels recommended by the FAO/WHO groups (see Table 1) are regarded by some as being unrealistically high, especially the allowances for pregnant and lactating women.

Deficiency may occur as a result of inadequate intake, malabsorption or vitamin D deficiency. Rickets is the classical disease in children. It is a condition in which growth is retarded, bowing of the legs is evident and softening of the other bones occurs. A similar condition of bone softening accompanied by weakness (osteomalacia) occurs in adults. As indicated above, osteoporosis occurs widely in elderly people.

The main dietary sources of calcium are milk and cheese. Tinned fish such as sardines, pilchards and herrings, where the bones are eaten, are also excellent sources. In Britain, non-wholemeal flour is fortified with calcium and this, too, markedly contributes to the diet. Added in the standard proportion of approximately 420 g/127 kg (14 oz/280 lb sack), it provides about 20% of the daily requirement.

Phosphorus

Phosphorus occurs extensively in the body in various forms such as phosphate, phosphoproteins, phospholipids, etc — in fact, it is second only to calcium as the most extensive mineral. It occurs widely in foods, particularly those that are high in calcium and protein, and no pathological dietary deficiency or toxicity of the element has been encountered. There have been reports of long-term use of antacids preventing absorption of ingested phosphates by the gut, but this is a rare situation. Symptoms of such iatrogenic deficiency are anorexia, bone pain and demineralization of the bone. This is accompanied by an increased urinary output of calcium. As stated previously, the calcium to phosphorus ratio in bone is 2:1 but, as the phosphorus requirements of other tissue are greater, the usual recommendation is that phosphorus intake should be equal to that of calcium. Rich sources of phosphorus are foods high in calcium (particularly milk and cheese), egg yolk and cereals, including enriched white flour.

Iron

Iron is present in all the cells in the body. It is stored in the liver and transported to the bone marrow where it forms an essential part of haemoglobin, the oxygen-carrying pigment of the erythrocyte. Only about 10–20% of ingested iron is absorbed by the body. Because of the cost of high-iron foods, deficiency of this element is a public health problem, particularly in underprivileged groups. Dietary needs increase with growth and also with menstruation due to losses in blood. During pregnancy needs are high, and as iron is so often deficient in the diet, oral iron is routinely given as a precautionary measure. The need for such supplementation can be determined by the nurse from a dietary history. A finger prick followed by a haemoglobin reading will irrefutably determine the patient's nutritional status with respect to iron. In infants the requirement is not easily met on a predominantly milk diet and the mother should ensure that food supplements are given after the first few months. Egg yolk is the most practical source.

Deficiency results in hypochromic anaemia (pale erythrocytes). Initially the main symptom is fatigue, but with severe deficiency palpitations, dizziness and ankle oedema may occur.

Toxic quantities may be ingested either by excessive supplementation or by accidental dissolving of the element from an iron cooking pot into an acid food. The result is a disease known as haemosiderosis, in which the blood pigment containing iron accumulates in the tissues, causing a distinct discolouration of the skin.

Rich sources of iron are liver, red meat, egg yolk and dried fruit, particularly raisins and apricots.

Magnesium

This mineral plays a role in neuromuscular transmission and is an activator of many enzyme systems. There is a strong correlation between its role in the body and that of sodium, potassium and calcium. In hypermagnesaemia the patient develops concomitant hypokalaemia. Parathyroid hormone secretion bears an inverse relationship to magnesium levels in the blood and there is also a strong correlation between the metabolism of magnesium, calcium and vitamin D. The highest concentration of magnesium is in the bone, liver and brain and the serum levels will not necessarily reflect a state of early deficiency. Hypomagnesaemia can result from excessive losses or from inadequate intake. While deficiency is not common, it has been seen following nasogastric drip and suction, and is a definite hazard of prolonged parenteral fluid administration and drainage. It has also been encountered in alcoholics and can occur as a result of diuretic therapy, hypercalcaemia and malabsorption. As detailed in Chapter 3, magnesium is needed in greater quantities by very active individuals. The reasons for this are

1. the essential role it plays, through enzyme systems, in the metabolism of carbohydrate, a major nutrient in the diet of these individuals;
2. the fact that magnesium is lost as a normal component of sweat.

Because of sweat losses, magnesium is also of particular importance in the diet of those living in very hot climates. Symptoms of deficiency are depression, irritability, convulsions, muscle weakness, hypertension, arrhythmias and tachycardia. Main food sources are dried peas and beans, nuts, wholegrain cereals and milk.

Iodine

Iodine is essential for the normal production and functioning of thyroxine, a hormone secreted by the thyroid, which has a vital overall effect on metabolism, energy output and mental and physical growth. Iodine is found particularly in products from the sea or nearby areas and thus fish and vegetables grown near the sea are the richest sources. Endemic dietary deficiency can occur in isolated inland communities. Goitre, i.e. enlargement of the thyroid, will occur as a physiological response to deficiency. Severe deprivation causes cretinism in children, a condition of retarded physical and mental development and slow metabolic rate, and myxoedema (a similar condition) in adults. Main features in the latter condition are deterioration of mental ability and sluggishness of movements. More common is non-dietary myxoedema resulting from reduced thyroid function due to ageing. This is treated with oral thyroxine supplements, not iodine.

Fluorine

This element is currently causing worldwide interest and debate. Small quantities occur in all foods and in tea leaves, but the major dietary contributor is water, various amounts being present in water from different areas. When fluorine is present in one part per million of water, the teeth of the inhabitants of the surrounding area become harder and there is a dramatic drop (up to 60%) in the incidence of dental caries. For this reason fluoride supplementation of water supplies in areas of low natural content is being widely practised in many countries including certain areas of Britain. The current controversy about its use does not relate to these well substantiated effects but rather to

1. the ethics of 'mass medication',
2. the fear of toxicity.

When water contains more than 2.5 parts per million of fluoride, the enamel becomes mottled, and progressively more unattractive with increasing amounts. Toxic doses of fluoride can also result in renal damage. Deficiency of the element causes an increase in dental caries. Reduced bone density is also prevalent in low-intake areas.

TRACE ELEMENTS

As stated earlier, the difference between mineral and trace elements is not well defined. The following elements constitute the major micronutrients in terms of the quantities present both in the body and in food.

Zinc

Research has identified the role of zinc in a diversity of metabolic processes. It plays a major role in various enzyme systems in the body. Like magnesium, zinc is lost in sweat, thus increasing the dietary requirements for sportsmen, miners and people living in hot climatic conditions. Deficiency is caused by inadequate intake, parasites in the gut causing long-term blood loss, and excessive sweating. Deficiency causes retardation of growth and sexual development, and impaired wound healing. The sense of taste is also reduced.

Major sources of zinc are most meat cuts, peas, egg yolk and cow's milk. Human milk is a poor source, as are rice, sugar, egg white and white bread.

As mentioned earlier, calcium and iron absorption may be impaired on a high-phytate diet. Zinc, too, whilst ingested in adequate amounts in a diet high in wholegrain cereals, may in fact have its availability reduced by the presence of phytate. It is also possible that fibre, which is present in wholegrain cereals in large amounts, may inhibit zinc absorption. The wide repercussions of this hypothesis are a subject of current research. In the first place, the consumption of a low-protein high-fibre diet in rural areas in Iran is being studied as a possible cause of low serum zinc levels and endemic retarded growth and sexual development. Secondly, the relationship of a high ratio of zinc to copper is being studied as a possible cause of coronary artery disease. There is a low risk of this disease in communities subsisting on wholegrain cereals and legumes and the low zinc to copper ratios are thought by some to have a protective effect. Typical diets eaten in communities where there is a high risk of corononary thrombosis have a high zinc to copper ratio. Zinc lost in sweat by strenuously exercising men is also proposed as the reason for their lower risk of developing the disease. The role of zinc is thus being widely scrutinized in an attempt to substantiate or refute various hypotheses currently presented.

Copper

It has long been known that there is an important relationship between iron and copper metabolism in the body, but it is only recently that the correlation between this relationship and diet-induced copper deficiency has received attention. Diet-induced copper deficiency has been encountered only in infants and appears to result from the consumption of an exclusively milk diet taken when the body is already depleted, i.e. following malnutrition or prematurity. Copper plays a role with iron in various enzyme systems and deficiency results in accumulation of iron in the liver and an anaemia which is not corrected by iron administration. The main sources of copper in the diet are liver, fish and green vegetables.

Chromium

Chromium has only recently been shown to be essential to Man. Its function is related to insulin output and utilization. In cases of deficiency there is reduced sensitivity of the tissues to insulin. Injections of insulin mobilize the chromium in the tissue and it is thought that long-term use of insulin injections may result in a minor deficiency. Dietary inadequacy may also cause deficiency manifested by low chromium levels in hair and abnormal glucose tolerance which is improved by supplementing the diet with chromium.

Vanadium

Recent work on the functions of this element has been of great interest, particularly with regard to its possible impact on public health. A study in which young men were given large doses of vanadium resulted in a significant drop in their plasma cholesterol levels. Other workers have correlated vanadium with dental caries, but much work still has to be done to substantiate these hypotheses. Food sources of vanadium have not been reliably established.

Tin

There is little information about the role of tin in the human body other than the fact that many ingested canned foods have a higher tin content than fresh food. Also, tin plating used inside food cans may be a cause of increased intake. However, the use of lacquer in tins and other forms of packaging for foods has reduced the hazard of toxicity which is unlikely to occur other than in exceptional circumstances.

Manganese, selenium, nickel and cadmium

All these elements are considered to be dietary trace elements. Their role in Man is not fully understood, but to date the dietary contributions of none of these elements appear to have a major effect in the body.

FIBRE

This is essentially the unavailable carbohydrate, found in natural food in the diet, which is unaffected by digestive enzymes but may be acted upon by colonic bacteria. Its main property is its bulk-forming capacity.

When combined with liquid, fibre reduces the transit time of excreta through the digestive tract, resulting in increased frequency of defecation. Recent work has correlated the increased incidence of several diseases of the gut, in particular cancer of the colon, with the change to refined foods and a reduction in the fibre content of the diet. The incidence of other diseases of sophistication has also been related to a change in eating patterns. The Department of Health and Social Security has stated that 'populations who eat a diet rich in fibre (particularly fibre from cereals and legumes) usually have a lower serum cholesterol concentration and a lower mortality from ischaemic heart disease than those who eat a Western-type diet relatively low in this kind of fibre'. Other studies have shown that fibre affects the metabolism of bile salts.

Modern processing of foods has resulted in reduced fibre intake and the nurse should emphasize to her patients the need for the inclusion in the diet of foods high in fibre. The housewife who depends on the expediency of farinaceous pre-prepared meals, the pensioner who eats mainly sandwiches due to the high cost of alternatives and lack of teeth, the single office worker who purchases convenience foods in preference to cooking, should all be made aware of the low fibre intake of their diet. Fresh fruit and vegetables and wholegrain cereals should be eaten daily. If this is impractical the diet should include daily dietary bran, the most effective class of fibre. This is an inexpensive product and light enough in weight for the elderly to transport it from the supermarket. Two or three tablespoons should be taken daily in the absence of generous helpings of other fibre. Bran can be combined with yoghurt or custard, sprinkled on cereal or soup, or used for coating fish before baking. As fibre combines with liquid in the digestive tract to provide bulk, it is of course essential to include ample amounts of liquid in the diet as well.

LIQUIDS

It is astonishing how many intelligent people, aware of the importance of correct nutrition, totally disregard the role of liquids in their diet. Water is the most essential dietary component in that a man deprived of water would die sooner than if deprived of any other nutrient. Water is the commonest single compound present in the body, constituting a higher proportion of body mass in lean and athletic people than in those who are inactive and overweight. It is the medium in which intracellular electrolyte processes occur and it is responsible for the transfer of elements at extracellular level. The functions of the blood stream are dependent on an adequate water intake and the elimination of waste products through the kidneys can occur only in a fluid medium. The control of body temperature occurs through evaporation of water: in hot weather heat stroke will result from inadequate fluid intake. The bulk-forming properties of fibre in producing faeces are dependent on the presence of adequate liquid.

Inadequate fluid intake can initially result in minor symptoms such as lethargy and constipation but under more extreme circumstances dehydration, ketosis and ultimately death can occur. To ensure adequacy, the recommended allowance of fluid (taken as water, tea, coffee, fruit juice, soup, etc.) is six to eight cups (1.5 litres) per day. In addition to this, the body will receive a further 1–1.5 litres of fluid from the metabolism of food. This 'water of oxidation' is derived from the metabolic breakdown of fat, protein and carbohydrates:

100 g of fat gives 107 ml of water
100 g of protein gives 41 ml of water
100 g of carbohydrate gives 55 ml of water

On this basis the water of oxidation in the diet markedly contributes to the body's water resources. Table 6 depicts the average obligatory daily water turnover of a 70 kg adult. This turnover is increased by increased uptake and subsequent excretion.

Various factors may influence the body's fluid requirements, for example:

1. climatic or environmental temperature and resultant sweat loss,
2. fever or increase in body temperature,
3. physical activity,
4. vomiting and/or diarrhoea causing excessive gastrointestinal loss,
5. severe burns causing a loss of extracellular fluid.

Table 6. Daily water turnover of a 70 kg adult.

Water intake (g)		Water output (g)	
Drink	650	Urine	700
Food	750	Skin	500
Oxidative	350	Faeces	150
		Lungs	400
	1750		1750

ELECTROLYTES

Some compounds, called *electrolytes*, when dissolved in solution, dissociate into simpler, electrically charged sustances. This characteristic determines the osmolarity of the solution; thus certain dietary components regulate the acid–base balance of the body and the osmotic pressure. For instance, sodium chloride (table salt) when dissolved in a solution, dissociates into two electrically charged ions: the positively charged to sodium (Na^+) ion and the negatively charged chloride (Cl^-) ion. Ionization also occurs with the salts of magnesium and potassium.

Sodium

The principal role of sodium is in extracellular fluids, particularly blood plasma, maintaining the optimum osmotic pressure of the fluids outside the cellular membranes. In this way, fluid balance in the body is also controlled through sodium.

The Western-type diet contains 12–14 g of table salt per day, an amount far in excess of the normal physiological need. The balance is exreted in the urine, in sweat and in small amounts in the faeces. Deficiency due to inadequate intake is therefore unlikely under normal circumstances. However, an increased intake may be necessary in exceptional conditions such as mining underground in high environmental temperatures or prolonged heavy physical activities. Furthermore, depletion may occur following extended exercise after consumption of a diet severely restricted in salt, or result from severe diarrhoea and excessive vomiting.

As acclimatization leads to a considerable reduction of the amount of sodium in sweat, sportsmen seldom need additional salt. Salt should not be taken during prolonged exercise, such as during a marathon race, because it can put an unphysiological load on the kidneys. This is discussed in Chapter 3 under 'Diet and physical activity' (pp. 107–111).

Dietary sodium is ingested mainly in the form of table salt and baking powder. The role of sodium in cardiac and renal disorders is discussed in Chapters 9 and 12. Briefly, there appears to be a correlation between a high salt intake and the incidence of myocardiopathy and hypertension. Increased amounts of sodium in the plasma, due to unsatisfactory elimination following cardiac and renal impairment, result in oedema due to changes in osmolarity.

Chlorine

This is found as the negatively charged chloride ion throughout the body in both intra- and extracellular fluid but in greatest concentration in gastric acid. Like sodium, it plays a major role in the fluid balance and acid–base balance in the body. Although unlikely to be deficient in the diet, depletion can occur with prolonged vomiting, and supplementation is sometimes necessary.

Potassium

Most potassium in the body is intracellular, potassium being an essential component of cell structure. A major function of the element is the regulation of intracellular osmotic pressure, but potassium also has a wide range of other roles throughout the body. It is essential for normal cardiac function, muscle contraction and the synthesis of protein. It is found in a variety of foods, especially fresh fruit and vegetables and those high in protein.

Dietary deficiency is unlikely to occur, but excessive loss due to vomiting, diarrhoea, burns or inadequate intake during parenteral feeding may cause deficiency. Muscular weakness, vomiting, cardiac arrhythmia and ultimately death may occur.

Hyperkalaemia (elevated blood potassium levels) can have equally severe consequences. Renal damage causing reduced elimination of potassium can result in serious cardiac arrhythmias. Patients are given a severely restricted intake excluding foods such as bananas, oranges, pineapples, tomatoes and soups, all of which are extremely rich sources of this element.

BIBLIOGRAPHY

Abt, A.F., van Schuching, S. & Enns, T. (1963) Vitamin C requirements of man re-examined. *Am. J. Clin. Nutr., 12*, 21.

Alhadeff, L., Gualtieri, T. & Lipton, M. (1984) Toxic effects of water-soluble vitamins. *Nutr. Rev., 42*, 33.

Anon. (1984) Recognizing and treating osteoporosis. *Consumer Res., 67 (6)*, 15.

Basu, T.K. (1979) Vitamins and cancer of epithelium origin. *J. Hum. Nutr., 33*, 24.

Burkitt, D.P., Walker, A.R.P. & Painter, N.S. (1972) Effect of dietary fibre on stools and transit-times, and its role in the causation of disease. *Lancet, ii*, 1408.

Buss, D.H. (1979) Some consequences of the new UK 'Recommended Daily Amounts of Food Energy and Nutrients' for evaluating food consumption surveys. *J. Hum. Nutr, 33*, 325.

Council of Foods and Nutrition (1963) Symposium on human calcium requirements. *J. Am. Med. Ass., 185 (7)*, 588.

Cravioto, J. & DeLicardie, E. (1971) The long-term consequences of PCM. *Nutr. Rev., 29 (5)*, 107.

De Bruin, E.J.P. (1970) Iron absorption in the Bantu. *J. Am. Diet. Ass. 57*, 129.

Department of Health and Social Security (1979) *Recommended Daily Amounts of*

Food Energy and Nutrients for Groups of People in the United Kingdom, 1st edn. London: HMSO.

Diem, K. & Lentner, C. (eds.) (1970) *Scientific Tables*, 7th edn., pp. 457–489. Basel: Geigy.

Flink, E.B., McCollister, R., Prasad, A.S., Melby, J.C. & Doe, R.P. (1957) Evidence for clinical magnesium deficiency. *Ann. Intern. Med., 47 (5)*, 956.

Hall, R.C.W. & Joffe, J.R. (1973) Hypomagnesemia: physical and psychiatric symptoms. *J. Am. Med. Ass., 224 (13)*, 1749.

Holemans, K.C. & Meyer, B.J. (1963) A quantitative relationship between the absorption of calcium and phosphorus. *Am. J. Clin. Nutr. 12*, 30.

Joint FAO/WHO Expert Group (1967) Requirements of vitamin A, thiamine, riboflavine and niacin. *Tech. Rep. Ser. WHO, 362*.

Joint FAO/WHO Expert Group (1973) Trace elements in human nutrition. *Tech. Rep. Ser. WHO, 532*.

Keller, W. & Fillmore, C. (1984) Prevalence of protein–energy malnutrition. *World Health Stat. Quart., 36*, 129.

Klevay, L.M. (1975) Coronary heart disease: the zinc/copper hypothesis. *Am. J. Clin. Nutr., 28*, 764.

MacIntyre, I. (1963) An outline of magnesium metabolism in health and disease. *J. Chron. Dis., 16*, 201.

Mahloudji, M., Reingold, J.G., Haghshenass, M., Ronaghy, H.M., Spivey Fox, M.R. & Halsted, J.A. (1975) Combined zinc and iron compared with iron supplementation of diets of 6- to 12-year-old village school-children in Southern Iran. *Am. J. Clin. Ntr., 28*, 721.

Mills, C.F. (1972) Some aspects of trace element nutrition in man. *Nutr. Lond., 26 (6)*, 357.

Palmisano, P.A. (1973) Vitamin D: a reawakening. *J. Am. Med. Ass., 224*, 1526.

Passmore, R., Nicol, B.M., Narayana Rao, M., Beaton, G.H. & Demayer, E.M. (1974) Handbook on human nutritional requirements. *Monograph. Ser. WHO, 61*.

Prasad, A.S. (1978) *Trace Elements and Iron in Human Metabolism*. London: Plenum.

Ronaghy, H.A. & Halsted, J.A. (1975) Zinc deficiency occurring in females. Report of two cases. *Am. J. Clin. Nutr. 28*, 831.

Schaumberg, H., Kaplan, J., Windebank, A., Vick, N., Rasmus, S., Pleasure, D. & Brown, M. (1983) Sensory neuropathy from pyridoxine abuse. *New Engl. J. Med.*, 309, 445.

Singleton, N. (1978) Vitamin D status of Asians. *Br. Med. J., 1*, 607.

Underwood, E.J. (1977) *Trace Elements in Human and Animal Nutrition*, 4th ed. London: Academic Press.

Waldbott, G.L. (1963) Fluoride in food. *Am. J. Clin. Nutr., 12*, 455.

Young, V.R., Taylor, Y.S.M., Rand, W.R. & Scrimshaw, N.S. (1975) Protein requirements of man. *J. Nutr., 103*, 1164.

2   Diet throughout the life cycle

FOOD GROUPS

While it is essential to understand the role of individual nutrients in the body and the foods in which they are encountered, it is quite impractical to design menus taking them into consideration individually. For simplicity, foods with similar composition are therefore classified in groups which are used as the basis for planning daily menus. In the past, seven basic food groups were used. Later this was reduced by reclassification to five, and today four basic food groups are generally used as the guide for optimum nutritional adequacy. These groups are shown in Fig. 3. They are:

1. the milk and cheese group,
2. the meat, fish and egg group,

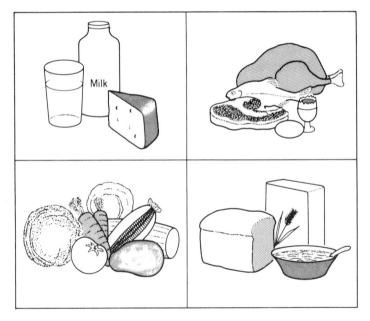

Fig. 3. *The four basic food groups.*

3. the vegetable and fruit group,
4. the bread and cereal group.

Interchangeable portions of these foods are used for variety in menu compilation and the nurse can also easily evaluate the daily intake of a patient to determine adequacy.

Group 1

A *standard portion* of this group is a cup of full or skimmed milk or yoghurt or 40–50 g cheese, either full fat or skimmed. An optimum intake for adults is two portions of this group per day, and young children and pregnant women require four portions per day. Lactating mothers should take six portions per day to meet their own and their babies' needs. This group of food provides complete protein, calcium and phosphorus, zinc, vitamins A and B_{12} and riboflavin; also fat if full-fat products are used.

Group 2

Two portions of this 'meat and fish' group should be eaten daily. Legumes, peanut butter and eggs should also be included several times per week by healthy individuals; vegetarians should replace their meat and fish portions with these equivalents, using one cup of peas, beans or lentils, four tablespoons of peanut butter or two eggs as an exchange for a main meal meat or fish portion. Those with a personal or family history of hypercholesterolaemia should include fish rather than eggs in their diet because of the presence of a large amount of cholesterol in egg yolks. Group 2 foods are necessary for their complete-protein content, iron (in meat and eggs), iodine (in fish), vitamin B complex (all exchanges except eggs) and vitamin D (in dark-fleshed fish). Meat, dark-fleshed fish and egg yolk also contain fat.

Group 3

Four portions from this group should be taken daily, including one serving of a fruit or vegetable rich in vitamin C, such as a citrus fruit, strawberries, tomatoes, a serving of raw cabbage or salad greens. This group in particular supplies carotene, vitamin C and cellulose to the diet.

Group 4

Four servings of this group are recommended daily, including at least one serving of a wholegrain product. A portion is made up of a slice of bread, half a cup of cooked cereal, noodles or rice, or 30 g ready-to-eat breakfast cereal. Although refined cereals provide little but starch, wholegrain products supply vitamin B complex, calcium, iron and cellulose to the diet.

Supplementary food

It can be seen that each group complements the others to ensure an optimal intake of most of the nutrients discussed in the previous chapter. However, if the recommended portions of these groups are used exclusively, the protein, fat and carbohydrate intake will be an inadequate energy source for active people, and the inclusion of fats (salad oil, butter, margarine, etc.) and additional carbohydrates (jam, biscuits, confectionery, etc.) will be a natural procedure for many individuals. The consumption of too much of this additional food will promote obesity: inactive overweight people will have to avoid them, reduce their intake of group 4 foods, and select skimmed milk products from Group 1 to cause weight loss. This regimen is discussed in detail in Chapter 5 (Overweight). With regard to the minerals and trace elements discussed in the previous chapter, it will be seen that only calcium, iron and iodine are enumerated above. It has been shown that adequacy of these nutrients in natural sources invariably ensures adequacy of the other minerals and trace elements.

COMPILATION OF MENUS

As indicated, the above food groups are used as a basis for scientific menu planning. However, there are several other factors which are of major importance when recommended allowances are converted into meals. Perhaps the most important nutritional aspect is to compare the recommended food groups with the meals that are in fact being served in Britain, and the advice given by experts to improve the British diet.

A recent (1979) report in the *British Medical Journal* (Passmore *et al*) recommends a 15% *decrease* in intake of fats and oils, in sugar consumption and meat intake. Pointing out that the quantities of alcoholic beverages consumed have risen steadily since 1960, they also recommend a reduction of 25% in alcohol intake.

Furthermore, the committee suggests a 15% *increase* in the consumption of potatoes, other vegetables and fruit and a 20% increase in the intake of grain products.

The recommendations include no change in intake in the consumption of dairy products (excluding butter), eggs and fish, pulses and nuts. Butter, of course, would fall into the fats and oils group in which a 15% decrease in intake is recommended.

In summary, therefore, when planning a menu, while the basic four food groups should be used as a standard of adequacy, recipe selection should take these considerations into account. Replacing fried foods with grilled or baked ones, serving fruit instead of rich desserts and sometimes substituting a pasta dish (preferably wholewheat) for meat are all practical measures that will help meet these recommendations.

Another important aspect of successful menu planning is *presentation*. Although the meal may be calculated to provide the optimum food value, the patient is unlikely to eat it with relish unless it is attractive. The inclusion of variety should be a major concern of the meal planner: difference in colour, texture and flavour all add enormously to the enjoyment of a meal. Hospital patients on full diets should be allowed a choice of menu items wherever practical, rather than the choice being made by the nurse who is occupied in serving meals from food trolleys onto plates. Hot foods should be served hot and cold foods chilled — this enhances palatability of the meal and inhibits the bacterial multiplication which can be rife in food at room temperature.

Each meal should include a high-protein food for both nutritional and satiety value. As protein takes a considerable time to digest, the feeling of fullness will be prolonged.

Breakfast

Breakfast is an important meal. The omission of breakfast is a common bad habit. The consumption of breakfast has been shown to increase mid- and late-morning efficiency, particularly if the meal includes some protein. Comparative studies on schoolchildren have shown that those who had consumed a breakfast containing a good source of protein had a better school performance and less late-morning fatigue or headache, and were less irritable than those who merely ate a high-carbohydrate snack, such as toast and marmalade, before leaving for school. This does not mean that bacon and eggs are necessary; a full-grain or combination cereal (such as muesli) with milk is a filling and nutritious breakfast.

The midday meal

If practical, the main meal may be served at midday and a third of the daily intake should be taken at this time. Meals followed by a small amount of exercise in the afternoon are more readily digested than those taken at night followed by sedentary relaxation. However, strenuous exercises should never be taken immediately after a large meal.

For most office workers and children the midday meal is either a canteen meal or a portable one packed before leaving home. Lunch is a necessary meal providing essential nutrients for a large proportion of the population, but the lunch box is frequently an extremely neglected aspect of our daily living. Even those who are not out at work frequently have a sandwich meal. The nurse should thus encourage intelligent attention to the preparation of this meal.

Lunch box preparation

In most cases bread will form the basis of the portable lunch. Wholewheat cereals contribute large quantities of vitamin B complex, iron and calcium, and should thus be used in preference to brown and certainly in preference to white bread. Nevertheless, some children have a phase of objecting to wholewheat bread and it might be better for the mother to use white bread instead temporarily, to ensure that the sandwiches are eaten and not discarded at school. As mentioned previously, protein is all-important in each meal and thus cheese, peanut butter, a meat spread or a hard-boiled egg are useful additions to the lunch box. Jam, honey or syrup are not recommended because:

1. They provide exclusively 'empty calories', i.e. they are foods which supply merely energy.

2. Concentrated sugars are rapidly absorbed and the feeling of satisfaction or fullness following consumption is for a very limited period.

3. Concentrated sugars create a medium conducive to the formation of dental caries.

A portion of fruit or carrots, a mixed vegetable salad or a few pieces of dried fruit all increase the nutritive content of the portable lunch.

Evening meal

For reasons of expediency this is usually the main meal of the day. It should cover the inadequacies of the other two meals, providing a variety of nutrients.

Snacks

For many people with a limited capacity for food, particularly children, snacks may provide an integral contribution to the daily requirement of nutrients. Sweets, refined confectionery and soft drinks should be kept to a minimum and replaced by foods with more nutritional value.

There are, however, several nutritional hazards in snack eating. In the first place, an excessive amount of kilojoules may unknowingly be taken by individuals oblivious to the fact that even very small quantities of food if taken too frequently throughout the day can lead to overweight. People may omit essential nutrients by filling up on mid-meal snacks of minimal nutritional value. Furthermore, snack foods are often far more expensive than those foods which make up a home-cooked meal. Dental caries are also promoted by frequent contact with food, particularly confectionery and other refined foods.

Fluids

Fluids are an essential part of the diet and should be included in adequate amounts. Six to eight cups are required per day, more in hot weather and more for people undertaking strenuous physical exercise. Tea, coffee, fruit juice and soup all contribute to the fluid requirement. Regrettably, in our sophisticated society there is a trend to minimize the importance of tap water as a drink. Children particularly should be educated to drink water as a routine practice in preference to sweetened drinks.

FOOD FADDISM

Not infrequently a patient will reject the nurse's attempts to guide him about sound principles of nutrition, embracing instead ideas based on emotional or misguided opinions. There are various factors which may prompt food faddism. Suspicion, fear of resultant disease (particularly cancer), morality or misguided religious fervour may all be responsible. Perhaps the biggest and most dangerous promoters of food faddism are health store assistants. From a position of strength behind the counter, these individuals, often with no other background than being food faddists, promote a viewpoint — and their wares — to gullible customers. There are many arguments against this practice. People may be dissuaded from seeking orthodox medical advice for symptoms requiring treatment. The propagation of nutrition misinformation and food quackery detracts from the vital role of scientifically substantiated information. People readily gain the impression that healthy foods are available only at inflated prices in a health store and not in a supermarket. Finally, the spending of money on totally unnecessary commodities is a waste that few can afford. Some of the nutritional ideas that faddists advocate to promote their ideas are considered below.

ORGANICALLY GROWN PRODUCE. There is no evidence to show that fruit and vegetables grown with the use of compost instead of fertilizer are nutritionally superior to ordinary commercially grown fruit and vegetables. The nutritional characteristics of a plant are genetically determined and are not affected by the environment, except in severely depleted soil which is unlikely to be used for commercial products as the crop yield, and thus the economic reward, is reduced in poor soil.

HONEY. Honey is recommended by many food faddists as being more healthy than sugar. This argument is unsubstantiated. Honey contains few minerals and vitamins and the price is out of proportion to the nutritional content.

RAW, UNPASTEURIZED MILK. Admittedly pasteurization does have a minimally detrimental effect on the nutritive content of milk. However, it also destroys pathogenic bacteria — a factor of vital importance to the consumer. The advantages of pasteurization unquestionably outweigh the disadvantages.

YOGHURT. This is made from skimmed milk to which microorganisms have been added to change the flavour and texture. The principal nutritional change is from lactose to lactic acid, which is relevant to those with lactose intolerance (as discussed in Chapter 8). Other than that, the composition of yoghurt remains essentially the same as the milk from which it was made.

FOOD SUPPLEMENTS. Under normal circumstances these are not necessary for healthy individuals who pay attention to their diet and include the four food groups as listed. Although supplements are justified in the diet of people undertaking extensive expeditions or those on an abnormally limited or depleted diet, the use of an assortment of pills as a regular precautionary measure is both unnecessary and wasteful. Furthermore, current research shows that massive doses of certain nutrients previously thought to be harmless may, in fact, have a detrimental effect on the body.

LIMITED DIETS. Some food faddists advocate a strictly limited dietary regimen. One of the most dangerous of these plans is the Zen macrobiotic diet. This eating pattern, initiated by the Japanese writer Georges Ohsawa, is based on the yin-yang theory. Yin foods are those which produce silence, calm, cold and diarrhoea; yang foods produce action, heat and light. Ohsawa claimed that a balance between yin and yang foods would promote health and harmony of soul, mind and body. The diet is based on ten progressively more stringent diets. It is said that as one works up to a higher diet one will achieve increasingly better health and well-being. Diet No. 7 is an exclusively cereal diet, whereas the lower grades of diet are more varied, including meat, salads, fruits, soup, etc. Needless to say, the diet becomes progressively more hazardous. Strict adherence to diet No. 7 can cause death due to a deficiency of nutrients. Referring to this diet, the American Medical Association's Council on Foods and Nutrition has stated 'It would be premature at this time to categorize all "unusual" dietary philosophies as hazardous without evaluating their nutritional contributions. But when a diet has been shown to cause irreversible damage to health and ultimately lead to death, it should be roundly condemned as a threat to human nutrition'.

VEGETARIANISM

The word 'fad' normally refers to a short-term craze and although vegetarianism for some people may be a short-lived exercise, for others it is a well researched, healthy way of living. There are two classes of vegetarians — the vegan and the ovolactovegetarian.

The vegan diet

The vegan rejects all foods of animal origin, including fish, eggs and dairy products. Adhering to a diet compiled exclusively of foods of vegetable origin, vegans encounter difficulty in achieving an adequate intake of certain nutrients. Children should be dissuaded from becoming vegans as a satisfactory intake of several nutrients, particularly calcium, is almost impossible due to the high requirements of childhood and the size of portion of vegetable sources needed to provide reasonable amounts.

PROTEIN. As indicated earlier, combinations of partially complete proteins (i.e. those which have a high proportion but not all of the essential amino acids) can result in a totally satisfactory intake. The vegan should include a portion of legumes or nuts each day as a main-meal meat replacement. Soya in particular has an excellent amino acid pattern and is versatile in the diet. A variety of acceptable dishes using the above foods, prepared as a casserole, salad or rissoles, ensures adequacy of diet in the adult.

CALCIUM. Although calcium is found predominantly in dairy products and fish bones, certain fruits and vegetables are also fair sources. The inclusion of large portions of dried figs, currants, raisins, cabbage, leeks and dried beans can effect a satisfactory calcium intake for adults. Wholegrain cereals, too, provide large amounts of calcium in the diet but the presence of phytate renders some of this inabsorbable and these products cannot therefore be regarded as reliable sources. The fermentation of yeast in bread dough destroys much of the phytate.

VITAMIN B_{12} (CYANOCOBALAMIN). This is found almost exclusively in foods of animal origin. Studies have shown that after 12–14 years vegans can develop subacute degeneration of the spinal cord — an irreversible condition due to vitamin B_{12} deficiency. There are commercially available supplements made from non-animal sources and vegans should be strongly advised to take these compounds in the recommended dosage.

IRON. Although iron is present in large quantities in wholegrain cereals and spinach, the presence of phytic and oxalic acids respectively reduces the relevance of them as major sources. Parsley, dried fruit and soya have a high iron content and should be particularly emphasized in the diet of vegan females, due to regular heavy losses in menstruation. It is also advisable that vegans, particularly females, have an annual check made on their haemoglobin level to ensure that it remains within normal limits in spite of their very restricted diet.

IODINE. This is found exclusively in fish and vegetable produce grown near the coast. Vegans living inland should use iodized salt to prevent a possible deficiency of this nutrient.

The ovolactovegetarian diet

If intelligent and selective in their choice of foods, these individuals have much less chance than vegans of developing nutritional deficiencies. Iron and iodine are the two nutrients most likely to be inadequate in this diet, but the regular consumption of eggs (supplying iron) and iodized salt will prevent deficiencies of these nutrients occurring in adults.

In spite of the inclusion of sources of essential calcium and phosphorus it is not advisable for children to become ovolac-tovegetarians unless the mother is aware of the nutritive compo-nents of food and of her child's requirements, and takes particular care in her choice of meals. Regrettably children are often coerced into this way of life by emotional and naïve parents influenced by unbalanced opinion and misinformed, unsubtantiated literature.

Protein foods in the vegetarian diet

Interestingly, studies done on ovolactovegetarians have shown that, in spite of the liberal inclusion of dairy products, these people suffer less than the standard population from coronary artery disease and various other diseases of sophisticated living.

TEXTURIZED SOYA PRODUCTS. It is largely as a result of the efforts of the Seventh Day Adventists that a variety of these products are available for vegetarians today. Soya has a good amino acid pattern and can be readily included both by vegetarians and by meat-eaters as an economy measure. Dried soya products are rehydrated and converted into stews. They are usually purchased in package form with the addition of various herbs and spices for added flavour.

BREWER'S YEAST. This is a particularly valuable food, 100 g supplying complete protein in greater quantities than that in 100 g of beef. The characteristic, pronounced, unattractive flavour precludes the use of large quantities of brewer's yeast in the diet, but small amounts can be put into soups and stews and added to loaves, thus making a substantial contribution to the otherwise limited protein intake of many vegetarians. As yeast readily ferments in a tepid medium, it should only be added immediately prior to serving or baking.

PULSES. Legumes of all sorts should play a prominent role in the vegetarian diet and be taken regularly as a main-meal meat replacement. The nutritive value of dried beans and lentils can be enhanced by soaking them raw in fresh water in a warm place for two or three days. Vitamins B and C are produced in considerable quantities in the sprouts, adding to the food value of the dish in which they are used.

YOGHURT OR KEFIR. These products are made from milk modified by the addition of microorganisms. They frequently play a major role in the diet of the ovolactovegetarian. They contribute the same food value as milk, and vegetarians should be dissuaded from assuming that they provide some mystical component with health-giving properties in the diet. Yoghurt first came into prominence at the turn of the century when Elie Metchnikoff, a Russian scientist, claimed that the longevity evident among the peasants in the Bulgarian Alps was due to the typical sour milk they drank. This was later disclaimed by other scientists who showed that genetic factors were responsible for the exceptional life-span of these people. However, food faddists today still make exceptional claims for yoghurt which are quite without substantiation.

Tofu. For the active vegetarian interested in overnight camping, tofu is of particular relevance. It is a curd made from soya milk, similar in texture to cottage cheese. It is made by souring soya milk by the addition of lemon juice and then separating the curd from the whey component by pouring it through a muslin cloth. The curd can be eaten with biscuits, sprinkled on salads or mixed with vegetables. Although simple to make at home (using 3 cups of water, 1 cup of soya flour and 25 ml of lemon juice) it is particularly useful for the hiker, who can carry a small quantity of soya flour and make an acceptable dish. Some vegetarians recommend the addition of a yeast extract, such as Marmite, to the milk before souring, for added flavour of the curd.

Peanuts. Peanuts contain approximately 26% of good quality protein on a par with cooked meat, which has a similar quantity, although a slightly better amino acid pattern. Other commonly eaten nuts have a slightly lower protein content. Nuts may be prepared in a variety of ways, including rissoles, roasts or loaves, and are useful and versatile inclusions in a vegetarian diet.

In conclusion, a word of caution about the vegetarian diet. Although few would deny that the intelligent vegetarian can select a healthy adequate diet, there is no doubt that the more restricted a diet becomes, the more difficult it is to consume a balanced diet. A common fault among vegetarians, for example, is to claim that in view of the fact that they do not object to eating eggs they are unlikely to develop iron-deficiency anaemia. However, the iron content of an egg is approximately 1 mg. As the recommended dietary amount is 10–12 mg/day and as only 10–30% of one's iron intake is absorbed, it is essential that good sources of iron are consumed several times a week. The vegetarian who merely eats the occasional dish which includes an egg as one of the ingredients should not be complacent.

The above remarks apply to calcium-rich foods and sources of protein, too. The value of protein depends on several factors including, not merely the amount we eat, but also the amino acid composition and the balance of amino acids that are eaten at the same time. It is therefore imperative that vegetarians have an intelligent interest and responsible attitude to their chosen way of life.

PREGNANCY AND LACTATION

Pregnancy is a period of extremely rapid cell production and anabolic activity. The growth of the baby, the increase in breast tissue and the retention of adequate reserves for labour and lactation are all major physiological changes. The production and function of the placenta, too, is a vital physiological process. This organ plays a dominant role in fetal nutrition, converting maternal nutrients to plasma proteins and haemoglobin characteristic of the fetus and quite different from those of the mother. These changes are dependent on a variety of nutrients and it is thus obvious that the well-being of the infant is largely dependent on the mother's diet. Over the years this has resulted in mass controversy and changes of opinion. It was originally thought that the fetus developed like a parasite on the mother and the expression 'a tooth lost for every baby' reflected this view of nutrition and the deficiency caused to the mother during pregnancy. In years gone by, people also held the false opinion that maternal 'cravings' for certain foods were a physiological mechanism to ensure adequacy of a specific nutrient for the infant. It was thought that the mother's selection of food during pregnancy would be guided by fetal needs.

More recently, several workers have reported studies of population groups which have related poor maternal diet with increased risk of prematurity and smaller infants. Immoderate consumption of alcohol and cigarette smoking have also been correlated with an increase in fetal deaths and retardation of infant growth. Increased numbers of premature and stillborn babies are also found in deprived communities. Brewer has done considerable research, emphasizing that the converse of this is equally true, i.e. that adequacy of maternal intake results in improved birth weight and a reduction in prematurity. These findings are supported by Singh *et al* who commented that because of the suspected relationship between overweight and pre-eclamptic toxaemia, women were unnecessarily advised to reduce their protein and energy intake. Both the above workers suggested that less emphasis should be given to the routine advice to pregnant women about not putting on too much weight, especially in socio-economic areas where patients depend on a limited range of low-cost foods for their nutrient intake. Reduction of these high-carbohydrate foods may reduce their intake of essential nutrients to inadequate levels.

Of enormous importance is the nutritional status of the woman when she becomes pregnant. The nausea and indigestion often seen in the early period may adversely affect the dietary intake during pregnancy but this will be of little nutritional relevance in women who have a history of sound nutrition and adequate reserves. By contrast, improved nutrition and supplementation must be to the advantage of both mother and baby, but it is unlikely to correct the effects of long-term poor eating habits.

Niswander *et al* found that birth weight is proportional to maternal body weight before conception and weight gain during pregnancy. He found that mothers of small stature who gained less than 10 kg during pregnancy have infants with an average birth weight of 2500 g. However, when larger women with a weight gain of 15 kg gave birth their infants weighed 3000 g on average.

On the basis of current research it is considered that the body, prompted by various hormonally induced changes, can adapt to a wide range of nutrient intake during this period. Although specific aspects which are enumerated below require particular attention, it now appears that the role of nutrition in pregnancy has previously been somewhat overstated. The suggested intakes of the essential nutrients have been stipulated in Table 1 on the assumption that the woman enters pregnancy with a satisfactory nutritional status. The malnourished individual will require a higher intake of deficient dietary components.

There are, however, specific aspects which should be considered. In the first place differences in dietary intake of mothers giving birth to babies with neural tube defects, in particular spina bifida, has raised the question of whether vitamin deficiencies could have some link with this disorder. In a recent study by Smithells *et al* there was a drop in incidence from 5% in the control series to 0.6% in the group who received multivitamin supplements. Other studies have confirmed this association and whilst the specific relationship between vitamin intake and neural tube defects is not fully understood, many clinics are today routinely giving large doses of vitamin supplements to women at risk.

Secondly, it will be noted from Table 1 that the protein requirement of a pregnant woman is surprisingly close to that of a non-pregnant woman. It should be emphasized that the amount recommended in Table 1 states the protein equivalent of egg or milk. Moreover, if ingested proteins of poor quality, they should be varied and improved. Thus, in general a woman should be advised that for the first half of her pregnancy she should merely adhere to the principles of a normal healthy diet based on the four food groups discussed in the previous chapter.

Nutritional recommendations during pregnancy

Energy intake and weight gain

The average weight gain during pregnancy is 10–13.5 kg, the rate of increase after the first 20 weeks being about 0.5 kg/week. During a normal pregnancy approximately 2 kg of fat will be deposited as a reserve for energy requirements and fat transfer to the infant in the last few months. Initial weight gain is largely due to fluid retention and expansion of blood volume. Later increase in weight results from the growth of the baby, uterus and liquor. An average fetus should gain 0.25 kg/week in the last eight weeks of pregnancy.

As mentioned earlier, there is a tendency today to lessen the emphasis on an optimal weight gain during pregnancy, particularly in underprivileged communities, to avoid restricting the intake of those already on a limited diet. However, it is often necessary to caution the patient not to eat excessively, warning her of the problems of weight reduction after delivery and pointing out that the increased energy requirement is extremely small — increasing from 700 kJ/day early to 1500 kJ/day during the second half of the pregnancy. The demands of the baby must outweigh the demands of self-improvement in the early months of infancy, and the overweight, unhappy, unattractive young mother is a common sight.

There are several reasons why women overeat during pregnancy. In the first place, the blood sugar level is often labile, resulting in increased appetitie and also possibly being the cause of 'morning sickness'. (This latter condition is frequently relieved by ingestion of lightly sweetened or high-carbohydrate foods.) There is an exaggerated response of blood sugar levels both to meals and to fasting resulting from hormone effects on the blood sugar. Another reason is that many women, normally controlled about their eating habits, regard pregnancy as demanding 'eating for two' and abandon all self-discipline with regard to food.

An important reason for weight control is that the pregnant woman has a higher risk of developing certain pathological conditions, which are in turn aggravated by weight gain. Diabetes, varicose veins and oedema all fall into this class.

The *rate* of weight gain is particularly important. During the

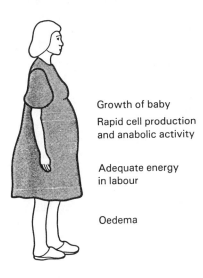

Growth of baby
Rapid cell production
and anabolic activity

Adequate energy
in labour

Oedema

Fig. 4. *Nutritional influences in pregnancy.*

second half of pregnancy a sudden increase in weight due to fluid retention may be related to the onset of toxaemia. The close monitoring of weight gain is thus performed nowadays principally as a check on the development of pre-eclamptic toxaemia. This condition can develop into a serious disorder including hypertension, albuminuria, convulsions, coma and ultimately death. The causative role of both dietary factors previously thought to be relevant, i.e. excessive weight gain and a high sodium intake resulting in increased fluid retention, is now in doubt. These two factors are regarded today as a manifestation, not a fundamental cause, of the condition.

On the other hand, failure to gain weight, particularly in the last ten or twelve weeks of pregnancy, may be an indication of poor placental function, leading to a 'small-for-dates' (growth-retarded) baby. This 'placental insufficiency' cannot be improved by increased dietary intake.

Sodium intake during pregnancy

Sodium retention occurs as a natural phenomenon during pregnancy. Progesterone secreted by the placenta promotes salt loss from the kidneys. The fact that sodium is *not lost* but retained in greater than normal quantities is due to the resultant compensatory mechanism which causes aldosterone to be secreted to counteract the salt-losing effect of the progesterone. This results in secondary fluid retention, adding significantly to the weight gain of pregnancy. Oedema may occur, resulting from reduced plasma osmotic pressure due to blood changes during pregnancy and also from pressure of the fetus on the vena cava causing increased capillary pressure in the legs.

The use of a low-salt diet for this condition is being questioned today, as reduction in the serum sodium levels results in compensatory increased levels of aldosterone, which promote sodium retention. For this reason sodium restriction is now seldom advised for hypertension of pregnancy. The patient is advised to have a normal but not excessive salt intake. She is also advised to reduce her kilojoule intake if there is excessive weight gain which appears to be the result of overeating.

Protein intake during pregnancy

One kilogram of additional protein is added to the 10 kg protein normally stored in the body of the adult female. To meet this 10% increase, additional protein intake is necessary. Half of the increase (i.e. 500 g) is taken up by the infant, 60 g protein is required by the placenta and the rest is needed for increase in lean body mass of the mother, enlargement of breast tissue and increase in blood volume. Furthermore, reserves are required for the demands of labour and milk production. 500 ml of extra milk per day will guarantee sufficient protein intake. This amount provides 17 g of protein, enough not only to meet day-to-day needs but to compensate for a possible previously restricted intake. Patients wary of potential weight gain from the increased milk intake should use skimmed milk.

Iron requirements in pregnancy

The need for routine oral administration of 30–60 mg of iron per day has recently been questioned, as the woman who has been well nourished prior to pregnancy and actively includes a high iron intake in her normal diet (with plentiful meat and eggs, and liver weekly) may well maintain a normal haemoglobin level throughout an uncomplicated pregnancy and delivery. Haemodilution occurs during pregnancy and a haemoglobin level as low as 10–12 mg/dl may be normal for some women. However, omission of iron supplementation is usually regarded as unwise due to the unpredictability of the course of the pregnancy. Excessive blood loss during delivery or the need for a Caesarean section will deplete the levels considerably. Furthermore, three or four months' reserve of iron is required during pregnancy for deposition in the fetal liver to compensate for the low iron content of milk. Thus supplements will ensure an optimal allowance for both mother and child.

Interestingly, the stores of iron and folic acid (see below) in the fetus are not dependent on maternal stores; i.e. even if the mother's diet is totally inadequate, parasitic demands of the infant will ensure adequate levels in the baby.

Calcium requirements in pregnancy

Calcium is an essential element for the production of bones and teeth in the infant. During the last three months approximately 25 g calcium are taken up by the infant, predominantly for the mineralization of the skeleton. It is also needed for various metabolic purposes, including blood clotting. Although one can adapt to a wide range of calcium intake and, as stated earlier, there is a hormonally induced increase in the deposition of bone during pregnancy, it seems unwise to be complacent about the situation. The recommended allowance in the second half of pregnancy is double the amount for the non-pregnant woman (see Table 1). This is achieved by the inclusion of an additional 500 ml of milk per day. Although the need is greater during the second half of pregnancy it is advisable to include this additional milk in the diet from the first trimester to ensure adequate reserves. Calcium salts as an alternative supplement are both unnecessary and less absorbable than the calcium present in milk. Furthermore, milk also provides other essential vitamins, and unless the patient is unable to tolerate milk for some reason such supplementation should not be considered. Should the patient prefer alternative foods as sources of calcium, she may replace 1 litre of milk with the same quantity of buttermilk or yoghurt, or approximately 150 g of yellow cheese.

Folic acid requirements in pregnancy

This vitamin is necessary for production of erythrocytes and may be routinely administered (300 µg/day) to prevent megaloblastic anaemia. Requirements increase during pregnancy and women who take minimal amounts of meat and vegetables are at high risk of developing a deficiency. In some areas, even among seemingly well nourished patients, anaemia due to folic acid deficiency may be encountered surprisingly often. Nurses should routinely advise pregnant women to take adequate amounts of green vegetables and women in low socio-economic groups should be advised to incorporate outer cabbage and lettuce leaves and the tops of carrots, turnips and beetroot in stews and soups for added folic acid.

Practical recommendations during pregnancy

1. Initially the nurse should take a dietary history to determine whether or not the basic diet provides satisfactory amounts from each of the four food groups.
2. The nurse should then discuss any nutritional inadequacies with the patient and modify her diet to meet her needs within the limitations of her budget.
3. An added 500 ml of milk or equivalent should be included in this diet to meet the increased needs for protein and calcium. Green vegetables should be emphasized to meet the requirements for folic acid and vitamins A and C, and the inclusion of liver once a week will contribute a large amount of iron and vitamin B complex.
4. In the absence of regular exposure to sunlight, vitamin D adequacy will be ensured by the weekly inclusion of dark-fleshed fish such as herring, kippers, sardines and salmon.

Complications of pregnancy

Nausea

Morning sickness may be caused by various factors. Although psychological reaction is sometimes blamed, there are usually basic physiological reasons, including hormonal changes and depressed blood sugar levels, for this reaction. Effective treatment will be the consumption of easily digestible carbohydrate foods (such as toast and plain biscuits) or sweetened foods (such as acid drop sweets) before rising in the morning. The avoidance of liquids at mealtimes is sometimes advantageous and in the event of repeated vomiting the consumption of foods supplying replacement electrolytes, such as Marmite and Bovril, is often helpful. Pyridoxine (vitamin B_6) is sometimes administered in therapeutic doses for this condition but its value is questionable. When severe long-term vomiting occurs the condition is known as *hyperemesis gravidarum* and the patient will usually need hospitalization. Here, under sedation, the feeding of small, easily digestible meals can be re-introduced.

Indigestion

Indigestion is a common and uncomfortable complication of late pregnancy caused by the pressure of the fetus on the abdominal contents and relaxation of the oesophageal–gastric sphincter. A degree of hiatus hernia may be present which is aggravated by the pressure of the uterus. This causes increased fermentation, regurgitation, acidity and heartburn. Various foods may be incriminated in such cases. Fresh bread is often a culprit (toast being better tolerated), and fried foods, fibrous fruit and vegetables and gaseous drinks may also precipitate indigestion. Eating too rapidly or chewing food for too brief a period can also result in discomfort. Generally, a diet containing less coarse roughage, eaten slowly and thoroughly chewed, is of great help. The situation may be further relieved by sleeping in a propped-up position.

Constipation

This, too, is a common complaint in later pregnancy due to the relaxing effect of progesterone on smooth muscle, dietary changes and limitation of exercise. It is sometimes aggravated by iron supplements.

The patient should be advised to take a large amount of *fibre* to assist the formation of bulk in the digestive tract. Examples of suitable foods are tomatoes, oranges, cauliflower and apricots, and wholegrain cereals such as wholewheat bread and all bran cereals. As these foods may give rise to indigestion, they should be carefully chewed and swallowed in small pieces to limit the effect.

Equally important is the adequate intake of fluid. Whilst *excessive* quantities will merely result in increased output of urine through the kidneys, the ingestion of *adequate* quantities is essential to combine with the fibre in the bowel helping to form bulk in the digestive tract, a point which should be remembered by all people advised to increase their fibre intake.

A third modification of the diet to counteract constipation is the inclusion of prunes and prune juice. These foods contain a component known as diphenylisatin which stimulates the gastro-colic reflex.

Discontinuation of iron supplements may also promote improvement of constipation. The nurse should advise the patient to try these basic dietary changes before resorting to potentially harmful laxatives.

Food cravings

Although frequently associated with emotional needs, such as apprehension or feelings of insecurity about the forthcoming birth, food cravings may be derived from a physiological need. The more labile blood sugar may drop to lower levels than normal, prompting a desire for food, particularly those items which are sweetened. Subconsciously supporting this increased need with the argument that weight control is less essential than usual, the patient may eat more than normal quantities.

Pica (the craving for unnatural articles of food) is a different situation. When it occurs in small children, especially the eating of sand, it is thought by many to reflect an iron deficiency. In pregnant women such abnormal cravings have not been correlated to specific needs.

Fetal alcohol syndrome

This chapter would be incomplete without some mention of this very relevant condition. Although as early as 1834 a report to the British House of Commons indicated that infants born to alcoholic mothers 'sometimes had a starved, shrivelled and imperfect look', it was only in 1973 that specific malformations in these infants were described. Growth defects, mental retardation, distinctive facial features and cardiac abnormalities are all seen in these children. The early months, in particular the month preceding the recognition of pregnancy, are crucial in this regard. Four or more drinks taken at one time or two strong drinks per day over a prolonged period increases the risk of the development of fetal alcohol syndrome. The risk increases with the proportionate increase in daily alcohol intake. Hence it is vitally important that pregnant women be cautioned about the hazards of immoderate or regular alcohol intake.

Lactation

The nutrient requirements of the mother during lactation are higher than at any other period of a normal healthy existence. The diet must be sufficient to provide the needs of both the infant and the mother. Since approximately 2 g of protein is required in the mother's diet to make 1 g of breast milk protein, the nurse should emphasize particularly the need for an adequate protein intake. When producing 850 ml milk/day, containing nearly 10 g protein, the mother requires an additional 20 g protein/day. There is also evidence that an inadequate intake of protein by the mother will result in a reduced volume of milk produced. In a study by Edozien *et al*, malnourished mothers who were given protein supplements during lactation produced larger quantities of milk during the period of supplementation.

Furthermore, 550 kJ (130 Cal) are required for the production of 100 ml of milk. This means that when the infant is receiving a daily intake of 850 ml of breast milk the mother requires 4200 kJ (1000 Cal) in addition to her basic needs. As 1 litre of cow's milk supplies both 2750 kJ (650 Cal) and 35 g of protein, a simple dietary modification is for the mother to add an additional litre of milk per day to her dietary intake. The nurse can easily remember to advise a pregnant woman to take an additional 500 ml and the lactating mother an additional litre of milk per day. Women who feel unable to consume such quantities of milk can replace it in part with cheese: approximately 150 g of cheese is equivalent to 1 litre of milk. This should be taken in addition to her own basic daily need of 500 ml of milk, or its equivalent.

Apart from the contribution of protein and energy, milk also provides a variety of other essential nutrients including calcium, which is required in large quantities during both pregnancy and lactation. It appears that during lactation a temporary physiological depletion of calcium may occur in the mother, but this is quickly replenished thereafter, providing the mother is on a reasonable diet. However, as the breast-fed baby obtains 0.5 g calcium/day in milk it is extremely important for the mother to maintain adequate available supplies. Although breast milk contains little iron (only 0.2 mg/day) these minimal amounts add up to approximately 36 mg over a six month period of lactation. Reserves may also be depleted due to blood loss during childbirth and foods such as liver, red meat, lettuce, etc., and other good iron sources should be emphasized at this time.

Certain *vitamins*, too, should be taken in increased amounts. As mentioned in the previous chapter, vitamin A is necessary for normal reproduction and lactation and should be taken in adequate amounts. Vitamin B complex, in particular thiamine, riboflavin and niacin, is also needed in greater amounts. The concentrations of these three vitamins in breast milk reflects dietary intake, and dietary supplementation to those breast-feeding mothers on an inadequate diet results in corresponding increases in their milk. In a study by Nail *et al*, levels of riboflavin in milk rose to levels ten times basal concentrations when supplements were administered. As mentioned in Chapter 1, both thiamine and niacin are required in proportion to the energy intake, so with the added energy requirements of lactation the need for these vitamins also increases.

Added vitamin C is also necessary at times of increased cell production, such as during lactation. Furthermore it has been shown that although breast milk is not a good source of vitamin C a higher consumption of vitamin C by the mother will result in a larger amount being secreted in the breast milk.

Of particular importance is the *fluid intake* of the lactating mother. Additional quantities of water, fruit juice, tea and coffee are essential to meet the increased requirements.

Lactation can be used as the ideal period for post-partum weight reduction by meticulous selection of the diet. An overweight mother can convert the excess kilograms carried over from pregnancy into a part source of her energy needs at this stage. Skimmed milk can be used in preference to full cream milk, thereby considerably reducing the energy intake. Foods providing merely 'empty calories' should be avoided and, providing the mother consumes adequate nutrients and fluid, the baby will suffer no harm. Where overweight is not a consideration the lactating mother should have a free selection of foods to make up additional calories. However, alcohol and certain other drugs may pass through into the milk and affect the infant, so the consumption of large quantities of alcohol should be avoided by all nursing mothers, and some may need to omit it altogether.

Finally, breast-feeding delays ovulation and while not a completely effective contraceptive measure it is a relevant one, especially in communities where other forms of contraception are seldom used. In Bangladesh, where breast-feeding is widely practised, lactational amenorrhoea (absence of periods) is 18.5

months. In that country only 9% of the women use contraceptives and McNeilly points out that should the practice of breast-feeding be limited to the extent that lactational amenorrhoea is reduced to six months, the use of contraceptives would have to be increased to 43% to hold fertility at its present rate. In another study on breast-feeding in Scotland it was found that lactating mothers ovulated on average 33 weeks after delivery, compared to 11 weeks in the bottle-feeding controls. In many parts of the world overpopulation and lack of available food resources is a mammoth problem and it is the responsibility of those who realize the many attributes of breast-feeding to promote it whenever practical.

INFANT FEEDING

It is not within the scope of this book to give more than a brief guide on infant feeding, as there are many excellent detailed textbooks available and the vulnerability of infants precludes the giving of specific advice for a baby without attention to his individual needs. In practice, there are probably more old wives' tales and misinformation about infant feeding than about any other aspect of diet, and this section will thus be directed at commonsense basic principles and their application. It is unfortunate that young mothers, already confused and often insecure about their new role, find themselves surrounded by a vast amount of contradictory information on the feeding of their babies. It is important that the nurse plays a supportive and understanding role at this stage, helping the mother to understand that it is relatively unimportant that one booklet tells her to introduce mixed feeding when her baby is six weeks old, whereas somewhere else she reads that six months is a more appropriate age. Dr. Spock, in his down-to-earth book *Infant and Child Care*, makes the following important comment: 'Don't be overawed by what the experts say . . . natural loving infant care that kindly parents give to their children is a hundred times more valuable than their knowing how to pin a diaper on just right or making a formula correctly.'

Breast-feeding

If at all possible the mother should breast-feed her baby. The milk is pure, readily digestible and free from contamination; the risk of infection is minimal provided the breasts are kept clean; and breast-feeding also saves time and money.

Furthermore, breast milk contains antibodies that protect the baby from infection during the early months. In particular, gastroenteritis, a major infectious disease in Great Britain, is largely absent in breast-fed infants. Other protective factors are also present in breast milk. Lactoferrin, an iron-based compound in milk, inhibits the development of pathogenic bacteria. As human milk, unlike cow's milk, does not contain the proteins to which young infants may be sensitive, breast-fed infants are far less prone to develop allergic reactions. Breast-feeding also promotes a feeling of contentment in both mother and baby and helps to establish a stable relationship. An indirect advantage, in our sophisticated society, is that the amount of milk taken — or rejected — is not obvious and the mother is thus less likely to become anxious if her baby drinks fluctuating amounts.

A note of caution: should breast milk be deficient in quantity or cause a reaction (e.g. in an infant who is lactose-intolerant or who reacts to the presence of certain allergens, for example cow's milk protein, consumed by the mother) the mother should be sympathetically but firmly advised to change to bottle-feeding. Although intial perseverance in breast-feeding is to be encouraged, the baby's well-being is all-important. Illness or her return to work may also prevent the mother from breast-feeding the baby and at this stage it is the nurse's role to reassure the mother and to emphasize that bottle-feeding can also be totally adequate.

On the other hand, Johnson *et al* demonstrated the importance of bedside teaching and guidance in breast-feeding success. The nurse's assistance is of great value to the inexperienced mother; her support, the way she discusses problems, even helping to put the baby to breast are major reasons why some mothers persevere and ultimately manage to feed their infants successfuly. Without this help some mothers resort to bottle-feeding more readily.

Nutrient considerations in infancy

Energy

In affluent societies where adult obesity is a public health problem, an important advantage of breast-feeding is the long-term control of overweight. It has been suggested that the adipose cells present in later life are established mostly in early childhood. A study by Taitz (1971) showed that at six months the weights of artificially fed infants were substantially higher than those of breast-fed infants, causing the former to be at higher risk for later obesity and associated diseases. Infantile overweight also results in increased incidence of respiratory infections. Artificial feeding often includes more energy per volume of feed, and as the bottle contents are visible the mother will be aware if the entire feed has not been taken. The nurse should assure the mother that, although she should give her baby feeds of, say, approximately 150 ml, this does not mean that the baby is expected to finish this quantity at every feed. If he is healthy, with a satisfactory weight gain, and normally takes an adequate amount, she should not persist in offering the balance if at some feeds he clearly indicates that he has had sufficient.

Immediate appeasement with food when the infant cries, the popular idea that an overweight baby is a healthy one, and the early inclusion of solids in an attempt to prevent the baby waking during the night for an additional feed, are all factors which promote an excess of energy intake and unnecessary weight gain. Taitz suggests that the 'restless, fractious, always-hungry baby' may well be one who is overfed with an overconcentrated artificial feed causing an increased thirst due to his need to excrete the excess electrolytes and urea.

The routine adding of cereal to bottle feeds is also to be discouraged. The baby who is old enough to require additional energy as cereal is old enough to take small quantities from a spoon.

Protein

When milk forms the basis of the diet an adequate protein intake will be assured. However, in underprivileged communities where milk feeds are sometimes replaced with diluted milk, tea or fruit-based concentrates diluted with water, the protein intake must be considered.

Breast milk provides 1.1 g protein/100 ml, whereas cow's milk contains three times as much. Cow's milk therefore results in an increased solute load on the kidneys, necessitating an adequate fluid intake. Whether in fact this is of any practical significance is not known, but it emphasizes the need for the accurate measuring of infant feeds when concentrates requiring dilution are used.

As the baby gets older and solids play an increasingly important role in the diet, the mother should be closely questioned to ascertain whether her choice of foods includes adequate protein: some mothers erroneously presume that the 'goodness' of a meat dish is concentrated in the gravy. As the milk intake is reduced, replacement with other forms of protein such as eggs, meat and fish should play a more prominent role.

Fluid requirements of infants

For about the first six months the infant will usually be given approximately 150–200 ml/kg body weight per day. Initially, most of this liquid will be given as milk, but as the baby gets older and takes more solid food, less milk will be given and more water and fruit juice should be included in the diet. The need for additional fluid in hot weather must be emphasized.

Carbohydrate requirements of infants

As mentioned earlier, milk is all-important in the infant's diet. Replacement of it in part by cereal or the addition of a thickening agent to the bottle is not justified for a young baby. The use of such cereals may result in an inadequate milk intake and gluten-containing cereals may induce earlier manifestation of coeliac disease (discussed in Chapter 8) in gluten-sensitive infants. The early introduction of solids in order to bring about a longer interval between feeds and encourage contentment in the baby is not advised. Mixed feeding may be introduced to increase the range of dietary components from the age of about four months.

In the United Kingdom, none of the modified or 'humanized' milks supplied for use by infants requires the addition of sugar, for such milk foods are manufactured with added carbohydrate. If, elsewhere, other milks are used, additional sugar is sometimes necessary in the proportion of one teaspoonful of sugar to each bottle feed, but in view of the fact that artificially fed babies are more prone to overweight this practice is seldom justified. Should constipation occur, the inclusion of a small amount of sugar, which will exert a hydroscopic effect, causing added volume in the digestive tract, may well produce a good result.

Diluted evaporated milk is not recommended for infants under 3 months; nor is fresh cow's milk, both because it may be a vehicle for pathogenic bacteria and because it is now considered that its protein content is dangerously high.

Vitamin requirements of infants

Routine supplementation of vitamins A, C and D is advisable during the first few months of life. In the United Kingdom all the modified milks made specifically for use by infants contain added vitamins, and the Department of Health and Social Security issues 'DHSS drops' which are available through welfare clinics at minimum cost and contain 1000 IU (300 μg) vitamin A, 400 IU (10 μg) vitamin D and 30 mg vitamin C.

Vitamin C

Although not essential for breast-fed babies when the mother has an adequate vitamin C intake, supplements are customarily given after the first fortnight of life. As vitamin C is water-soluble, early inclusion is usually advised as mild overdose of this vitamin will merely result in excretion of the excess in the urine. The daily requirement of 30 mg is met either by a daily dose of 'DHSS drops' or 60–90 ml of orange juice. The baby is usually started off with half a teaspoon of juice mixed with half a teaspoon of water. The quantities are then progressively increased until the baby is getting six teaspoonfuls of each. The water is then decreased until the baby is taking the recommended amount of pure juice. With the gradual introduction of mixed feeding, other sources will naturally be included. The nurse should emphasize to the mother that vitamin C is readily destroyed by heat and light; the juice should therefore be prepared immediately before use and not boiled or exposed to the air for long periods. As some babies tend to be allergic to orange or tomato juice during the early months, rosehip juice or pharmaceutical concentrates are sometimes more suitable sources of vitamin C.

Vitamin D

Breast-fed babies, or those on a non-supplemented proprietary brand of milk, are usually given vitamin D in controlled amounts during the first few months. Later, when more milk and other foods are being taken and more exposure to sunlight is practical, a vitamin concentrate is less necessary. The nurse should emphasize the prescribed dosage to the mother, as hypervitaminosis can be caused by over-enthusiastic mothers giving their babies toxic amounts of vitamin D. Furthermore, the safe margin between the necessary and the toxic doses of this fat-soluble vitamin appears to be narrower than formerly thought. Cod-liver oil is a rich source of vitamin D.

Iron in the infant's diet

Full-term infants are born with a reserve of iron adequate for the first few months of life, but from about the age of three months iron supplements should be given, the most natural and digestible being egg yolk. Initially only the yolk is given, as the white can cause an allergic reaction.

Sodium in the infant's diet

The role of this electrolyte in the aetiology of hypertension in later life has been widely discussed for several years. The inclusion of salt in processed infant foods to satisfy the taste of the mother rather than the baby has been repeatedly criticized. However, until the role of sodium as an environmental factor in the induction of hypertension has been substantiated, there seems little reason to do more than caution mothers not to add more than the minimum amount of seasoning to their infant's food. Formulas must be accurately diluted: hypernatraemia is a greater risk to infants than to adults as the former do not have free access to water for elimination.

Fluoride in the infant's diet

In areas where the fluoride content of the water is inadequate, fluoride supplementation should be commenced soon after birth.

The mother should be cautioned to administer the precise dose required and *not* to enthusiastically feed her baby excessive (and extremely hazardous) quantities.

FEEDING FROM BIRTH TO THREE MONTHS

For a full-term baby, milk forms the basis of the diet for the first three months of life, breast-feeding being most desirable. Should artifical preparations be necessary, modified milk is usually given for the first three to six months.

The infant is usually given 150 ml milk/kg body weight per day. Initially this is divided into six feeds per 24 hours but this is soon reduced to five feeds (omitting the 2 a.m. feed).

Bottle-feeding ingredients

Modified milks are those which most closely resemble breast milk in composition and they are the food of choice for all young infants. Powdered milks are usually given in the proportions indicated on the tin. Initially, the baby may be given a partially skimmed variety, to which carbohydrate is often added by the manufacturer to bring the composition more in line with breast milk. After the age of three months, most infants receive full-fat milk. Evaporated milk, if used for young infants, is reconstituted in the ratio of two parts of milk to three parts of water, although hungry babies are sometimes given equal parts of evaporated milk and water. As previously mentioned, liquid cow's milk is seldom advised for the first few months.

Sugar is occasionally added, 5 ml per feed. In view of the previously mentioned problems of overweight encountered in artificially fed babies, the addition of sugar should not be a routine applied regardless of weight. The use of glucose instead of sugar in babies' feeds is unnecessary: the added cost is not justified and the extreme sweetness of glucose may be detrimental to the infants' later food preferences.

Up to the age of three months, the water used in the formula should be boiled. Thereafter, this practice may be discontinued in cities where the water is subject to stringent regulations regarding purification. However, in areas where the cleanliness of the water is doubtful or where water is carried some distance and allowed to stand in unsterilized containers before use, water should be boiled until the infant is at least one year old.

FEEDING FROM THREE TO SIX MONTHS

Mothers often wish to know about the advisability of including pasteurized dairy milk at this stage. While it is simple and saves money to do so, it is not now considered advisable because of the possibility of contamination. Pinholing of the foil bottle-top may allow entrance to bacteria even while the top is ostensibly still closed, and contamination may also occur during handling after opening the bottle. If fresh milk is to be included in the diet, boiling directly before use should be recommended as a routine.

Although hungry babies may be given supplementary refined cereals from as early as two months, this is seldom advisable and it is usually only from about four months that food other than milk has a role in the infant's diet. Starting mixed feeding is necessary not only to provide those nutrients which are inadequately supplied by milk, but also to accustom the infant to a variety of new flavours and textures in food. Mixed feeding is usually commenced with the inclusion of refined cereal. Those fortified with iron are to be recommended as during this period the infant's iron reserves will become depleted. This is quickly followed by egg yolk (to provide iron), puréed vegetables and fruit (for additional vitamins and minerals), finely ground meat, including liver (for iron and vitamin B complex), fish (providing iodine) and milk desserts. All these are important additions to the diet.

The nurse is frequently asked about the relative value of freshly prepared puréed vegetables and fruit, as opposed to the widely produced bottled product. The advantages of the bottled foods are many — they are easy to use, portable and hygienic. The nutritive value of many of the foods is quite satisfactory, although much of the vitamin C may be destroyed with processing and long-term storage and by exposure of the bottle to light. However, bottled foods are expensive if used routinely and have the added disadvantage of uniformity of texture. Mothers who wish to include these products should be advised to intersperse them with freshly prepared products and to progress to the 'junior' range, which has a coarser texture, as soon as practical.

The nurse should advise the mother to bear certain considerations in mind when commencing with supplementary food:

1. In the beginning, foods should be very bland and semi-liquid in texture.
2. Only one food at a time should be introduced, to enable the mother to gauge any specific reaction.
3. Initially, very small quantities should be given.
4. Strongly flavoured foods should be avoided, as an infant's palate is very sensitive.
5. Foods with little nutritive value (such as marrow, jelly, etc.) should be used infrequently: only those foods which make some nutritive contribution to the diet should be selected.
6. New foods should be introduced at the beginning of the meal while the infant is still hungry.
7. During hot weather the infant's main requirement is fluid; at such times new flavours should be introduced in the form of liquids such as soup or custard rather than as dry food (such as toast) which may be rejected simply because the baby is thirsty.

FEEDING FROM SIX MONTHS TO A YEAR

During this period the infant's rate of weight gain will gradually slow down. One can expect an infant of average birth weight approximately to double his weight in the first six months of life and to triple it by the time he is a year old. During this time he is being educated in the eating habits of his culture. Foods from the family table will be included with increasing frequency and his food habits will slowly become established. The mother may question the necessity of optimum cleanliness of bottles and nipples at this stage when the infant is coming into contact with floor dust and contaminated furniture as he crawls around his environment. It should be stressed that the need to continue sterilizing of bottles until the child is one year old results from the relative ease of contamination which can occur with milk. Small deposits of milk left unnoticed in the bottle can constitute a serious hazard the following day when the bottle is re-used. With the commencement of weaning towards the end of the first year, and the use of a cup far more suited to satisfactory hand-washing than a bottle, sterilization may obviously be terminated.

During the second six months of his life, the baby's milk intake will be reduced to about 800 ml/day and his average diet will be similar to that appearing below.

Sample menu

On awakening
 200 ml milk

Breakfast
 fruit, yoghurt or porridge with a little grated apple
 180 ml milk

12 noon
 minced meat or fish with mashed carrots or cauliflower tops
  and potato moistened with a little stock or gravy
 180 ml milk

Mid-afternoon
 orange juice and a rusk

Supper
 scrambled egg mixed with a little cereal or banana custard
 buttered toast
 180–200 ml milk

This diet supplies approximately 3800 kJ (900 Cal) which is the baby's energy requirement at this stage. Adequacy of energy intake can be readily checked with a simple calculation. The infant's requirement is approximately 2100 kJ (500 Cal) when one month old and this slowly increases at the rate of approximately 400 kJ (100 Cal) every two months until he is taking 4200 kJ (1000 Cal) at one year.

Nutritional complications in infancy

Gastroenteritis

If the infant's diarrhoea persists longer than 24 hours medical help should be summoned; sooner if the diarrhoea is very severe. As soon as diarrhoea occurs, all solid foods and milk should be stopped for 24 hours. The infant's main need is for fluid which should be given as soon as possible. The usual feed consists of equal quantities of Darrow's solution and boiled water mixed with two teaspoonfuls of sugar per bottle. If Darrow's solution is unavailable, the infant is given a solution of half a teaspoonful of salt and 5 teaspoonfuls of sugar in one litre of boiled water as frequently as possible until medical help is obtained. After 24 hours of the above regimen, feeding is recommenced, whatever the state of the stool, using skimmed milk initially. The Darrow's solution or substitute is given between feeds to replace fluid lost in the stools.

Constipation

The frequency of bowel movement in the infant is often related to the type of milk used in feeds: generally, those babies taking cow's milk have less regular bowel actions than those on breast milk. It is thus important that when a mother complains about the constipation of her infant the normal habits of the baby should be ascertained. Some infants will regularly have a daily bowel action while others might have an interval of several days between bowel movements.

Certain dietary factors play a role in this problem. In the first place, the feed should be checked to ensure that the *proportions* used are correct. The inclusion of too much milk powder may cause constipation. The addition of a small amount of *sugar* to the feed will increase fluid retention in the gut and promote a bowel action.

Fat has a lubricating effect and the infant on skimmed milk may thus become constipated due to the low fat intake. A change to full-cream milk or the inclusion of a small quantity of butter or margarine on the vegetables may improve the situation.

Ascertain that the baby is taking adequate fluids; in hot weather this requirement is greater. Some mothers, when changing to a mixed diet, reduce this essential component of the baby's intake.

The *roughage* content of the diet is also important; the residue of vegetables and fruits, combined with liquid in the gut, are required to form the necessary mass to promote a bowel action. The inclusion of *slightly* coarser vegetables and fruit than previously and an increase of fluid may rectify the situation.

Prune juice or puréed prunes provide a factor which stimulates a gastrocolic reflex.

The overweight infant

As mentioned earlier, overweight in infancy is a serious problem which should be treated. This is often difficult in view of the attitude of parents that 'bouncy babies' are cute and healthy. Overweight infants are more prone to bronchial infections and eczema and are at greater risk of becoming overweight adults with concomitant complications of ill-health. The mother should be given immediate advice to omit sugar from the diet and to replace full milk with skimmed milk. She should clearly understand that she should not merely give her infant less of his usual feed diluted with water as this will obviously reduce his protein and calcium intake. At meal-times starchy porridges, potatoes and toast should be given in limited quantities, and margarine and fatty gravy should be severely restricted.

Mashed yellow and green vegetables such as carrots, spinach, marrow and pumpkin are useful 'fillers' providing few kilojoules and are recommended for overweight babies who have a large appetite. Naturally, fruit, mince, egg and cereals should still retain a prominent role in the diet to ensure adequacy of essential nutrients.

The underweight baby

As indicated in the sample menu, fruit juices are usually included in the mid-afternoon. The reason for this is the length of time required to digest milk. If milk were given at 3.30–4 p.m., the infant would be unlikely to be hungry for his 6 o'clock feed. However, if previous gastroenteritis or other illness has caused a weight loss to below normal limits, additional energy in the form of an extra milk feed mid-afternoon may be indicated. Lunch is then given at noon, the milk feed at 3.30 and supper at 6.30–7 p.m.

FEEDING TODDLERS AND PRE-SCHOOL CHILDREN

During the period from one to three years of age, increased muscle tissue is deposited and increased mineralization of bone and teeth occurs. The daily energy requirement increases slowly, from 4000 kJ (1000 Cal) to only 5800 kJ (1400 Cal). The mother should be aware that a reduction in appetite occurs over this period and that the rejection of certain previously acceptable foods is characteristic of this stage of growth. The inclusion of 600–700 ml of milk as a drink or in made-up dishes each day will ensure adequate protein and calcium intake.

Although doubts have been raised about the advisability of milk for toddlers, the evidence against milk has so far not been widely supported. It appears that there is a gradual diminution of lactase activity after the third or fourth year of age, but this does not justify the widespread discouragement of milk-drinking in young children. It is of interest that a study undertaken in the USA comparing lactose inolerance in black and white children showed that such intolerance was demonstrable in half of the black children who rejected milk in a free feeding programme. It would seem that black children are more susceptible to a deficiency of the lactase enzyme and the nurse should be cautious about encouraging children, particularly black ones, to drink milk if they complain about abdominal discomfort or mild diarrhoea following milk ingestion.

During the toddling phase eating habits are established and the development of the child as an individual results in an increasing feeling of independence. The child learns to eat without assistance and the mother should realize that manipulation of cutlery is, initially, a time-consuming and demanding exercise. Encouragement from the mother is important in establishing normal interest in meals; the mother who repeatedly reprimands her child about his spilling, messing and speed of eating promotes a negative attitude to food in her child. Bite-size pieces to allow the handling and independent consumption of food, the serving of small portions to encourage the consumption of all food presented, the use of deep bowls and manageable mugs; all are helpful in assisting the child to come to terms with his new independence. Foods should not be routinely mashed together but rather served separately so that the child can appreciate different flavours and textures of food. Also, small portions of new foods should be served with known foods. If these are rejected it is usually advisable not to persevere too much but rather to reintroduce the unknown food after a short period, without fuss.

During these years the child will continue to need mid-meal snacks because of his limited capacity for meals. Timing of snacks and the types of food given at these times are important factors to consider. Large quantities of concentrated sweetness will reduce the appetite for the next meal. The routine daily serving of sweetened synthetic drinks to young children should be avoided. From an early age children should be made aware that water is a palatable and necessary part of their diet.

Environmental stimuli play a valuable part in the child's development at this stage and the well nourished child has a particular advantage in that he can be optimally receptive and reactive to these stimuli. The malnourished child is doubly handicapped. In the first place, normal brain development is directly attributable to an adequate food intake; sufficient protein is particularly important. Secondly, the lethargy and disinterest that accompany malnutrition prevent the child from responding and reacting to normal environmental stimuli.

The need for protein and calcium will be met by the daily inclusion of 600 ml of milk and the child's need for iron and vitamins A and C will be met by the regular ingestion of meat, fruit and vegetables. During these years the child should begin to understand that there is a correlation between his diet and his health and that selection of foods is important. A varied diet including very limited quantities of sweet foods and confectionery will help prevent overweight and dental caries. Fruit such as apples and pears, which have an abrasive action on the teeth, are useful inclusions as mid-meal snacks or desserts to help remove particles of food remaining between the teeth and promoting decay.

Several problems may arise during this period. Some children tend to use their meal-times as weapons to achieve other ends and the nurse should firmly make the mother realize that food should not be used as a bribe, nor meals as an attention-getting mechanism by the child. This should be stressed particularly to the inexperienced mother.

Children at the toddling age should be encouraged to take regular meals, as the habit of constant nibbling is difficult to break if once established. Indulgent relatives should be dissuaded from repeatedly giving sweets to children. An interesting Swedish study has inversely correlated the educational level of parents to their children's intake of sweets and confectionery; the higher the socio-economic group, the lower the consumption of these foods.

Another study undertaken on nursery school children pointed to the fact that children's eating habits could be changed by association. While being told an exciting, graphic story, the children were informed that the heroine drank a special drink which they, too, could enjoy. With relish they then swallowed an unappetizing mixture. Thereafter they were told that the villain drank a distasteful drink, and the children refused to drink a mixture that they had always enjoyed in the past!

The concern of anxious and over-conscientious mothers that their child's repeated rejection of meals will result in an inadequate intake and disease is usually unfounded. Disregard of this negative attitude to food will often defuse the situation and the nurse can play a major role by plotting the child's height and weight on the normal percentile chart to reassure the mother. However, whether or not the child's weight is within the limits of normality, the reasons for the continued disinterest in food should be identified. The consumption of too many sweets and confectionery, sitting too long at table waiting for the meal and becoming restless, distraction by siblings, television or family rows at table; all may cause disinterest in food. Overtiredness may also play a major role.

Young children have a keen sense of taste and only minimal amounts of seasoning should be added to their food. The routine use of sauces and condiments masking the taste of the meal should be discouraged.

Liquids in adequate quantities remain an essential part of the diet. Although by this stage the child will be toilet-trained the mother should regularly confirm that the child is having regular bowel actions of normal consistency, as a hard, dry stool may be the result of too little liquid in the diet.

FEEDING SCHOOLCHILDREN (SIX TO SIXTEEN)

Many children lose their formerly healthy appetites while adjusting to a new environment. Breakfast is often omitted due to tension and apprehension about the day ahead and the school lunch may be left untouched due to the child's preoccupation with group activities. Nourishing school meals can contribute a major proportion of the child's daily nutrient requirements. The preparation and service of these meals should be well supervised to ensure both optimal retention of nutrients during cooking and the consumption of adequate amounts by the children. The impact of unappetizing institutional meals, served in an unattractive way, is a memory familiar to most of us from some stage of our childhood. In these days of inflation and high costs it is imperative that school meals should be both nourishing and enjoyable to ensure minimum waste.

Irregular eating is another dietary aspect which should be considered. The lack of adult supervision at home and the independent preparation of meals and snacks by children can result in various problems. The regular inclusion of unsuitable foods, the consumption of snacks just before meals, spoiling the appetite, and the over-consumption of snack foods, causing overweight, can all result from an undisciplined parental approach to nutrition.

Of particular nutritional importance is the provision of a suitable late-afternoon snack for children returning home from school. This can, for example, be milk, crackers and fruit, soup and a cheese sandwich, or sausage and salad. Such snacks not only provide valuable nutrients, but reduce the desire for constant nibbling, an unhealthy and unnecessary habit encountered in many schoolchildren.

Nutritional requirements

The recommended allowances of nutrients are stated in Table 1. The protein requirement gradually increases as puberty approaches, boys requiring more than girls to build increasing muscle mass. During the growth spurt of puberty, calcium requirements also increase in both sexes due to the growth of bone. With the onset of menstruation, the iron requirement of girls increases. Due to added energy requirements, particularly in boys, the need for vitamin B complex increases. Studies on children have demonstrated that disadvantaged children are liable to suffer from inadequate intakes of several nutrients, in particular iron, calcium and vitamins A and C. When determining nutritive adequacy the nurse should confirm whether there is a daily intake of meat, fish, legumes or eggs, milk, and fruit or vegetables. Although during this stage of life no foods need be avoided, the most common error of feeding is an excess of refined carbohydrate-rich food, particularly as the child gets older.

Elementary school children are usually better nourished than older ones where the problem of 'group identification' plays a progressively more important role. Initially this has little impact other than the desire of younger children to have the same varieties of spread on their sandwiches as their friends or for non-Jewish children to eat matzos during Passover. However, poor eating habits may be aggravated in the teenager with the onset of a feeling of independence and reliance on the opinions of friends. The purchase of large amounts of 'junk foods' (sweets, confectionery and cool drinks) or the spending of much time — and money — at the local store which is a meeting place for groups of friends can result in the consumption of a predominantly carbohydrate diet. Parental interest and understanding of nutritional values and the supervision of the child's diet are thus essential factors in establishing a sound eating pattern. The increasing numbers of working mothers have resulted in progressively more children returning to empty homes after school and their greater dependence on their own — often unsound — selection of foods from those available at home or from convenience foods en route. This important environmental influence is discussed further in Chapter 3.

Nutritional complications

Overweight

Overweight may be caused by excessive intake of food or inadequate exercise, resulting in the conversion of surplus energy to adipose tissue. It has been suggested that not only is lack of physical exercise relevant, but the overweight child is also more efficient in the use of muscles and execution of movements. Hence, less energy is expended than by his peers. Added to this, the child with a history of overweight in infancy has a greater tendency to become obese later, as will be discussed in Chapter 5. There are diverse causes of excessive intake and the identifying and treatment of these is often of assistance in the therapy of these children. Undisciplined family eating habits, lack of parental supervision and example, parental replacement of love or time with preferred foods or an attempt by parents or grandparents to win affection via food are all factors which promote poor eating habits. Children who feel insecure often overeat and those who fail to be accepted adequately by their peers may also project their attention to food. Overweight children also frequently have limited eating habits, refusing vegetables and salads, and eating exclusively concentrated foods.

Obesity can be successfully treated only if the child is motivated to lose weight. The nurse can often encourage the child with arguments of increased agility, improved appearance and clear complexion. The keeping of a graph depicting weight loss is usually a helpful visual stimulus to older children: weight is plotted in ½ kg losses down the left-hand side of the page and the dates at three-day intervals across the base of the graph.

A dietary history is taken and the diet should be modified to fit in as far as possible with the family eating pattern. The intake should be divided into three meals per day, or four if only a light snack is taken at school and the child returns home mid-afternoon. Often, the avoidance of all foods sweetened with sugar or prepared with fat and reduction in the intake of starchy foods to one or two portions per meal is sufficient modification. It is advisable to allow young people to have one portion of normally disallowed food per week as a 'treat', as the thought of severe dietary restriction for an indefinite length of time is even more depressing and demoralizing to the young than to adults. It is strongly advised that a programme of daily exercise should be part of the weight reduction plan. This can be taken as jogging, timed exercises in the privacy of the bedroom, or regular visits to a gym or exercise class. The expected weight loss will depend on the extent of the obesity and the age of the child, although certain workers consider that younger children should merely retain their weight and, with time, 'grow into it'. This approach may have a demoralizing effect on the child who, if motivated, expects to see results. For this reason, others consider that a weekly weight loss ranging from 400–500 g in younger children to a maximum of 800–1000 g in obese older children is desirable.

The current serious increase in the development of *anorexia nervosa*, particularly in teenagers, is a situation which cannot be ignored in the treatment of overweight and the nurse should exercise extreme tact in her attitude to young people.

Anorexia

Anorexia, meaning a loss of appetite (as differentiated from anorexia nervosa, a serious psychological condition, discussed in Chapter 6) is a common occurrence among children or teenagers, usually for a brief period. Although it may be precipitated by one of the common children's diseases or other organic disorder, it may be due to a preoccupation with schoolwork or sport. It may also occur as a reaction to parents' insistence about the types or quantities of foods which should be eaten. The child may merely not have an appetite for such food at that stage or, alternatively, may enjoy the attention received as a result of the rejection of food. Reassurance about the absence of organic cause should be coupled with advice to the mother that her first approach should be to hide her concern and disregard her child's rejection of food. Eating between meals should be strictly controlled and sweets should be withheld. Should the situation be prolonged and result in loss of weight, medical opinion should be sought in an attempt to prevent the condition progressing to anorexia nervosa.

Voracious appetite

A ravenous appetite occurs particularly during the pubescent growth spurt in boys, often being aggravated by the considerable amount of exercise done at that age. The daily intake of a balanced diet and the inclusion of a litre of milk will satisfy the needs for protein and calcium. Added energy needs can be met by increased quantities of wholewheat bread, which also provides vitamin B complex which is necessary for the utilization of energy. Other wholegrain cereals such as brown rice and oats may be included in large amounts to meet energy needs. Unfortunately, the habit of eating large amounts of food may remain after the need has passed and the child should be cautioned not to become overweight.

Acne

Contrary to popular belief, diet plays a surprisingly unimportant role in the development of this skin disorder. Suggestions that carbonated drinks, sweets and chocolates are responsible have been unsubstantiated. A study in which patients were fed a special bar containing ten times the amount of chocolate present in the average chocolate bar indicated that there was no effect. Reports that a high-carbohydrate, high-fat diet may be responsible for an increased output of sebum (the greasy secretion of the sebaceous glands in the skin) are also unconfirmed.

However, one food which may occasionally aggravate acne is milk. Because of the hormonal content of milk, an effect on the skin may be precipitated and teenagers with acne consuming large quantities of milk should drastically reduce their intake temporarily to see if an improvement occurs.

Otherwise, a normal varied diet, including adequate fluid, is advisable. The condition is alleviated less by a change of diet than by regular cleaning to prevent clogging of the ducts of the sebaceous glands, by avoiding having greasy hair or make-up in contact with the skin, and by refraining from picking or scratching the area of acne.

THE OFFICE WORKER'S DIET

The main problem for those away from home for lunch each day is the provision of a satisfactory lunch. In the absence of suitable institutional canteens the most satisfactory and economical arrangement is the packed lunch. A few basic principles should be applied when compiling this meal, possibly the most important of which is to regard it as an important part of the daily intake. The packed lunch should not be just a snack thrown together in a few minutes preceding departure from home, but should be remembered when earlier meals are prepared. The preparation of an additional meat rissole or individual chicken pie when making supper or the making of cheese scones or toasted cheese sandwiches for variety all encourage the consumer to eat his lunch in preference to buying an unsuitable, expensive snack. The production of a month's supply of sandwiches which are frozen until required is often a useful manoeuvre.

A portion of a *protein* food should always be included. This not only provides necessary nutrients but has the added advantage of having a high satiety value, preventing early hunger after the meal. This high-protein food may take the form of cheese, cold meat, peanut butter, boiled egg, etc. Meat, yeast and fish extracts or spreads are of little value in this respect as only small quantities are used in sandwiches, making little contribution to the protein content of the meal.

Wholewheat bread is far superior to white or brown. It provides vitamin B complex, extra proteins and fibre, which is of a particular importance to the sedentary worker in preventing constipation, and should always be used in preference to white bread.

Salads or a thermos flask of *soup* made from low-fat stock with the addition of a large proportion of leafy green and yellow vegetables are of value as fillers, particularly for the individual wanting to control weight or lose it. Soup can be varied with tomato paste, onions or mushrooms. Those less concerned about their weight may add barley, potatoes or legumes to produce a rich substantial soup which can form the basis of a meal.

People who live alone tend to have less incentive to cook a meal on return from work. For a variety of reasons (being too tired or lacking cookery expertise, shortage of money or inadequate cooking facilities) single people often eat snacks rather than nutritious meals. Fruit juices, although healthy, do not supply fibre for bulk in the digestive tract; cheese is a nutritious snack but very fattening if taken in excess; convenience foods are often farinaceous, relatively expensive and low in fibre.

A routine of three balanced meals is imperative for health. Minimal effort is required to prepare a breakfast of muesli, a nourishing packed lunch and a dinner of fish or meat and a potato with salad and fruit. However, many 'singles' need encouragement and guidance to initiate an orderly eating pattern.

THE HOUSEWIFE'S DIET

The two main problems confronting the full-time housewife are related to the proximity to food as an occupational hazard. Firstly, there may be lack of self-discipline regarding food consumption at meal-times. There may be diverse causes for this attitude, including:

1. frustration at having to contend with family and domestic obligations instead of involvement in a chosen career;
2. inability to cope with extensive demands made on her time, resulting in snack eating instead of attention to balanced meals;
3. financial difficulties causing self-deprivation at meal-times and the subsequent consumption of high-carbohydrate snacks;

4. constant contact with and orientation towards food and feeding in her role as caterer for the family.

Whatever the reason, the situation usually results in overweight and frequently promotes deficiency of certain necessary nutrients.

The second difficulty for housewives is that, having become overweight, they often lack the motivation to cook separately for themselves or even modify their method of food preparation to solve the problem. It is important for the nurse to take a firm no-nonsense attitude to these patients who need assistance to achieve any long-term change of attitude. Many of these individuals can benefit enormously by being referred to supportive organizations such as Weight Watchers, which provide a programme of regular reinforcement of goals.

THE ELDERLY

A recent survey showed that Great Britain had more than 7.5 million inhabitants over the age of 60. Regrettably, the nutritional needs of these people are often neglected by the community. The nurse should be aware that, even in good health, the elderly patient has specific food requirements that must be met for continued well-being. With ageing, various physiological changes occur. The nutritional implications are diverse and modify the requirements of the individual. Nutritional deficiency states such as anaemia and scurvy are not uncommon in elderly patients.

One of the major factors to be considered is reduced energy requirement and resultant obesity. At 65 years of age the basal metabolic energy needs are 29% lower than at the age of 25. Energy utilization is further reduced by the frequent lack of incentive for physical exercise and impaired activity due to joint disease or other physical debility. Unwise dietary selection and an emphasis on high-carbohydrate food readily promote obesity as energy intake exceeds energy needs.

The *kidneys* are also affected by ageing. Reduced efficiency of renal filtration may occur, resulting in uraemia. This is often coupled with nausea, impairing the appetite and curtailing the intake of food. The situation may be aggravated by the fact that due to lessened bladder control only minimal quantities of liquid may be taken from early afternoon in order to avoid having to get up at night to pass urine. This can result in dehydration and extrarenal uraemia in elderly people. They should be advised to take adequate liquid, especially early in the day.

Degenerative diseases, such as atherosclerosis and diverticulosis, may add further complications to the eating pattern of the elderly person. The advice to adhere to a low-cholesterol or high-fibre diet may radically affect long-standing eating habits. It is stressed that theoretical requirements should be carefully weighed against practical implications when advising elderly people to modify their eating habits.

The lack of his own teeth or the use of ill-fitting false ones often accounts for the individual's lack of interest in fresh fruit and vegetables and his dependence, instead, on sandwiches. Added to this, impaired sense of smell and taste may reduce the desire for a varied diet.

Constipation is a frequent complication of ageing. Reduced muscle tone and diverticulosis (which is said to occur in 40–50% of elderly people) may be prime causes. The common pensioner's diet of predominantly refined carbohydrate foods, with a limited intake of fruit, vegetables and fluid, will aggravate the condition. The advice to patients to include two to four tablespoonfuls of millers' bran on their food each day and drink eight or ten glasses or cups of liquid per day usually alleviates constipation. The elderly should ensure that vegetables, salads and/or fruit — although not necessarily the accompanying pips and rough skins — are included in the diet daily. Regular exercise is also an important consideration in the prevention of constipation.

Added to these physiological changes, environmental and psychological factors markedly influence the nutritional status of the elderly person. The reduction in income is frequently a major problem. Pensions which fail to keep abreast of the rising cost of living and the escalation in cost of fuel and transport are factors which may result in dependency on a cheaper high-carbohydrate diet. Concurrent debilitating diseases, however, may cause increased protein needs.

Individuals may be restricted in their shopping by the distance between the shops and their home and the difficulty of carrying large packages of fresh produce any distance. The death of a spouse may remove the incentive for cooking, and depression from this or other causes may further reduce the motivation for food preparation. Forgetfulness and senility also markedly affect the selection, preparation and consumption of meals. All too frequently the eating pattern of the elderly person is reduced to a monotonous and deficient diet of bread and tea. Various organizations are assisting in these problems in a number of ways. 'Meals on Wheels' plays a vital role in improving the nutritional status of the elderly, particularly those who are less mobile. Another move in the same direction is the recent initiation of cooking classes for the aged being conducted by the staff of the Department of Dietetics at Queen Elizabeth College, London. The director of the Geriatric Nutritional Unit, Dr. Louise Davies, has also written two cookery books especially for the elderly — *Easy Cooking for One or Two* and *More Easy Cooking for One or Two* (Penguin).

It is often necessary for the nurse to advise elderly people not only about their nutritional requirements and how to include them in suitable foods, but also how to budget their finances to ensure a balanced diet. The community nurse can play a particular role in this area by introducing a communal 'meals club'. This involves assembling a number of single elderly people (usually about five) living within a short distance of each other and organizing a weekly meal roster. Each of the people concerned is responsible for one meal for all participants each week within a stipulated budget (possibly laid down with the diplomatic advice of the nurse). From Monday to Friday, all gather to eat each day at a central venue, usually the home of the day's 'cook'. There are several advantages to this type of scheme. In the first place, the consumption of meals in congenial surroundings is a social activity many people enjoy. The purchase and cooking of the meal once a week is a mentally stimulating challenge. Many elderly people have a transport arrangement or help with shopping once a week which can conveniently fit in with their day for cooking.

The community nurse, in particular, should be aware that the elderly patient, particularly the single person living alone, needs regular encouragement to continue with the regular preparation of balanced meals. Prompted by less efficient digestion or ill-health, the elderly are particularly susceptible to the claims of food faddists, which in many cases further undermine their health. The elderly should be encouraged to rely on the sympathetic assistance of the nurse in this regard.

Finally, is there a correlation between nutrition and longevity?

This question is sometimes raised by people wanting to know whether dietary modifications can be made to ensure a longer life-span. Morrison discusses this subject in a recent review article and concludes with the comment: 'There is conflict between nutrition that enables maximum growth and physical capacity, nutrition that reduces risk from degenerative disease, and nutrition that produces maximum longevity . . . optimum human life is not an institutional abstraction but a multiplicity of sets of idiosyncratic personal preferences. It may be that, as far as nutritional manipulation is concerned, full youthful vigour is incompatible with a healthy ripe old age. If we want a lot of one, we may have to settle for a bit less of the other'.

BIBLIOGRAPHY

American Academy of Pediatrics, Committee on Nutrition (1974) Salt intake and eating patterns of infants and children in relation to blood pressure. *Pediatrics, Springfield, 53(1)*, 165.

American Academy of Pediatrics, Committee on Nutrition (1974) Should milk drinking by children be discouraged? *Pediatrics, Springfield, 53(4)*, 576.

Boysen, S.C. & Ahrens, R.A. (1972) Nutrition education and lunch surveys with second graders. *J. Nutr. Educ., 4*, 172.

California Diet Association (ed.) (1973) *A Dozen Diets for Better or Worse*. Los Angeles: California Diet Association.

Coutts, J. (1972) Current feeding practices at the Royal Manchester Children's Hospital. *Nutr. Lond., 26(5)*, 293.

Darden, E. (1972) Sense and nonsense about health foods. *J. Home Econ., (Dec.)*, 4.

Davies, L. & Holdsworth, M. (1978) The place of milk in the dietary of the elderly. *J. Hum. Nutr., 32*, 195.

DHSS Working Party of the Panel on Child Nutrition (1974) *Present Day Practice in Infant Feeding. Report on Health and Social Subjects (9)*. London: HMSO.

Edozien, J.C., Rahim Khan, M.A. & Waslien, C. I. (1976) Human protein deficiency: results of a Nigerian village study. *J. Nutr., 106*, 312.

Eyal, F., Maayan, C. & Godfrey, S. (1978) Heart failure apparently due to overfeeding in a neonate. *Archs. Dis. Childh., 53*, 908.

Foote, R.G. & Ludbrook, A.P.R. (1973) The use of a liberal salt diet in pre-eclamptic toxaemia and essential hypertension with pregnancy. *N.Z. Med. J., 77*, 242.

Hayden, M.R. (1981) *Foetal Alcohol Syndrome*. Brochure, Dept of Health, Welfare and Pensions, RSA.

Hepner, R. & Maiden, N.C. (1971) Growth rate, nutrient intake and 'Mothering' as determinants of malnutrition in disadvantaged children. *Nutr. Rev., 29(10)*, 219.

Jamieson, S.R. (1972) Infantile gastroenteritis — a preventable disease. *Royal Soc. Health J., 92*, 211.

Jelliffe, D. & Jelliffe, P. (1979) *Human Milk in the Modern World*. London: Oxford University Press.

Jelliffe, D.B. & Patrice, E.F. (1972) Lactation, conception and the nutrition of the nursing mother and child. *J. Pediat., 81*, 829.

Jivani, S. (1978) The practice of infant feeding among Asian immigrants. *Archs. Dis. Childh., 53*, 69.

Johnson, C., Garza, C. & Nichols, B. (1984) A teaching intervention to improve breast feeding success. *J. Nutr. Educ., 16*, 19.

Jones, R., Lacey, J., Chadbund, C., Crisp, A., Whitehead, J. & Stordy, J. (1978) Common mistakes in infant feeding: survey from a London borough. *Br. Med. J., 2*, 112.

Jones, R., Lacey, J., Chadbund, C., Crisp, A., Whitehead, J. & Stordy, J. (1978) Variation in energy intake of adolescent schoolgirls. *J. Hum. Nutr., 32*, 419.

Journal of the American Medical Association (1972) Cooking classes help older Britons eat better. *J. Am. Med. Ass., 222*, 532.

Kohrs, M. (1984) New perspectives on nutritional counselling for the elderly. *Mod. Med., 5*, 81.

Maclean, G.D. (1977) An appraisal of the concepts of infant feeding and their application in practice. *J. Adv. Nurs., 2*, 103.

McNeilly, A. (1979) Effects of lactation on fertility. *Br. Med. Bull., 35*, 151.

Morrison, S. (1983) Nutrition and longevity. *Nutr. Rev., 41*, 133.

Nail, P., Thomas, M. & Eakin, R. (1980) The effect of thiamins and riboflavine supplementation on the level of those vitamins in human breast milk and urine. *Am. J. Clin. Nutr., 33*, 198.

Nel, E. (1976) Fads and fallacies of diet. *S. Afr. Nurs. J., 4*, 7.

Nichols, B.L. & Nichols, V.N. (1983) Nutrition in pregnancy and lactation. *Nutr. Abstr. Rev., 53*, 259.

Niswander, K.R., Singer, J., Westphal, M. & Weiss, W. (1969) Weight gain during pregnancy and prepregnancy weight. *Obstet. Gynecol., 33*, 482.

Oakes, G.K., Chez, R.A. & Morelli, I.C. (1975) Diet in pregnancy: meddling with the normal or preventing toxaemia. *Am. J. Nurs., 75(11)*, 1135.

Ounsted, M. & Sleigh, G. (1975) The infant's self-regulation of food intake and weight gain. *Lancet, 1*, 1393.

Passmore, R., Hollingsworth, D. & Robertson, J. (1979) Prescription for a better British diet. *Br. Med. J., i*, 527.

Robson, J.R.K., Konlande, J.E., Larkin, F.A., O'Connor, P.A. & Hsi-Yen Liu (1974) Zen macrobiotic dietary problems in infancy. *Pediatrics, Springfield, 53(3)*, 326.

Sarat Singh, N. & Borkotoky, R.K. (1975) Weight gain in pregnancy. *J. Indian Med. Ass., 64(3)*, 53.

Smithells, R.W., Sheppard, S. Schorooh, C. & Seller, M. (1980) Possible prevention of neural-tube defects by periconceptual vitamin supplementation. *Lancet, 1*, 339.

Taitz, L.S. (1971) Infantile overnutrition among artificially fed infants in the Sheffield region. *Br. Med. J., 1*, 315.

Thomson, A.M. (1959) Diet in relation to the course and outcome of pregnancy. *Br. J. Nutr., 13*, 509.

Wharton, B. & Berger, H. (1976) Bottle feeding. *Br. Med. J., 1*, 1326.

Young, M. (1976) The accumulation of protein by the fetus. In: Beard, R.W. & Nathanielsz, P.W. (eds.) *Fetal Physiology and Medicine*, pp. 59–79. London: W.B. Saunders.

For further reading the nurse is referred to the following monographs on the subject:

Storrs, A. (1985) *Geriatric Nursing*. London: Baillière Tindall.

Nutrition and Health in Old Age (1979) DHSS Report on Health and Social Subjects, No. 16. London: HMSO.

Korhs, M. & Kamath, S. (eds.) (1982) Symposium on Nutrition and Aging. *Am. J. Clin. Nutr., 36*, 735.

Harper, A.E. (1982) Nutrition, aging and longevity. *Am. J. Clin. Nutr., 36*, 737.

3 Environmental influences affecting diet

INTRODUCTION

Our eating habits today are markedly influenced by our life-style, including the pressures of work, community demands and limited time. For many people one-third of their daily food intake is taken outside their homes. Added to this, religious, cultural and traditional demands are extremely relevant influences on food choices. Snack eating (one of the causes of the widespread incidence of dental caries), dining at ethnic restaurants and eating on-the-run (a situation which has resulted in the coining of the term 'traveller's diarrhoea' caused by contaminated food) are all practices which are directly attributable to the way of life of our society in the latter years of the twentieth century, and they affect the eating habits of the patients in our care as much as our own.

CONVENIENCE FOODS

For a variety of reasons progressively more meals are consumed outside the home. Due to vast sales and the greater ease with which these convenience foods are prepared, the cost difference between them and home-cooked meals is becoming less — hence the greater incentive to depend more heavily on them. Low-cost canteen meals at places of employment have been a further cause of this phenomenon. The breadwinner often has his or her main meal at work and this results in the serving of a snack meal in the evening, often to the rest of the family as well.

Regarding current terminology, *convenience foods* are those in which a greater or lesser amount of preparation has been done prior to the sale of the food item or made-up dish. *Fast foods* refers to the speed of service with which the consumer receives the food in a ready-to-eat form after ordering it. *Junk foods* have been defined by the United States Department of Agriculture as a food which does not provide at least 5% of the Recommended Daily

Allowance for protein, vitamin A, vitamin C, thiamine, riboflavin, niacin, calcium or iron per 100 kcal serving. From this definition one can see that this term is often erroneously used merely to describe take-away foods such as hamburgers or milkshakes!

It seems unlikely that our society will ever be able to implement the recommended routine of having three well balanced meals freshly cooked at home. It is also preferable to take the main meal at midday as it is then followed by exercise which assists the circulation of blood and the digestive process. However, our life-style seldom allows this. Hence it is more beneficial to look at those meals and snacks consumed outside the home and intelligently select food items which make some nutritional contribution to one's diet.

The most sensible and economical snack meal is obviously the portable lunch taken to work, for which suggestions have been included in Chapter 2. Alternatively, a serving of muesli mixed with a few tablespoons of milk powder and carried to work in a small plastic container with a well fitting lid can form the basis of an excellent lunch; chop in an apple and stir in cold water just before eating. This meal is not only delicious and easy to prepare but, unlike most of the snacks discussed below, contains a lot of fibre, which is largely absent in most take-away foods.

When purchasing a snack meal, be sure that it contains some protein, not only for its nutritional contribution but for the feeling of satiety which will prevent one needing another snack before the next meal. Foods which are predominantly sugar (for example, sweets and chocolate) or starch (for example, crisps) will have only a short-term effect in alleviating hunger. Yoghurts and milk, too, although protein foods, are rapidly absorbed and should be taken with a snack, not instead of one.

This does not mean that all sweetened foods are necessarily *bad* and salted forms *good*. For example, 'health bars' made from cereals, nuts and sugar both satisfy the sweet tooth and have a long-term satiety value resulting from the combination of the other ingredients. Similarly, hot dogs and hamburgers are portable, satisfying meals for individuals with a higher energy requirement than just a health bar. A toasted cheese sandwich and fruit, a cup of pea or bean soup and a salad roll, a small packet of peanuts and a yoghurt are all nutritious snack meals.

Too many kilojoules you say? Assuming that one's energy needs are 10 000 kJ (2400 Cal) and that one-quarter of this requirement is taken in the lunch-time snack meal, one may consume 2500 kJ (600 Cal) at this meal. Naturally, those who wish to lose weight should take less kilojoules; those with a higher energy output need more.

Table 7 is given as an estimated guide for snack eaters. It shows that take-away foods are often high in fats and low in fibre and many are concentrated sources of kilojoules but have become an integrated part of our life-style. Regrettably, reduced energy expenditure in the form of physical exercise has also become part of the sedentary pattern of life of many people today. It is emphasized that whilst intelligent dietary selection is of major importance, increased physical activity to expend the kilojoules obtained from some of the more concentrated snack foods is of equal importance to healthy individuals.

Table 7. Approximate protein, kilojoule and calorie content of some common snacks.

Food item	Protein (g)	Kilojoules	Calories
Hamburger, McDonald's*	12	928	221
Hotdog	11	1345	320
Cornish pastie (200 g)	16	2780	664
Toasted cheese sandwich	9	1385	330
Pea or lentil soup (200 g)	9	830	198
Salad roll	6	1050	250
50 g peanuts, roasted, salted	12	1200	285
50 g chocolate, plain	2	1095	262
Cheese and tomato pizza (200 g)	19	1965	468
Yoghurt, low fat, fruit (200 ml)	10	798	190
Milkshake, McDonald's* (300 g)	11	1580	376
Beer, canned, bitter (250 ml)	1	330	80
Milk, full-cream (250 ml)	9	714	170
Orange juice, sweetened (200 ml)	1	434	102
Coffee, 2 tablespoons milk, 2 teaspoons sugar	1	252	60

(Adapted from Paul, A.A. & Southgate, D.A.T. (1978) *McCance and Widdowson's The Composition of Foods*. London: HMSO.)
*From Appledorf, H. (1974) Nutritional analysis of foods from fast food chains. *Fd. Tech., 28*, 50–55.

RELIGIOUS INFLUENCES

The religious and traditional practices related to eating habits are magnified in people when they are ill, away from home or elderly.

Such conditions increase the need for the security and comfort of one's environmental heritage. The nurse should make every effort to understand the relevance of eating practices to the patient, as dietary recommendations must always remain within the framework of acceptable foods. Those cultural patterns most frequently encountered in Britain are summarized below.

Jews

Eating habits are affected by both religious and traditional laws. The word 'kosher' means pure or clean. It is used to describe the practice of slaughtering meat — in which the animal is not stunned before being bled to death — and its cleansing before use. The meat is salted, allowed to stand to promote drainage of the blood from the tissue, and then washed several times to remove all surplus blood.

Other kosher stipulations date back to the Levitican code in the Old Testament and relate to the selection of meat. Only the forequarters of the animal are used, and animals with cloven feet (pigs, deer, etc.) must be avoided. Fish with scales are permitted but crustacea (lobster, prawns, etc.), which are regarded as scavengers, may not be eaten. Meat and milk may not be served at the same meal: in strictly orthodox homes, separate crockery is kept for 'meat' and 'milk' meals. Vegetables, fruit, cereals and fish may be served at all meals. Strictly orthodox individuals may object to using hospital crockery and cutlery which is washed with soap made from animal-based fat and used for both meat and milk products. They may also object to eating ordinary cheese as this is prepared with rennet obtained from the stomach of animals.

In areas where there are many resident Jews, hospitals may cater for the dietary needs of these patients. Alternatively, patients may receive dispensation from the Rabbi allowing them to eat non-kosher food in hospital, but some of the more orthodox patients may choose to avoid meat altogether whilst away from home, unless it is prepared in a strictly kosher environment.

Roman Catholics

Catholics were formerly forbidden to eat meat on Fridays. Although this is no longer required by Papal decree, many Roman

Catholics still traditionally eat fish on Fridays and the nurse may need to bear this point in mind when counselling or feeding patients.

Seventh Day Adventists

Members of this group are usually ovolactovegetarians. Children often become vegetarians at an early age and the nurse should confirm that the child's intake of nutrients, particularly iron and calcium, is satisfactory. Wise selection of foods can result in a well balanced diet with adequate amounts of nutrients, but lack of interest or ability in the mother may preclude a satisfactory balanced diet. Supplements are sometimes necessary to ensure sufficient intake, particularly for children. However, Seventh Day Adventists often have a sound understanding of their nutritional needs and the possible shortcomings of their diet, which is an integral part of their way of life.

Hindus and Moslems

These have been included in the following section under the headings 'Indians' and 'Pakistanis' respectively for ease of reference. However, the eating habits of these peoples are determined more by their religious than their cultural origins.

CULTURAL INFLUENCES

The nurse must avoid the tendency to deprecate food patterns which do not conform to her own: such bias can only reduce rapport with the individuals concerned and hinder her efforts in health care. The comments that follow are generalized, intended only for guidance.

Arab eating practices

Most Arabs embrace the Islamic faith and therefore eat no pork. Traditionally, the main meal is served on the Tibsy (round tray) around which the family sit to eat. A classical dish is the *seeleek*, a platter consisting of rice, which is boiled in milk and then mixed with oil, on which the meat is arranged. Mutton is the preferred meat and this is eaten in large quantities. Other meat dishes enjoyed are *shish-kebabs* (sticks threaded with cubed roast mutton), *samoosas* (triangular pastry cases, filled with meat and fried) and *maghliyah* (meat rissoles eaten with a piquant sauce and a type of raw grass). The light meal in the evening may comprise white cheese, olives and bread. Food is usually taken in the hands to eat and although younger people may readily adapt to the cutlery of Western society, others may prefer to use their hands, which are usually well washed and immaculate before a meal.

Indians

Most Indians are Hindus, although there are also Moslems, Buddhists and Christians in India.

For more than 3000 years Hindus have venerated the cow. The practice may have originated partly as a practical measure to protect the milk supply, but today it is part of the religious tradition and Hindus will naturally eat no beef.

One of the main philosophies of Hinduism is the sanctity of life. Depending on how strictly this is applied, Hindus may or may not be strict vegetarians. Some eat all meat other than beef, although less emphasis is placed on meat than in British homes, even in affluent sectors of society. Some Hindus eat fish, eggs and milk as their only animal derivates, others restrict themselves exclusively to milk.

It is said that it is more than sheer chance that highly spiced dishes originated in hot climates. Spices were necessary to help combat deterioration of perishable foods and salt was essential to replace that lost in sweat.

Foods included in the diet are *dhal* (lentils), *chapattis* (un-leavened wheat cakes) and *ghee* (clarified butter). *Roti*, a flat round bread which is lightly fried, and *pilaau* (rice) are eaten with *curries* and *breyani* (a mixture of meat, fish or poultry mixed with rice, lentils, potatoes and spices). The meal will often begin with a sweet dish in some form *(soji, vermicelli halvah* or sweet rice). Tea is usually made by boiling the water and milk together, and then adding tea leaves and spices.

Regrettably, Indians and the Pakistanis (discussed below) often live under poor economic conditions and have been found in practice to be affected by nutritional deficiencies more than other immigrant groups. It is the nurse's duty to ensure that recent immigrants are aware of the availability of health services and welfare foods.

Pakistanis

Being Moslem people, Pakistanis avoid pork. Much oil and *ghee* are used in the cooking of their spiced and curried foods. No alcohol is consumed. Instead, large quantities of black tea are served, often with mint, or black coffee with cardamom seeds. The festival of *Ramadan*, a period of rigid daily fasting for the ninth lunar month of the Islamic year, is a period during which Moslems neither eat nor drink from sunrise to sundown. In the evening the *ifta*, or evening breakfast, is eaten and special delicacies are often made for the nights of social eating. The festival of *Id Al-Fitr* follows the fasting, and celebrations may continue for up to three days.

West Indians

West Indian cooking is largely based on fish and the produce of rich tropical soil. The staple dish is rice and 'peas' (what we call beans), of which several varieties are grown. These legumes are also used for soups and in other vegetable mixtures. *Salt fish* and *akee* are also commonly eaten. *Akee* is a fruit which, when cooked, gives dishes the flavour and appearance of scrambled egg. Much West Indian food is spiced and strongly flavoured and immigrant patients may find British food insipid and miss their multitude of tropical fruits such as pawpaws, pineapple, mangoes and soursop, a large prickly fruit used to make a tart drink. Commonly used vegetables are the versatile breadfruit and plantains, which are large banana-like fruit, usually sautéed in butter or mixed with meat or chicken.

The African diet

People coming from rural areas in underdeveloped countries, particularly African states, are often accustomed to eating a diet consisting primarily of unrefined foods. The inclusion of large quantities of fibre is thought to protect them from various diseases prevalent in Western societies, such as cancer of the colon, diverticulosis, etc. Because of the relatively low concentration of nutritive value in these foods, and the high content of indigestible fibre, such people are sometimes accustomed to eating enormous quantities of food to meet their nutritional needs. They are thus dissatisfied with smaller British portions of more concentrated refined foods and may need to be served additional portions of vegetables, cereals, etc.

IMPLICATIONS OF PHYSICAL ACTIVITY

It is particularly the industrial nurse who may be called upon to be involved in this type of health care. It should be emphasized straight away that the individual who plays a social game of football, tennis, hockey or cricket only once or twice a week will have his dietary needs adequately covered by the average high-protein, high-energy Western-type diet. In fact, this energy expenditure is for many people an essential component in maintaining normal body weight. The effect of occupation on 24-hour energy expenditure is shown in Table 2. However, persons involved in *regular, physically demanding exercise* should be aware of certain dietary needs.

Energy requirements

The amount of energy utilized during different forms of physical exercise depends on both the type of physical activity undertaken and the weight of the participant. The energy requirements for specific sports are listed in Table 8.

Sportsmen who are of normal weight should weigh themselves at the start of the training season and then at monthly intervals

Table 8. Energy requirements for various sports.

Sport	Average energy expenditure (kJ/h)
Golf	900
Tennis	1700
Cycling (up to 20 km/h)	1800
Swimming, squash and football	1500–2500
Running or jogging	2600

thereafter to ascertain whether their kilojoule intake remains adequate for their increased requirements. The overweight sportsman places unnecessary additional strain on his heart, muscles and joints and should avoid rigorous exercise until his weight is within normal limits, meanwhile taking only moderate exercise and adhering to a weight reduction diet.

Fluids

During strenuous exercise, body heat production is increased and unless this additional heat is lost body temperature rises. If it exceeds 41°C, heat stroke becomes imminent. To prevent this rise in body temperature, heat is lost from the body by sweating. If the sweat lost is allowed to exceed 3% of body weight, physical performance is impaired. Loss of 5% of body fluids results in heat exhaustion. During prolonged exercise, like marathon running, fluids should be taken regularly every 12–15 minutes. Cold water (4°C) is usually tolerated best and small amounts of sugar may be added for energy metabolism (see below). Carbonated cool drinks may be more acceptable but should be 'degassed' to prevent distension. The recommended intake is 200–250 ml each time, depending on environmental temperatures.

Carbohydrates

These assume major importance in the diet because the athlete's prime concern is the production of energy from carbohydrates and fats. However, body carbohydrate reserves (glycogen) are much less than body fat stores and become readily depleted, thereby impairing performance after as little as two hours of strenuous exercise. Body carbohydrate reserves must therefore be kept well stocked. The work of a group of Swedish physiologists has led to the practice of carbohydrate loading to increase endurance prior to prolonged exercise. These physiologists suggested that for about a week before a race carbohydrate reserves should be depleted by the consumption of a high-protein, high-fat, low-carbohydrate diet. For the last three days prior to the race, a high-carbohydrate diet was recommended to ensure optimum repletion of glycogen stores.

However, recent research suggests that the depletion phase is unnecessary and today many athletes merely consume the high-carbohydrate diet for three days before the athletic event. A further advantage of carbohydrate loading is that glycogen is stored in combination with water. As the glycogen is converted into energy, it releases this water which helps to offset that lost by sweating during the race. Carbohydrate loading is effective only in events lasting more than one hour and is of no value for short-duration events like sprints. During an endurance activity, 30 g of glucose or sucrose dissolved in one litre of fluid represents a physiologically sound drink.

As a *pre-game* energy source, a maximum of 50 g sugar should be taken. This should be consumed not less than two hours before the start of the competition, or performance can be impaired. This is because the sugar causes insulin to be released into the blood stream. A high blood insulin level will in turn inhibit the release of glucose from the liver for energy, and muscle glycogen has to be used instead. Early depletion of glycogen reserves results in premature fatigue.

Fats

In sports like mountaineering or long-distance hiking, where concentrated foods are required to ensure a satisfactory energy intake, fat is the most important food, yielding 38 kJ/g: twice as effective as an energy source as protein and carbohydrates. However, the primary need is always for carbohydrates as carbohydrate reserves become depleted early, whereas body stores of fat provide an almost inexhaustible source of energy.

Protein

It is fallacious to imagine that, because muscle tissue is primarily made of protein, large quantities of meat must be consumed by the athlete who wants to develop muscles. The athlete who includes a normal portion of a protein food (meat, fish or cheese) at each meal and 500 ml of milk per day will ingest at least 78 g of protein per day, which is adequate. The consumption of large amounts of high-protein foods at the expense of carbohydrates is not only costly but leaves the athlete with reduced glycogen stores.

Vitamins

A satisfactory intake of *vitamin B complex* is necessary to metabolize the high-carbohydrate diet mentioned earlier. It has also been shown that mild deficiency of vitamin B complex — thiamine in particular — impairs physical activity. For this reason adequate amounts of wholewheat bread, wholegrain cereals, meat, liver, dried beans, peas and soya beans should be included.

Vitamin C plays an essential role in the manufacture of intracellular material which maintains tissue integrity and is important for tissue repair. It may thus be particularly valuable in body contact sports.

Minerals

From a physiological point of view, there is seldom justification for increasing salt intake when participating in sport. In most sports, such as football, hockey and squash, active participation occurs for only one or two hours. During intense sweating the body will at most lose 3–5 g of salt per hour. However, the normal Western diet provides 12–15 g/day and this greatly exceeds the normal physiological requirement of 0.5–1 g/day, allowing more than enough to cover the needs of the athlete during less than three hours of strenuous exercise. Many workers feel that the normal intake is adequate to cover even prolonged activity like marathon running, cycling or mountaineering. Added to this, the salt consumed to increase the palatability of food during the last three days of carbohydrate loading adds considerably to the sodium intake. Potatoes cooked with salt, sweetcorn, soup, bread, etc., will all ensure adequate reserves except at a very high temperature and humidity. The consumption of salty drinks during a race is not recommended as it can cause an unphysiological load on the kidneys.

POTASSIUM. Carbohydrate loading undertaken during the last few days before an athletic event should be accompanied by a sufficient potassium intake. Potassium is required for the process of depositing glycogen in the muscles and liver, and high-potassium foods such as fruit juices, bananas, pineapples, tomatoes and soups made with meat should be included in the diet.

MAGNESIUM. This mineral is lost in sweat and has been found to be depleted in some sportsmen involved in heavy training. Magnesium activates some of the enzymes in carbohydrate metabolism and is thus of particular importance for those on the high-carbohydrate diet. Foods which are good sources of magnesium are cereals, legumes, meat, fruit and nuts.

Sample menu (carbohydrate loading)

The following diet is suggested as an example of a carbohydrate-loading regimen for three days prior to long-duration exercise.

Breakfast
  orange juice, stewed dried peaches, porridge, milk and sugar
  wholewheat toast, margarine and jam as desired

Mid-morning
  bananas, dried fruits, glucose sweets

Lunch
  chicken pie and chips
  fruit yoghurt

Mid-afternoon
  fruit juice and sweet biscuits

Dinner
  thick barley soup with roll and margarine
  lean pork chop
  roast potatoes, peas, beetroot salad, canned fruit and custard

Bed-time
  cup of cocoa with sugar and sweet biscuits

BACTERIAL CONTAMINATION

Travel has become an integral part of life today. This may take the form of commuting from one suburb to another for purposes of employment, or travelling to another country by boat or air on vacation. This situation has resulted in a dramatic increase in food poisoning. 'Traveller's diarrhoea' is extremely difficult to pinpoint and can occur for a variety of reasons. Individuals may eat a food a long distance from where they have bought it having conveyed it in a temperature conducive to bacterial multiplication. Alternatively, food may be eaten in a boat or aeroplane and because passengers disperse at their destination the cause and widespread incidence is never located. Another problem is the lack of knowledge of the principles of hygiene often evident among the managers of small outlets of take-away foods. In areas where there is inadequate surveillance this, too, can be a major source of contaminated food.

It is often the responsibility of the industrial or school nurse to supervise kitchen activities. For this, a basic knowledge of bacterial contamination of food and the essentials of sanitation are necessary.

The two most common types of bacterial food poisoning are due to *Salmonella* and *Staphylococcus*.

Salmonella

Salmonella is found primarily in animals, and this type of food poisoning will usually be encountered in products of animal origin. Silliker comments that the most frequent cause of outbreaks is consumer mishandling of poultry, meat and dairy products. Symptoms (nausea, vomiting, headache and diarrhoea) can appear from 4 to 36 hours after ingestion of infected food. The long delay may be due to the fact that the toxins develop in the digestive tract and only then cause symptoms to occur. Freezing of meat does not preclude or destroy contamination with *Salmonella* bacteria. Bland foods are excellent vehicles for this type of organism: custard fillings, cream puffs, chicken mayonnaise or croquettes which have been insufficiently cooked or have been subjected to too much handling and kept luke-warm for a long time are excellent sites for the development of these bacteria.

Staphylococcus

Staphyloccocci are readily destroyed by cooking but the toxins which produce the symptoms of food poisoning are destroyed only by prolonged high temperature. Gastroenteritis follows 1–5 h after ingestion of contaminated food.

Staphylococcal food poisoning is often caused by kitchen

workers, as the organism lives most frequently in Man. About 60% of the general public have this organism in the interior of their nose, and although not all strains cause food poisoning, nose-pickers can cause enormous damage in an institutional kitchen. Fig. 5 shows a *Staphylococcus* culture originating on a kitchen worker's unwashed hands. As with *Salmonella*, bland foods are most often affected. The bacteria multiply very readily at room temperature and in warm weather.

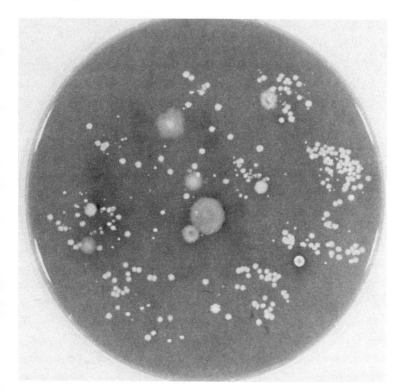

Fig. 5. *Staphylococci cultured from the uwashed hands of a kitchen worker.*

Clostridium botulinum

A much less common type of bacterial food poisoning is caused by a potent toxin produced by *Clostridium botulinum*, which is found in soil all over the world. This bacterium particularly contaminates vegetables, rather than fruit which are too acid. On contamination a toxin develops *in the absence of air* (i.e. it is an anaerobe), and thus inadequately sterilized home-canned vegetables can be dangerous. Food will not necessarily taste or smell bad, but the can will be 'blown' which will be the danger signal to the consumer. All blown cans should be discarded, although in most cases this phenomenon will be due to a harmless 'hydrogen swell'. In an emergency, the contents can be heated for approximately 15 min at 80°C and then consumed. To ensure that the middle of the can reaches this temperature and is adequately sterilized, the food will need to be boiled for much longer, a process which often destroys the more delicate flavour of food. Furthermore, as 1 g of the toxin of *Clostridium botulinum* is sufficient to destroy the entire population of the USA, it would seem advisable to discard the blown tin and not take a chance.

Ptomaine poisoning

The term 'ptomaine' was used particularly in the latter part of the 18th century and comes from the Greek word '*ptoma*', meaning a dead body. Ptomaines are nitrogenous products formed in the latter stages of food decomposition, when food is so obviously spoilt that people will refuse to eat it. This type of poisoning does not therefore pose a problem in our society.

KITCHEN HYGIENE

There are four cardinal rules for caterers to apply in the kitchen:

1. Frozen meat and poultry must be completely thawed before cooking and kept separate from other foods to prevent cross-contamination. Inadequate thawing and subsequent unsatisfactory heating has been the cause of more than one widespread outbreak of food poisoning. Cook all meat thoroughly — rare meat encourages the development of bacteria.
2. Use separate surfaces, utensils and equipment for raw and cooked foods if possible. Wash tables and small equipment with a good detergent and hypochlorite (approximately 250 parts per million) for disinfectant purposes. All surfaces and

equipment must be well dried. Taps and sinks should be cleaned regularly and cloths should be boiled at the end of each day.

3. Keep food, particularly meat, fish, cream and mayonnaise either *hot* or *cold*. Room temperature encourages the growth of bacteria.

4. If possible, avoid the use of leftovers. When they are used, reheat them thoroughly before use.

Equipment

The following points related to large-scale equipment should also be borne in mind:

1. The optimum heating of the water in a dishwasher is essential. The temperature of the washing water should be not less than 60°C, and for effective elimination of bacteria the final rinse water should be not less than 82°C.

2. Cold rooms should remain constantly at approximately 4°C, a temperature low enough to inhibit the growth of contaminating organisms.

3. The oil in the deep-fat fryer should be changed regularly. Repeated heating causes breakdown of the oil resulting in irritating fractions which have been found to be carcinogenic in rats. Thus oil should not just be topped up if insufficient, but frequently drained and discarded.

4. The meat slicer should be washed with freshly made-up hypochlorite solution and paper towelling after use. The damp cloth so often in evidence in kitchens can be a major source of contamination.

5. Uninformed kitchen workers are a serious threat to hygiene in an institution. They should be told repeatedly to wash their hands after visiting the toilet and the supervisor should ensure that soap and disposable towels are always available for this purpose. Infected lesions on the skin should be reported immediately and food should at all times have minimum contact with hands. Nose-pickers and those with colds or throat infections should be aware that they are a potential hazard. Regular talks to kitchen workers, incentives such as certificates for having undertaken a short course

in kitchen sanitation and food hygiene, and the use of eye-catching posters which are regularly replaced, all help to maintain a high standard of food service hygiene. It is unfortunate that the essential service of food production is all too often left in the hands of unschooled and disinterested workers.

DIET SELECTION AND DENTAL CARIES

Plaque is the soft, tenacious bacterial deposit which forms on the surface of the teeth as a precursor to tooth decay. It is the medium in which the oral bacteria, of which *Streptococci* are the major genus, thrive and multiply. If plaque is not removed, this will result in penetration of the dental enamel and development of caries.

Tooth decay starts with pathogenic bacteria colonizing vulnerable sites on the teeth, especially pits and fissures of the crown. In addition, there must be sufficient carbohydrate in the diet to produce plaque and acid. Susceptibility to caries is dependent on several factors, including heredity, anatomical positioning, intake of minerals — especially fluoride and calcium in water — and other dietary components. Until some years ago sugar was the only factor universally implicated in causing tooth decay. However, recent research has pinpointed several other dietary factors. While findings do not suggest that the level of sugar intake is unimportant, they indicate that total sugar intake is not the only, nor necessarily the principal, cariogenic factor in modern diets. Refined carbohydrate, fat, fibre and foods affecting the acidity of the mouth are important in this respect, and so is the frequency of intake, i.e. the pattern of eating.

SUGAR. In a recent study by Hacket *et al* it was found that the total sugar intake of a group of 11- to 14-year-old English children was 118 g/day. This constituted approximately 21% of their total energy intake. Confectionery was the largest single source of sugar with a large amount of the sugar taken between meals — both important factors in the causation of dental caries — as discussed below.

Sucrose and glucose cause more acid production in the plaque than any other commonly eaten food items. In this way the development of caries is accelerated by the enhancement of the bacterial substrate. Although there appears to be little correlation between the quantity of sucrose eaten and the severity of tooth decay, the vehicle in which the sugar is consumed is of major importance. Interestingly, it has been shown that food containing salt is retained in the mouth for a shorter period than foods which are unsalted. Thus for controlling both weight and dental caries there is merit in advising people to select salty food items in preference to sweetened ones. However, due to the possible correlation between salt and hypertension, this advice has controversial implications. The length of time that foods remain in the mouth has been shown to be of great importance and thus, contrary to popular opinion, carbonated beverages are preferable to diluted cordials which stay longer in the mouth.

It also appears that sugar is cleared from the mouth more rapidly when taken in liquid than in solid forms, indicating that cool drinks are theoretically preferable to sweets. Nevertheless, ordinary tap water is, of course, superior to all types of synthetic, sweetened drinks and children in particular should be taught to appreciate it as a necessary and refreshing drink.

OTHER CARIOGENIC FOODS. There are certain other foods, particularly those comprising a large proportion of refined carbohydrate, which accelerate the development of tooth decay. Thus white bread, pastries, scones and other confections are all potentially cariogenic. This potential is increased if the food is sticky: doughnuts and jam tarts, for example, are considerably worse in effect. Aristotle, who wrote what is thought to be the first comment on the aetiology of dental caries, attributed the condition to sweet figs adhering to the teeth!

The *fat* content of foods also plays an important role in this area by limiting time of contact with the teeth. For example, chocolates and caramels are cleared from the mouth more readily than boiled or jellied sweets, and are therefore preferable.

The *roughage* content of foods plays a role due to its abrasive action on the teeth: emphasis on wholegrain cereals, fruit and vegetables will assist in the cleansing of the teeth, and the consumption of a fruit at the end a meal is a routine that the nurse should encourage in her patients.

EATING HABITS. Frequency of intake is another important factor. Snack eating aggravates the situation, particularly when high-carbohydrate foods predominate. Within 13 min of eating carbohydrates, the pH of the dental plaque drops from 6.0 to 5.0 owing to increased bacterial activity. Assuming that the teeth are exposed to acid for approximately 20 min each time food is consumed, one can readily understand how caries are produced if foods which promote cariogenicity are eaten regularly during the day. A further implication is that if sweets or confectionery are to be eaten, it is far better to eat the total amount at one time than to spread the consumption over the day.

ACIDITY. Finally, the pH of the mouth is relevant. Studies have shown that acid drops, orange suckers and fruit cake all increase acidity in the mouth, thus enhancing the cariogenic effect of the foods eaten. As mentioned earlier, carbohydrate foods increase the amount of acid in the mouth. Megadosage tablets of vitamin C have also been incriminated by some workers for the deleterious effects they have on the teeth. These chewable tablets are extremely acidic and may significantly contribute to the incidence of caries.

In conclusion it is emphasized that, having discussed the cariogenicity of various food items and dietary components in a positive way, the relative importance of each factor is still, however, questionable. In a recent review article on the subject, Walker ends his commentary with the statement: 'Finally, it is humbling to have to admit after a century of caries research . . . information is inadequate to satisfactorily answer the salient question posed, namely, are meaningful reductions in dental caries by voluntary dietary means practicable? It is equally humbling that, when widespread improvements do occur, as they have occurred, there is uncertainty over the factors responsible.'

Fluoride

Today opposition to the widespread administration of fluoride in areas where the water supply is deficient is largely based on emotion. Much of the feeling is directed at the lack of freedom of choice by the public rather than the effects of the added mineral.

Well substantiated reports estimate that a drop of 60–65%

occurs in the incidence of caries in children when water supplies in deficient areas are supplemented, due to the hardening effect of fluoride on the teeth. It is important that fluoride administration begins early in infancy for optimum uptake by the teeth. Previously, supplementation began prenatally but today it is generally accepted that the placenta is a highly effective barrier to the fluoride ion and administration from the first few weeks of life is advised for deficient communities. In Britain, water is fluoridated in some cities and the normal intake by persons in these municipal areas will be adequate. In other areas intake may be deficient and the nurse should be conversant with public health practices in the community in which she works.

Interestingly, there is a drop in incidence in dental caries in communities both with and without fluoridated water, possibly as a result of an increase in fluoride intake in processed foods. For example, the use of fluoridated water for canned vegetables, additions in baby foods and formulas, and the widespread use of fluoridated toothpaste may well play a role in the improved situation.

A word of warning: fluoride in excess is potentially extremely dangerous to health. In areas where water is fluoridated, mothers should be seriously cautioned about administering excessive fluoride to their children by additional supplementation. Given an excess of fluoride, tooth enamel becomes pitted, mottled and discoloured, bone structure will become abnormally dense, and irreversible kidney damage may occur.

Dental health: conclusions

In conclusion it is stressed that tooth decay is one of the few diseases which, at least in part, can be controlled by ourselves. Everyone, particularly children, should be aware of the role that they can play in minimizing decay of their teeth. The environmental factors involved are summarized below:

1. *Oral hygiene*, particularly mechanical removal of plaque.
2. *Control of diet* as discussed above.
3. *Control of bacteria*, by chemicals such as fluoride which inhibit absorption of plaque on the tooth surface, or by antibiotics. Much thought is currently being given to the use of immunization against cariogenic bacteria and the presence

of antibodies in caries-free subjects. However, this research is still in the experimental stage.

4. *Tooth protection*: fluoride taken systemically makes the enamel more resistant to the effects of bacteria. The use of epoxy to fill fissures in the teeth has also been found to be most effective in protecting against decay.

BIBLIOGRAPHY

Appledorf, H. (1981) Nutrition for the New Generation. In: Ellenbogen, L. *Controversies in Nutrition*. London: Churchill Livingstone.

Bibby, B.G. (1975) The cariogenicity of snack foods and confections. *J. Am. Dent. Ass., 90*, 121.

Committee on Nutrition Misinformation, National Academy of Sciences Research Council (1974) Water deprivation and performance of athletes. *Nutr. Rev., 32(10)*, 314.

Druker, D.B. (1979) Sweetening agents in food, drink and medicine: cariogenic potential and adverse effects. *J. Hum. Nutr., 33*, 114.

Edgar, W., Bibby, B.G., Mundorff, S. & Rowley, J. (1975) Acid production in plaques after eating snacks: modifying factors in foods. *J. Am. Dent. Ass., 90*, 418.

Grivetti, L.I. & Pangborn, R.M. (1974) Origin of selected Old Testament dietary prohibition. *J. Am. Diet. Ass., 65(6)*, 634.

Hackett, A., Rugg-Gunn, A., Appleton, D., Allinson, M. & Eastoe, J. (1978) Sugar-eating habits of 405 11–14 year old English children.

Harties, R. (1967) Carbohydrate consumption and dental caries. *Am. J. Clin. Nutr., 20*, 152.

Hewetson, J.M. (1979) Diet and the control of dental disease in normal children: practical applications. *J. Hum. Nutr., 33*, 111.

Huskisson, J.M. (1978) A bacteriological study of roast chickens sold in Cape Town. *S. Afr. Fd. Rev., 5(4)*, 21.

Johnson, N.W. (1979) Aetiology of dental disease and theoretical aspects of dietary control. *J. Hum. Nutr., 33*, 98.

Leverett, D. (1982) Fluorides and the changing prevalence of dental caries. *Science, 217*, 26

Ludwig, T.G. & Bibby, B.G. (1957) Acid production from different carbohydrate foods in plaques and saliva. *J. Dent. Res., 36*, 56.

Mayat, Z. (1970) *Indian Delights*. Durban: Women's Cultural Group.

Mayer, J. & Bullen, B. (1960) Nutrition and athletic performance. *Physiol. Rev., 40*, 394.

Pether, J.V. & Gilbert, R. (1971) The survival of *Salmonella* in fingertips and transfer of the organisms to food. *J. Hyg., Camb., 69*, 673.

Piggott, J.R. (1979) Food preferences in some United Kingdom residents. *J. Hum. Nutr., 33*, 197.

Roberts, D. & Hobbs, B. (1974) Feeding the traveller. *Royal Soc. Health, 3*, 114.

Schafer, R. & Jetley, E.A. (1975) Social psychology of food faddism. *J. Am. Diet. Ass., 66(2)*, 129.

Silliker, J.H. (1982) The *Salmonella* problem: Current status and future direction. *J. Fd. Protection, 45*, 661.

Tank, G. & Starvick, C.A. (1964) Caries experience of children one to six years old in two Oregon communities. I: Effect of fluoride on caries experience and eruption of teeth. *J. Am. Dent. Ass., 69*, 749.

Thomas, M. Noah, N.D., Male, G.E. Stringer, M.F. Kendall, M., Gilbert, R.J., Jones, P.H. & Philips, K.D. (1977) Hospital outbreak of *Clostridium perfringens* food poisoning. *Lancet, 1*, 1046.

Walker, A.R.P. (1984) How practical are meaningful reductions in dental caries by dietary means? *Nutr. Abstr. Rev., 54*, 211.

Wolfe, L. (1971) *The Cooking of the Caribbean Islands*. Amsterdam: Time-Life International.

II Diet in disease

4 Nutritional Care of Patients

by Vivien Coates

The first section of this book has considered the principles of normal nutrition and the second part will review the needs of patients who require therapeutic diets. During the course of this chapter it is intended to discuss the role of the nurse in the nutrition of hospital patients. Patients taking either the standard hospital or one of the special oral diets (e.g. diabetic or reducing diet) are often in need of thoughtful nutritional care, and this is an aspect of the nurse's role which has become increasingly under-valued. In this chapter some aspects of hospital nutritional care that have been found to be inadequate will be mentioned; possible consequences of an inadequate diet and ways in which nursing intervention can help improve patient nutrition will be considered. The terms 'enteral' and 'parenteral' nutrition will be explained, and these topics will be briefly reviewed. Included in this chapter there is also a summary of methods of nutritional assessment.

MALNUTRITION AMONGST HOSPITAL PATIENTS

As discussed in Chapter 13, recent research has clearly indicated that a high percentage of hospital patients are malnourished, with the situation worsening during their stay in hospital. Research studies that have investigated the nutritional status of random samples of patients in general hospitals have found that many patients can be said to be suffering from some degree of protein-calorie malnutrition. In America Bistrian *et al* (1974, 1976) found that approximately 50% of surgical patients and 40% of medical patients were malnourished. Similar results were obtained by Hill *et al* (1977) after nutritional assessment of samples of English patients.

These research studies illustrated that there were many patients in hospital whose nutritional status was wrongly assumed to be adequate. Subsequent research has indicated that the nutritional status of patients will often deteriorate further whilst the patient is in hospital (Weisnier *et al*, 1979; Johnston, 1980).

Possible consequences of inadequate nutritional status

It is important that patients are adequately nourished as it has been found that the nutritional status of patients may have an effect upon the course of their illness. Some areas in which nutritional status is known to have an effect are mentioned below.

IMMUNE RESPONSE. Patients who are malnourished tend to be more susceptible to, and suffer more seriously from, infection (Blackburn, 1980). Furthermore, infection predisposes the individual to malnutrition.

WOUND HEALING. Patients whose nutritional status is poor and who are catabolizing rather than synthesizing tissue are likely to suffer delayed healing. Surgical wounds, ulcers or fistulae may not repair, and complications such as wound dehiscence or pressure sores may occur.

WEIGHT LOSS. This is perhaps the most commonly accepted sign of tissue catabolism. It is associated with an increased rate of morbidity. The rate of weight loss is as important as the amount of weight lost. Prolonged uncomplicated weight loss of 40% of body weight is fatal and if rapid wasting occurs the loss of 25% carries a poor prognosis (Woolfson, 1978).

THERAPY. The response to treatments such as antibiotic therapy or chemotherapy is known to be compromised in the malnourished patient. Conversely, repletion of surgical patients has been found to reduce morbidity and mortality. Goode and Hawkins (1978) found that malnourished patients' recovery from surgery was prolonged; Mullen et al (1980) demonstrated that feeding patients pre- and postoperatively reduced surgical complications; while Wilmore (1977) found that morbidity was lower in patients who were receiving nutritional support than in those who were not.

Thus the consequences of overlooking the importance of the nutritional status of patients may be great. For any one of the above reasons the recovery of malnourished patients may be prolonged or severely impaired.

Possible causes of impaired nutritional status of hospital patients

Clinical

Many of the illnesses that necessitate admission to hospital wards affect the patient's normal intake, digestion or absorption of food, or their metabolic needs and, therefore, place the patient at risk of impaired nutritional status. Some examples are given below.

INFECTION. This can increase patients' nutritional needs via an increase in metabolic rate. Infection increases body temperature which causes an increase in body energy expenditure. Therefore the basal metabolic rate increases according to the severity of the infection.

RESPIRATORY DISEASE. Many patients suffering from respiratory disease are found to be malnourished. Difficulty in breathing may reduce the patient's inclination to eat as chewing and swallowing may increase dyspnoea. Symptoms such as increased sputum production or frequent coughing may also contribute to anorexia. Cancer may (for reasons as yet unknown) cause an increasing resting metabolic expenditure (Shils, 1976) and thus will require an increased nutritional intake to maintain nutritional status, whilst the illness may predispose the patient to reduced intake. Depending upon the situation and type of the cancer a variety of nutritional problems may be induced. Local problems may include reduced intake due to obstruction of part of the gastrointestinal tract. Malabsorption of nutrients may occur, e.g. protein may be less efficiently absorbed in patients with pancreatic neoplasm and resulting insufficiency of pancreatic enzymes.

DISEASES OF THE GASTROINTESTINAL TRACT. Any diseases that alter the ability of the body to absorb nutrients or which affect metabolism, e.g. Crohn's disease or ulcerative colitis, may also increase the risk of protein-calorie malnutrition.

PARALYSIS OR MUSCULAR WEAKNESS. Patients suffering from paralysis or muscular weakness, such as following a cerebrovascular accident, may be susceptible to nutritional problems as they may be unable to manipulate cutlery, hand–eye–mouth co-ordination may be poor, and food once in the mouth may not be chewed or swallowed efficiently. The loss of dignity which may accompany feeding difficulties may render the patient less inclined to eat.

PAIN OR ANXIETY. Regardless of origin, pain or anxiety may induce anorexia to the extent that the patient is unable to eat enough to maintain his body weight. Surgery or other trauma, such as accidental injury, may greatly affect body metabolism. The response has been termed 'the metabolic response to trauma' (see Chapter 13). The severity of the response correlates well with the magnitude of the injury and typically results in a proportionally increased metabolic rate, and thus energy requirements (Elwyn *et al*, 1981).

The brief review above serves to indicate that many patients on general wards may have nutritional problems which are not immediately obvious but may, nevertheless, require careful nutritional management.

Hospital practice

In addition to the unavoidable problems mentioned above, hospital practice may also contribute to the development of nutritional problems. Some examples are given below.

Lack of nutritional awareness has been mentioned previously. It is known that malnutrition may be undetected as assessment of patients' nutritional status or intake is rarely undertaken. The advent of the trolley system of meals enables patients' food to be both distributed and re-collected without anyone being aware of what the patient has eaten. It is potentially dangerous, therefore, to equate nutritional nursing care with no more than serving the patient with his meal tray. Nutritional care is usually given low priority when in competition with other medical treatments. Whilst attention may readily be given to the use of rapid treatments such as surgery or medication, a long-term rather nebulous therapy such as nutrition is often accorded lowly status.

Intake may be repeatedly restricted for diagnostic procedures, whilst meals missed because of the timing of treatment or doctors' rounds may deplete a borderline patient further.

Lack of communication between patient and nurse or between hospital personnel may contribute to nutritional neglect.

Responsibility for nutritional care is often divided between doctors, dietitians and nurses. If responsibility is vague and no personnel are accountable for nutritional care, it may not be adequately undertaken by anyone.

Summary

This section has so far noted that a significant number of hospital patients are malnourished and that this situation may be detrimental to their recovery. It is known that many patients on general hospital wards suffer from diseases which will predispose them to an inadequate nutritional intake and therefore eventually compromise their nutritional status. It has also been stated that hospital practice may contribute to patients' nutritional problems.

NURSING INTERVENTION AND NUTRITIONAL EDUCATION

This section will consider areas in which nursing practice can play an important role in patient nutritional care.

Nurses have a unique advantage in hospitals as they are the only personnel who are with the patients throughout the day. This enables them to observe and assess patients in a way that is often not possible for other hospital staff such as doctors or dietitians.

Nutritional assessment

On admission, estimation of nutritional risk should be routinely undertaken as follows:

1. Accurate height–weight measurements should be taken and noted.
2. The patient should be questioned regarding relevant food preferences and dislikes (e.g. milk) and special dietary needs.
3. Mouth problems, e.g. lesions or lack of saliva due to administration of specific drugs, should be identified, and presence and state of teeth and whereabouts of dentures established. (All too often, an elderly patient is fed less appetizing, sloppy foods for a prolonged period because family or friends have not been alerted to fetch the necessary dentures from the patient's home where they were forgotten

in the stress of the emergency admission to hospital. Even worse, dentures may be left unused, in the handbag next to the patient's bed, having been forgotton by the senile person.)

When a nurse has measured a patient's weight and height, has made a clinical visual assessment of his body and is aware of his diagnosis and social circumstances, she has enough information to decide if a dietitian should be asked to assess the patient more fully. As the dietitian works on many wards she may be unable to see all patients routinely and may therefore rely upon ward staff informing her of patients who may need her attention.

Assessing patients' intake

While in hospital the nurse has the opportunity to observe and assess the situation further.

1. While working with the patient, i.e. in the bath, doing dressings, etc., she can judge the condition of his skin and the presence of dehydration or skin lesions.
2. Where practical, routine monitoring of weight should occur in hospital. In exceptional circumstances, the prostrate patient can be weighed in bed on a platform scale in the Stores Department.
3. The presence of diarrhoea or vomiting will markedly affect the patient's nutritional status. If these are prolonged, the patient will enter hospital deficient in nutrients, and dehydrated. If fully conscious, the patient may be extremely thirsty due to fluid losses but too exhausted and lethargic to ask repeatedly for fluids to replenish his losses. If permissible (e.g. if not required to be 'nil per mouth' for imminent surgery) a jug instead of a glass of water at the bedside is appropriate. Erratic weight gain may result from rapid rehydration and continued losses from the GI tract.
4. Appraisal of food intake. If patients are eating independently, close observation (and routine charting if in doubt about adequacy of intake) is essential to determine whether they routinely finish their meals, obtain food from visitors or have little appetite. In paediatric wards the sweets, cold drinks, etc., brought by relatives and friends are a particular

problem; children sometimes hide forbidden foods to prevent confiscation. (The diplomatic routine checking of
bedside lockers will often bring to light hidden items for
consumption: alcohol stored by the alcoholic, sweets and
biscuits kept by the diabetic or individual on a weight
reducing diet, laxatives by the patient with anorexia nervosa
or other purgative addict, or potato crisps for the hypertensive patient rebelling against eating a low-salt diet.)

Helping patients to eat

Nurses need to check that patients are able to eat their meals.
Some patients will need help to reach their meals and careful
positioning (for example of patients who are hemiplegic) may be
necessary. Patients who eat slowly or who are confused may need
to have each course given out separately to ensure that they get
hot food and that they eat an acceptable quantity. Patients with
poor sight or little manual dexterity may need to have plate covers
or clingfilm removed. Plate guards or adapted cutlery may be
necessary and it is the nurse who will usually assess whether a
patient needs utensils or aids and order them. This topic will be
discussed more fully below.

The position of the patient will greatly affect his ability and
inclination to eat his meals. This is particularly important for
patients who are eating in bed. Patients who are too low down in
the bed, turned on to one hip, unable to reach their tables, or
perhaps slumped to one side in the case of very weak or hemiplegic
patients, will obviously encounter difficulties when trying to eat.

The practice of routinely checking around the ward to ensure
that each patient was suitably positioned prior to meal-times had
much to recommend it. More recently, however, nursing has
moved away from routine practice and this, coupled with wards
which are often subdivided into bays and cubicles, has meant that
it is easy to forget the needs of patients who are not readily visible.

Dependent patients will need to be fed by a nurse. This can
often prove to be a lengthy task and therefore time must be
allowed to do this when planning nursing care. Feeding patients
can often require considerable skill and should not always be
allocated to the most junior nurses.

As protein malnutrition is the most likely deficiency to occur in a hospital ward (particularly as patients are often routinely given vitamin and mineral supplements), the foods which are high in protein should be fed to the patient first. Cottage pie, milky puddings, cheese and egg dishes and nutritious soups (i.e. those made with a basis of milk or legumes) are often well received and supply considerable nutritional value. The nurse must also ensure that the meal is attractively served to the patient, as presentation may influence whether the patient eats or refuses his meal. Many hospitals now let patients choose their own meals according to a menu system and the nurse may need to help patients fill in their menus, or check that they are ordering acceptable meals for themselves.

Although most of the suggestions above would appear to be common sense it is known that patients have eaten clingfilm, that patients have been unable to eat because no-one checked if they had any teeth, that meals have been removed untouched because the patient was unable to reach his tray; and therefore it would seem necessary to remind nurses that they must undertake to check these often very small details. If the nurse is not responsible for them it is unlikely that anyone else on the ward would help the patient with difficulties such as those mentioned above.

Interruption of meals

Patients may be unable to eat their meals because of other ward activities. Any treatment that the patient finds unpleasant or painful, such as having a dressing changed or having physiotherapy prior to his meal, may impair his appetite. Therefore if possible his care should be planned to ensure that he has recovered from such ordeals prior to his meal-time.

Alternatively, following meals with a drugs' round or by care of pressure areas may be unacceptable to many patients and may mean that they feel rushed or are unable to finish their meals. Ward domestics may be under pressure to clear the trays as soon as possible and this may also result in patients feeling hurried. Nurses must also rememember that patients who are off the ward at meal-times must have food saved for them, and that it will need to be reheated.

Nursing care of patients taking special diets

The nutritional care of patients taking special oral diets such as reducing, diabetic, low-fat or high-protein, has also been investigated and found to be inefficiently managed at ward level. At the conclusion of her study Evans (1977) states that the special diets for the hospital patients in her study were managed so inadequately that she was doubtful whether the use of dietitians and diet kitchens could be justified.

The particular requirements of patients who need a special diet are usually determined by the dietitian, often in conjunction with the doctor. According to her instructions the catering staff will then prepare food specifically for the patient. Once in the ward, however, it is the nurse who must ensure that the patient receives the correct meals and that his diet is well managed. Some aspects of special diets for which the nurse should be responsible are mentioned below.

If the aim of dietary care is either to reduce or increase a patient's weight the nurse is usually responsible for weighing and monitoring the patient's progress. If the results are to be accurate the nurse must be aware of what the patient is wearing when weighed, that he is weighed at the same time each day, that the bladder is emptied, that the same scales are used and that the results are correctly charted. Nurses can also assess whether patients prescribed special diets are eating the correct food. Nurses and domestic staff need to be aware of patients' individual needs to prevent such common errors as added sugar to diabetics and those having a weight-reducing diet, too much milk for those on a low-protein diet and full-cream milk instead of skimmed milk to those on a low-fat diet. Diabetics may leave food and need to be offered alternative sources of carbohydrate. The intake of patients taking reducing diets needs to be monitored. It may also be necessary to check the type of food and drink they have on their lockers and of that brought in for them by relatives. Patients taking a high-kilojoule or high-protein diet may need help to take the large volume of food prescribed for them. If they are merely given large meals the patients may be 'over-faced' by the amount of food on their plates. The nurse may therefore need to be prepared to offer supplements and between-meal snacks to these patients. It is the responsibility of the nurse to ensure that cartons of supplements and snacks are distributed to the patients rather than allowed to accumulate in the ward refrigerator.

Patient education

Patient education is an integral part of the rehabilitation of the sick. Beginning on the day of admission, the nurse's responsibility should extend beyond the immediate needs of the patient. The stress of hospitalization, changed routine and a new awesome environment may affect the patient's emotional response and attitude to many aspects of life, in particular food intake. The warmth and comfort which accompanies the serving of a 'special' cup of tea, out of routine, or a 'treat' (e.g. ice-cream) to the insecure, unhappy patient is at times far more important than the coincidental nutritional value.

As patients are prescribed special diets, or nutritional support is initiated, family members should be informed and involved as long-term management is often their responsibility.

But patient education need not be confined to those on special diets. The widespread incidence of constipation among hospital patients is often unnecessarily treated with laxatives. Guidance about increasing fibre and fluid intake would be far more valuable to many patients in the long term than resorting to the regular use of potentially harmful laxatives which is continued after discharge from hospital. Nurses have a unique advantage in hospitals as they are the only personnel who are with the patients throughout the day. The serving of meals can be used as a practical demonstration. Merely by being encouraged to observe the items on the plate, the diabetic can learn about equivalent portions of interchangeable foods; the patient on a weight-reducing diet will understand the role of salads and vegetables as 'fillers' and the patient on a normal trolley diet will confirm the value of attractive presentation.

The serving of small portions with the placing of different foods in a colourful arrangement, using flowers left by discharged patients to brighten the trays, enhances presentation and acceptability.

Thus the extent of care that nurses can give to patients taking ordinary or therapeutic oral hospital diets is a singular responsibility. In isolation, many of the ways in which a nurse can help seems small; however, her care overall ranges from assessing and monitoring patients' status and nutritional needs, assisting them to eat and liaising with other hospital personnel to teaching patients about their diets and, as such, nurses can make an enormous contribution to patients' nutritional care. Although not solely responsible for the extent of malnutrition in hospital discussed at the start of this chapter, nurses have in the past been criticized for not undertaking their responsibilities in this area of care (Jones, 1975; Johnston, 1978). If nurses do become more aware of the extent of the contribution they should be making to patients' nutrition, they have the potential to help improve the nutritional status of their patients.

PRACTICAL HELP FOR HANDICAPPED PEOPLE

It is always preferable for patients to undertake as much of their personal care as is possible. For patients with physical disabilities there are many specially designed utensils which may enable them to increase their independence. Some aids have been developed which will allow patients to feed themselves despite disabilities which would otherwise prevent them from doing so. If nurses are aware of the availability of such tools it may help them to increase an individual's independence whilst in hospital, and also promote their chances of being able to cope at home. Some examples of these implements are shown in Fig. 6.

Persons who find it difficult to angle spoons to their mouths due to stiff joints may benefit from cutlery angled to their requirements (Fig. 6a). Wrist extensor splints (Fig. 6b) or a leather cuff (Fig. 6c) may facilitate the holding of cutlery. Large wooden or sponge handles (Fig. 6d) may help people with an inadequate grasp to hold cutlery. If only one hand can be used, a combined spoon/fork with a cutting edge may be helpful. Clip-on plate guards may help people who find it difficult to pick food off the plates as they provide a surface for the food to be pushed against. Non-slip place mats, suction plates, cups with two handles to grip, etc., will provide greater stability for crockery.

For people unable to use any cutlery, food can be put on a special turntable plate which is at mouth height and food can be eaten directly from the plate. Insulated cups are available and may help people who drink slowly or prevent someone without

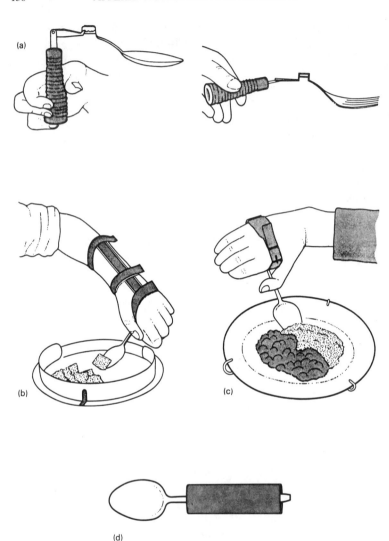

Fig. 6. *Examples of specially designed utensils for handicapped patients.*
(a) Spoon and fork that can be angled to suit the individual.
(b) Wrist extensor splint with pocket for spoon or fork.
(c) Leather and elastic webbing cuff with pocket to hold spoon or fork.
(d) Sponge rubber tubing used to build up the handle of a spoon.

sensation from getting burnt. Heated plates can be used to keep food hot for people who eat slowly.

The aids mentioned above and many others are commercially available. It is also possible for patients to have utensils tailor-made to their unique requirements. Further information about equipment for the disabled can be obtained from the following addresses:

Equipment for the Disabled
2 Foredon Drive
Portslade
Brighton

Home Management Booklet
Equipment for the Disabled
Mary Marlborough Lodge
Nuffield Orthopaedic Centre
Headington
Oxford OX3 7LD

ENTERAL AND PARENTERAL NUTRITION

Although the majority of patients can with suitable help be adequately nourished by consuming an oral diet there are some patients for whom other methods of nutrition are needed. For these patients the alternatives are either enteral or parenteral nutrition.

'Enteral' feeding is the provision of nutrients to the alimentary tract by mouth, nasogastric tube, oesophagostomy, gastrostomy or duodenostomy. Enteral feeds are liquid and may be blended whole foods or commercially produced solutions. The patient can drink the feed if it is sufficiently palatable, or it can be delivered by tube to the stomach or small intestine. The feed may be taken to supplement the oral diet or it may be the only method of nutrition.

'Parenteral' nutrition is the term applied to the method of providing nutrients to the body by a route other than the alimentary tract. Although subcutaneous and rectal infusions of nutrients may be administered, parenteral nutrition today is almost exclusively used to describe the intravenous administration of nutrients. 'Total parenteral nutrition' is the term used when the individual is receiving all his nutrients via a parenteral route.

When nutrition is partially supported by parenteral feeding the term 'supplementary parenteral feeding' is used (Moghissi and Boore, 1983). Fig. 7 illustrates how it is decided whether an individual needs nutritional therapy and, if so, whether enteral or parenteral nutrition is the treatment of choice.

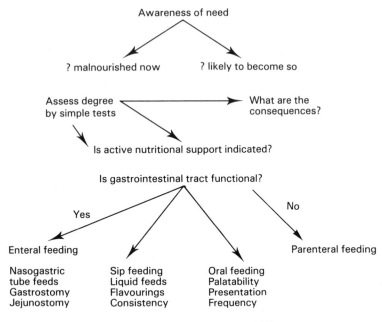

Fig. 7. *Nutritional therapy (Lee, 1979).*

Enteral feeding will always be chosen in preference to parenteral feeding if the patient can tolerate it as it is a simpler, safer and less expensive method of patient feeding. For enteral feeding to be possible the patient must be able to digest, absorb and metabolize the nutrients delivered to the alimentary tract.

Enteral feeding is indicated if patients are found to need a greater intake of nutrients than they could normally consume; this may be due to oesophageal obstruction, short bowel syndrome, granulomatous disease of the gastrointestinal tract, gastrointestinal tract fistulae, malabsorption syndromes, preoperative bowel preparation or preoperative 'building up' of patients. Failure to provide enough nutrients to meet a person's needs may either predispose the person to malnutrition or worsen a pre-existing state of malnutrition. The possible consequences of an inadequate nutritional status have been discussed above.

The choice of enteral feed to be given to the patient will be influenced by the metabolic condition of the patient, his existing nutritional status, his diagnosis and whatever further medical or surgical treatment he will require.

The feeds are usually manufactured (rather than blended whole food) and are a solution of carbohydrate, fat and whole protein. A simpler type of nutrients may be given in an 'elemental diet' in which nutrients made up of essential parts of the foods, such as simple carbohydrates, fatty acids, amino acids and minerals are used (Moghissi and Boore, 1983). Table 9 shows the composition of some of the commonly available enteral feeds.

Although this route of nutrition is comparatively simple (when compared to parenteral feeding), both the patient and the administration of the feed will need careful management. The patient will need to be nutritionally assessed so that baseline data is available from which to monitor subsequent changes. The dietary needs of the patient will need to be calculated before the choice of preparation, and the quantity required can be ascertained. The above two aspects are usually undertaken by the doctor and dietitian. However, the administration of the feed is largely a nursing responsibility. Insertion of nasogastric tubes is a nursing duty and is done in accordance with the policy of the hospital in which it is undertaken. Insertion of tubes such as gastrostomy tubes is a medical procedure. Once the tube is in position nurses usually care for the tube, check and, if necessary, dress the site of insertion, and also maintain all the utensils and equipment used in the administration of the feed. Once the feed is started the patient's tolerance to it must be noted and any side-effects treated. The main complications of enteral nutrition are:

1. unpalatability of feeds to be drunk,
2. ulceration if large or inflexible nasogastric tubes are used,
3. aspiration of feed, especially in elderly or comatose patients,
4. nausea, vomiting, cramps,
5. diarrhoea.

The nurse may also need to help the patient adjust psychologically

Table 9. The composition of some of the commonly available enteral feeds.

Feed	Packaging	Content						Energy Value	
		Protein (g)	Fat (g)	Carbohydrate (g)	Na (mmol)	K (mmol)		kcal	kJ
Clinifeed 1875 ml Iso	5×375 ml	53	77	245	29	72		1875	7875
Clinifeed 1875 ml Protein Rich*	5×375 ml	150	55	350	64	108		2500	10500
Ensure 1880 ml	8×235 ml *or* bottle	70	70	270	61	61		1920	8064
Ensure Plus 1880 ml	8×235 ml can	103	100	375	90	92		2720	11424
Express Enteral Feed 2000 ml Standard	4×500 ml carton *or* 2 litre pouch	63	96	253	55	65		2064	8669
Express Enteral Feed 2000 ml High Energy	4×500 ml carton *or* 2 litre pouch	117	128	404	85	87		3134	13163
Fortison 2000 ml Standard	4×500 ml bottle	80	80	240	70	76		2000	8400
Fortison 2000 Energy Plus	4×500 ml bottle	100	130	358	70	76		3000	12600
Isocal 1896 ml	8×237 ml can	65	83	252	44	64		2008	8438
Nutrauxil 2000 ml	4×500 ml sachet	76	68	276	66	64		2000	8400
Triosorbon 200 ml water+ 5 sachets Triosorbon	5×85 g sachet	81	81	238	85	85		2000	8400

All figures rounded off to nearest whole number.

to an artifical mode of nutrition. As meal-times and food are often sources of pleasure the patient may feel he is deprived of this enjoyment whilst being enterally fed. Enteral nutrition is more fully discussed by Johnston (1979).

Patients who are unable to tolerate enteral feeds must be considered for parenteral feeding. The primary indication for parenteral nutrition is gastrointestinal failure. Table 10 indicates the main conditions which may necessitate the use of total parenteral nutrition.

Table 10. Indications for complete parenteral nutrition.

1.	Preoperatively, e.g. malnutrition secondary to carcinoma of the upper gastrointestinal tract, pyloric stenosis, ulcerative colitis.
2.	Gastrointestinal disorders — granulomatous conditions, e.g. Crohn's disease, malabsorption syndromes, short bowel syndrome, ulcerative colitis.
3.	Postoperatively — after major gastrointestinal surgery complications, such as fistulae, obstruction, peritonitis.
4.	Hypercatabolic states — e.g. burns. Intensive care unit cases — e.g. road traffic accidents with complicated trauma, chest, skull injuries. Complicated acute renal failure.
5.	Cachexia, e.g. malnutrition from whatever cause; severe anorexia nervosa; some cases of malignant disease; chronic renal failure, reversible liver failure.

(Lee, 1979)

The choice of feeds to be given to the patient and the rate of infusion are governed by the nutritional status of the patient and the reasons for which the patient is being fed. To illustrate the possible variations in patients' requirements Table 11 shows the estimated daily protein and calorie losses in patients not receiving any nutrition.

Once again it will be necessary to assess the nutritional status of the patient prior to starting nutritional therapy and then to monitor the patient both physically and biochemically throughout the feeding regimen. Administration of the feed and care of the infusion site and equipment are critically important. As this method of feeding is potentially dangerous a thorough knowledge of the side-effects and possible complications is necessary for anyone involved in this aspect of patient nutrition. The main complications of which to be aware are those of catheter displacement, air embolism, infection and metabolic disorders.

Once it is decided that a patient is to be parenterally fed it will take the combined skills of medical, dietetic, nursing and pharmaceutical staff to ensure that the feed is effectively administered.

Table 11. Estimated daily protein and kilojoule losses in patients not receiving any nutrition.

	Protein (g)	kJ
Medical patient (without temperature or injuries)	45–75	6 300– 8 400
Postoperative (uncomplicated)	75–125	8 400–14 700
Hypercatabolic state (e.g. major burn, multiple injuries)	100–300	14 700–21 000

(Lee, 1974)

Intravenous feeds are usually given through a central rather than a peripheral vein, and it is the doctor who must insert a central venous catheter. Once the catheter is known to be in the correct position (confirmed by an X-ray) it is the nurse who must maintain it. The catheter must be kept free of any kinks, the site of insertion must be checked regularly (hospital policy varies) and, when necessary, re-dressed according to the dictates of the hospital; all connections in the system must be kept airtight and clean. The nurse must ensure that the correct feed is being infused at the correct rate and that this information is documented. Care of the infusion equipment such as giving sets, feed containers and drip counting machines (if used) is also important. The nursing staff must also constantly observe the patient for the development of any complications associated with this method of feeding. Six-hourly urinalysis is usually undertaken to check that the patient has not developed glycosuria (an indication that too much glucose is being infused). Blood sugar may also be directly measured. Daily weight is recorded to monitor signs of fluid retention. Further assessment tests such as levels of blood urea, electrolytes and proteins, and urinary urea, electrolytes and nitrogen will be regularly undertaken (by medical staff) to monitor the effect of the feeding. The range of tests and the frequency with which they are undertaken will vary according to hospital practice.

However, monitoring the effect of the feed on the patient is usually a combined medical, dietetic and nursing responsibility.

The role of the nurse in the care of patients receiving parenteral or enteral nutrition has been more fully discussed elsewhere (Jones, 1975; Moghissi and Boore, 1983; Allen, 1984).

THE NEED TO ASSESS THE PATIENT'S NUTRITIONAL STATUS

The need to assess the nutritional status of patients has been referred to several times in the course of this chapter. The nutritional support required by individual patients will vary. The previously well nourished patient who has no problems of ingestion and absorption can withstand a reduced intake of short duration. However, as has already been discussed, if a patient is unable to absorb enough food to sustain himself and is unlikely to do so for some time, attention must be given to ensuring that his nutritional needs are met. Determining patients in need of support and the efficiency of that support can only be achieved by nutritional assessment. This allows the status of the patient to be established and monitored, an estimate of the patient's nutrient requirements to be made, and any subsequent nutritional plan to be evaluated.

Methods of nutritional assessment

As both fat and protein reserves need to be assessed it is necessary to use a variety of methods of assessment. The methods currently available will be briefly reviewed below. Assessment of nutritional status by clinical visual appraisal and by information gained from the patient has already been discussed on page 130.

Nutritional assessment by physical measurement

BODY WEIGHT. This allows a composite measure of body mass to be made. Although this method is an imperfect guide to fat tissue reserves if the patient is oedematous or particularly muscular, it is thought to give a good reflection of the changes in body mass in an individual over a given time. Weight alone allows a baseline to be established on admission which may then be used to indicate change in overall nutritional status, but not where the change has occurred. The patient's normal weight in health must be taken into consideration. In conjunction with height, weight allows the determination of ideal weight for the individual and the prediction of the energy requirements of the body (Platt *et al*, 1963).

ASSESSMENT OF BODY FAT USING SKINFOLD THICKNESS MEASUREMENT. Skinfold thickness measurements are used to assess the fat reserves located in the subcutaneous tissue. It can be assumed that the subcutaneous fat reflects the energy reserve of the body. If this method of assessment is to be employed the assessor must use acceptable calipers, for example Harpenden calipers, and they must be able to locate the sites to be measured accurately. Possible sites include triceps, biceps, subscapular, supra-iliac, thigh or medial calf.

ASSESSMENT OF BODY PROTEIN USING MID-ARM CIRCUMFERENCE AND MID-ARM MUSCLE CIRCUMFERENCE. Protein tissue, which is often described as the lean body mass, may be assessed by measurement of body muscle size. Muscle mass is most easily assessed in clinical practice using mid-arm muscle circumference. The above can be calculated by measuring upper-arm circumference and subtracting an allowance for the surrounding skin and fat. The site of measurement is the circumference of the arm at the level of the triceps skinfold thickness (Grant *et al*, 1981).

Nutritional assessment by biochemical analysis

BLOOD. Serum transport proteins synthesized by the liver can be measured. Synthesis is reduced as the body stores of protein are depleted; therefore a low serum protein indicates a reduction in body protein reserves. The most commonly used transport proteins are albumin and transferrin. There are, however, many variables which will affect the protein concentration.

URINE. Urinary analysis to measure the levels of waste products following metabolism of protein tissue can also be used to indicate nutritional status; for example, creatinine height index and 3-methylhistidine excretion.

Nutritional assessment by tests of immune function

TOTAL LYMPHOCYTE COUNT. Protein-energy malnutrition is known to compromise the response to infection. A reduction in the peripheral lymphocyte count is associated with depleted cellular immunity (Goode, 1981). A total lymphocyte count of 800–1200 mm^3 is indicative of moderate protein-energy malnutrition whilst less than 800 mm^3 indicates severe deprivation.

CELL-MEDIATED IMMUNITY. This is an important host defence against infection. For the purposes of nutritional assessment the skin test recall antigen may be used. An intradermal injection of, for example, *Candida* sp. streptokinase should produce a skin weal 5 mm wide in 1–2 days. If no such response occurs the patient is said to be anergic. The situation is reversed when the patient is adequately nourished (Blackburn, 1980).

For a detailed review of methods of nutritional assessment see Grant *et al* (1981).

BIBLIOGRAPHY

Allen, D. (1984) Patient care in hyperalimentation. *Nurs. Times, 80,* (18), p. 28.

Bistrian, B.R., Blackburn, G.L., Hollowey, E. & Heddle, R. (1974) Protein status of general surgical patients. *J. Am. Med. Ass., 230 (6),* 858.

Bistrian, B.R., Blackburn, G.L., Vitale, J., Cochran, D. & Naylor, J. (1976) Prevalence of malnutrition in general medical patients. *J. Am. Med. Ass., 235,* 1567.

Blackburn, G.L. (1980) The bottom line in sepsis . . . interconnections between sepsis, immune competence and malnutrition. *Emergency Medicine, 12,* 72.

Elwyn, D.H., Kinney, J.M. & Askanazi, J. (1981) Energy expenditure in surgical patients. *Surg. Clin. N. Am., 61(3),* 545.

Evans, E. (1977) Special diets in hospital. *Nurs. Times, 26,* 795.

Goode, A.W. (1981) The scientific basis of nutritional assessment. *Br. J. Anaesthesia, 53 (12),* 161.

Goode, A.W. & Hawkins, T. (1978) In: Johnston, I.D.A. (ed.) *Advances in Parenteral Nutrition,* p. 557. Lancaster: MTP Press.

Grant, J.P., Custer, P.B. & Thurlow, J.T. (1981) Current techniques of nutritional assessment. *Surg. Clin. N. Am. 61 (3),* 437.

Hill, G.L., Blackett, R.L., Pickerford, I., Burkinshaw, L., Young, G.A., Warren, J.V., Schorah, C.T. & Morgan, D.B (1977) Malnutrition in surgical patients — an unrecognised problem. *Lancet, 1,* 689.

Johnson, I.D.A. (1980) The relevance of nutritional care to the hospital patient. *Acta Chirurgica Scand., Suppl. 507,* 289.

Johnston, I.D.A. (1978) Panel discussion. In: Johnston, I.D.A. & Lee, H.A. (eds.) *Developments in Clinical Nutrition,* p. 112. Tunbridge Wells: Medical Congresses and Symposia Consultants.

Jones, D.C. (1975) *Food for Thought*. London: Royal College of Nursing.

Lee, H.A. (1974) *Parenteral Nutrition in Acute Metabolic Illness*, pp. 312–313. London/New York: Academic Press.

Lee, H.A. (1979) Why enteral nutrition? In: Johnston, I.D.A. & Lee, H.A. (eds.) *Developments in Clinical Nutrition*, p. 16. Tunbridge Wells: Medical Congresses and Symposia Consultants.

Moghissi, K. & Boore, J. (1983) *Parenteral and Enteral Nutrition for Nurses*. London: William Heinemann Medical Books.

Mullen, J.L., Buzby, G.P., Matthews, D.C., Smale, B.F. & Rosato, E.F. (1980) Reduction of operative morbidity and mortality by combined pre-operative and post-operative nutritional support. *Ann. Surg., 192 (5)*, 604.

Newton, G.M. & Andrewes, C. (1984) *Medical Nursing*, 10th edn. London: Baillière Tindall.

Platt, B.S., Eddy, T.P. & Pellett, P. (1963) *Food in Hospitals*. Oxford: Nuffield Provincial Hospital Trust.

Shils, M.E. (1976) Nutritional problems induced by cancer. *J. Med. Clin. N. Am., 63 (5)*, 1009.

Silk, D.B.A. (1980) Clinical nutrition in hospitals: Principles. *Hosp. Update, 6 (8)*, 761.

Weisnier, R.L., Hunker, R.N., Krumdieck, M.D. & Butterworth, C.E. (1979) Hospital malnutrition — a prospective evaluation of general medical patients during the course of hospitalisation. *Am. J. Clin. Nutr., 32*, 418.

Wilmore, D.W. (1977) *The Metabolic Management of the Critically Ill*. New York/London: Plenum Medical.

Woolfson, A.M.J. (1978) Metabolic considerations in nutritional support. In: Johnston, I.D.A. & Lee, J. (eds.) *Developments in Clinical Nutrition*, p. 35. Tunbridge Wells: Medical Congresses and Symposia Consultants.

5 Overweight

'We are unanimous in our belief that obesity is a hazard to health and a detriment to well-being. It is common enough to constitute one of the most important medical and public health problems of our time, whether we judge importance by a shorter expectation of life, increased morbidity or cost to the community in terms of both money and anxiety' (James). This was the opening statement of a recent expert group on obesity in the UK who discussed this widespread community problem at length and deliberated on its effects.

Obesity represents an imbalance between energy intake and output, resulting in a surplus of energy which is converted to fat and stored as adipose tissue. Individuals whose weight is 10–20% above the desirable weight for their age, sex and frame are defined as overweight. When the weight exceeds 20% more than the desirable weight a person is regarded as obese.

In the presence of overweight there is an increased tendency to develop a variety of diseases. Diabetes mellitus, cardiovascular disorders, gallstones, osteo-arthritis of the weight-bearing joints, varicose veins, flat feet and several other complications (Fig. 8) occur predominantly in the obese. These individuals also constitute an increased surgical risk and may have to pay increased life insurance premiums. In general, the medical risks of obesity, including excess mortality, increase proportionately to weight gain. Yet in spite of widespread and well substantiated warnings about the hazards of overweight and the trend in Western society to regard the human body as more attractive if slender, obesity remains the biggest challenge to medical practice today. The abundance of a wide range of food, the effect of highly specialized advertising and the change in eating habits over the past decade all contribute to the enormity of this public health problem.

Progress in technology has resulted in increased emphasis being placed on the consumption of processed foods, in particular highly refined and predominantly carbohydrate products. These represent a high energy yield per portion. Coupled with this, advances in home appliance and transport development have caused a

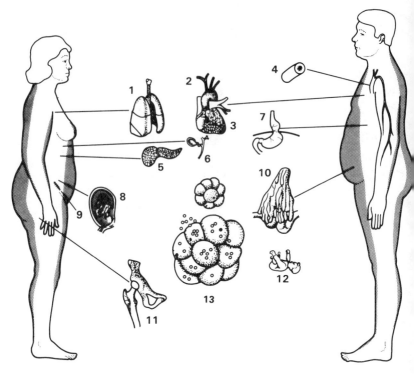

1 **Lungs** — restricted breathing
2 **Raised blood pressure and its complications** — due to increased load
3 **Heart** — greater strain with greater body mass
4 **Atherosclerosis** — causes rupture in the blood vessels
5 **Pancreas** — diabetes
6 **Gallbladder** — gallstones
7 **Hiatus hernia** — stomach displaced into chest cavity
8 **Pregnancy** — prolonged labour
9 **Surgery** — technically difficult
10 **The omentum** — fat accumulates in abdominal cavity
11 **Joints** — increased wear and tear
12 **Baby fat** — obese babies become obese adults
13 **Adipose tissue** — found throughout the body

Fig. 8. *Health risks of obesity.*

reduction of energy output. This high energy intake and low output has, not surprisingly, been to the physical — and often psychological — detriment of a large portion of our society. For example, the consumption of just a snack of 1000 kJ (230 cal) per day in excess of requirement will result in the slow deposition of excess adipose tissue. As mentioned earlier, 37 kJ is equivalent to 1 g of fat, and one can simply divide the excess kilojoule intake by 37 to determine the approximate theoretical weight gain that can be anticipated with this amount of excess kilojoules. In one year the weight gain will be

$$\frac{1000 \times 365}{37} = 9.9 \text{ kg}$$

The nurse can point out to the patient that the theoretical anticipated weight gain will be nearly 10 kg (24 lb) per year, should such excess be routinely consumed. Portions of common snack foods yielding 1000 kJ include:

    a slice of custard tart
    a small (75 g) helping of suet pudding
    a small (50 g) sausage roll
    a few cheese straws (40 g)
    1.3 pints (780 ml) of beer

CONTROL OF ENERGY INTAKE

Garrow has commented: 'feeding behaviour in Man is a very complex subject and the situation is becoming steadily less clear'.

Unlike lower animals we do not have the adaptive capacity to balance our energy intake and utilization over a short period. In a fascinating study undertaken by Wooley *et al*, it was shown that subjects were incapable of determining the energy content of food consumed. They were not able to judge whether they had been overfed or underfed compared to a standard intake and were thus unable to make appropriate compensations in the short term.

With increased sophistication of eating, our responses have become confused and today we are unable to correlate taste with nutritive value of foods. Other studies have reinforced the opinion that voluntary food intake is only minimally related to energy content as judged by the appearance of the specific food.

In the long term there appears to be a tendency to regulate energy intake but it is doubtful whether this is a voluntary measure due to increase in girth or whether it occurs spontaneously as a result of physiological compensation.

ESTIMATION OF OVERWEIGHT

In spite of the high incidence of this condition and its detrimental effects, there is still a surprising amount of controversy about the estimation of overweight in individuals. Although tables giving the desirable weights for people of specific heights are widely published (see Table 12), the concept of frame size must be accurately applied to obtain precise conclusions. The subjective determination of frame size by merely judging the circumference of one's wrist is not an accurate assessment. Added to this, the range of weight given for each frame size is often too wide to give the unequivocal value that individuals wish to use as reference. Skinfold thickness is another measure of overweight. Several sites are used and, using calipers and a set of tables which relates skinfold to body fat, conclusions can be drawn about the individual's ideal mass. However, variability in clinical observation, differences in calipers used and complicating factors in patients, such as ethnic differences in fat distribution and the inability to measure very obese subjects, detract from the total reliability of this method. Various other anthropometric measurements may be made with greater or lesser accuracy but, for many of us, merely looking at our image in the mirror or reflecting back on our food intake over the past few months and the fact that clothes are pulling is sufficient incentive to encourage a moderate weight loss to previous comfortable levels!

AETIOLOGY OF OVERWEIGHT

Certain hypotheses have been advanced to explain the reason why some people become overweight and others maintain their weight within narrow limits without much apparent effort. Extensive research has resulted in many conflicting explanations. However, there are certain factors which appear to play an important role and the nurse should take cognizance of these when interviewing patients.

Table 12. Metropolitan Life Insurance Co. height and weight tables.

Height	Small frame	Medium frame	Large frame
	⟵————————————lb————————————⟶		
Men*			
5′ 2″	128–134	131–141	138–150
5′ 3″	130–136	133–143	140–153
5′ 4″	132–138	135–145	142–156
5′ 5″	134–140	137–148	144–160
5′ 6″	136–142	139–151	146–164
5′ 7″	138–145	142–154	149–168
5′ 8″	140–148	145–157	152–172
5′ 9″	142–151	148–160	155–176
5′ 10″	144–154	151–163	158–180
5′ 11″	146–157	154–166	161–184
6′ 0″	149–160	157–170	164–188
6′ 1″	152–164	160–174	168–192
6′ 2″	155–168	164–178	172–197
6′ 3″	158–172	167–182	176–202
6′ 4″	162–176	171–187	181–207
Women†			
4′ 10″	102–111	109–121	118–131
4′ 11″	103–113	111–123	120–134
5′ 0″	104–115	113–126	122–137
5′ 1″	106–118	115–129	125–140
5′ 2″	108–121	118–132	128–143
5′ 3″	111–124	121–135	131–147
5′ 4″	114–127	124–138	134–151
5′ 5″	117–130	127–141	137–155
5′ 6″	120–133	130–144	140–159
5′ 7″	123–136	133–147	143–163
5′ 8″	126–139	136–150	146–167
5′ 9″	129–142	139–153	149–170
5′ 10″	132–145	142–156	152–173
5′ 11″	135–148	145–159	155–176
6′ 0″	138–151	148–162	158–179

*Weights at ages 25 to 59 based on lowest mortality. Weight in pounds according to frame (in indoor clothing weighing 5 lb, shoes with 1″ heels).
†Weights at age 25 to 59 based on mortality. Weight in pounds according to frame (in indoor clothing weighing 3 lb, shoes with 1″ heels).
1 ft ≈ 0.3 m. 1lb ≈ 0.45 kg.
Courtesy of Metropolitan Life Insurance Company.

Body type

Body type is unquestionably of importance. Although in a family of obese individuals the overweight is largely due to familial cooking and eating patterns, or restricted activity, genetic body shape may also play an important role. Allen's rule states that large slow-moving people are usually found in colder climates and thin active people with long arms and legs are encountered in the tropics. The Bushmen are well known for their ability to store fat in their buttocks as a method of adaptation to conditions. Thus certain people utilize their food intake extremely efficiently and others may refer relatively small excesses of energy intake to fat deposits on their hips. While such people would do admirably in a situation of stress and starvation, circumstances in affluent Western society demand enormous self-control.

A recent comparative study on energy intake is of relevance here. Two groups of subjects were selected, one group being relatively lean and the other group overweight. The latter group required a diet containing far less energy than the thin group in order to lose weight. Conversely, on a higher energy intake, those who had been initially overweight returned much more rapidly to this level than those who started in the lean group. The thinner subjects needed a much higher energy intake to become overweight. Whilst Hirsch's theory of fat-cell production in childhood (discussed below) may well play a role in this phenomenon, there is little doubt that genetic determinants are also of major importance.

Overweight in infancy

In obesity there is abnormal enlargment of the adipose tissue mass. This may occur as a result of the formation of additional fat-cells (hyperplastic obesity) or by an increase in the amount of fat stored in existing fat-cells (hypertrophic obesity). Studies undertaken by Hirsch have suggested that in early life multiplication of cells may be the predominant factor responsible whereas later an excess of energy results in the expansion of individual fat-cells. Although it is not clear exactly when the change in adiposity occurs, it would seem that during childhood and particularly during the early months of life, fat-cell production probably reaches a peak. The final fat-cell number seems to be reached at approximately 20 years of age, after which the individual will respond to an energy excess or deficiency by expansion or shrinkage of the fat-cells present. According to

Hirsch's theory (as this has become known), it is imperative to prevent infants and children from becoming overweight and thus increasing their vulnerability to obesity and its sequelae in later life. The control of overweight in children is discussed in Chapter 2.

Environmental aspects

The housewife involved in planning and cooking her family's meals is more prone to undisciplined and excessive eating than her husband, who is preoccupied and away from temptation for most of the day. Conversely, many businessman are involved in extensive social eating and drinking in the course of their duties. The lavish functions used to execute business arrangements are a distinct hazard to the longevity of the participants. Children, too, are affected by environmental stimuli. In this age of permissiveness, there is often an attempt to compensate for the lack of a satisfactory home environment by an abundance of pocket money, and sweets, snacks and cold drinks may play too prominent a role. The child who is given food to compensate for absent parental love, or time, is encountered frequently in our materialistic society.

Energy output

In our age of technical advance, machines frequently do the work previously done by people. Even the typist who changes from a mechanical to an electrical typewriter will theoretically show a weight gain of 4 kg/year if she does not limit her diet accordingly! Without regular exercise, an increase in body weight is almost inevitable with the continued consumption of a diet providing optimum amounts of nutrients. Energy requirements at 65 years of age are 29% lower than at the age of 25 and thus there is an ever-increasing surplus to be used for exercise, or to be converted to adipose tissue if the food intake remains the same.

Drug-induced weight gain

This may occur but perhaps not as commonly as many of our patients would like to think. Contraceptive pills can result in a small increase in weight due to fluid retention, but this is unlikely to account for more than 2–3 kg. The overweight person can thus be assured that a reduction in energy intake will still readily reduce her weight although she may possibly level out at a slightly heavier weight to compensate for the oedema.

Long-term cortisone treatment presents a dual problem. People on large doses not only retain fluid but frequently have the further problem of developing a voracious appetite. This is fortunately a reversible condition, but weight gain can readily occur during the period of cortisone administration and careful attention to diet is imperative. It should be emphasized that these side-effects occur particularly with large doses of the drug, and the patient who claims resistance to techniques of weight reduction due to administration of cortisone in the distant past is hoodwinking herself.

Pleasure, greed, enjoyment or self-indulgence

Pleasure cannot be neglected when looking for the causative factor in obesity. It is a common response to indulge unnecessarily when a delectable food is served. The pattern of food intake is also important: Fabry *et al* reported a study in which men eating one or two large meals per day were heavier with thicker skinfolds than controls eating three or more smaller meals per day. Thus the importance of self-discipline as an essential component of weight control must not be ignored. To many people this becomes a life-long challenge, and for those who tend to become readily overweight self-denial is an essential aspect of weight maintenance.

Genetic and hormonal abnormalities

Genetic and hormonal abnormalities have been correlated with overweight in experimental animals. In Man, glucose tolerance and insulin, cortisol and growth hormone response differ between lean and overweight people. However it is not yet known whether these are causal or resultant factors in obesity. Regrettably, many overweight individuals rely on unsubstantiated stories of hormonal causes and adopt a fatalistic attitude towards their problem as a result. It should be pointed out to them if any known endocrine disease were responsible for their overweight other symptoms of the disorder would also occur and the patient would be in no doubt about the presence of an organic illness.

Brown fat and thermogenesis

The possible role of brown adipose tissue in obesity is currently being studied in depth. Brown fat, so called because of its extensive blood supply and oxidative pigments which lend colour to the tissue, contains many large mitochondria. It is found predominantly in animals and plays a major role in the regulation of body temperature. This occurs because of the stimulation of the sympathetic nervous system which causes thermogenesis, i.e. energy production in the form of heat in a cold environment. Thermogenesis is also effective in maintaining weight in animals. This is known as dietary-induced thermogenesis, i.e. the loss of excess kilojoules consumed as heat. It is not known how much brown tissue is present in human beings, but some researchers find a reduced capacity for dietary-induced thermogenesis to play an important role in obese people.

THERAPY

The most effective method of weight reduction is dietary modification, i.e. by restricting energy intake and relying on fat deposits in the body for energy utilization. A wide range of diets, formulas and invasive procedures are available to assist the overweight individual to reduce weight. Well advertised, brightly packaged products, regimens and pills promoted with supportive literature are sold to desperate fat people in nearly every supermarket or chemist, and the fads and gimmicks suggested in women's magazines appeal to gullible readers. Yet all overweight individuals as well as those who work with them will agree that obesity rapidly recurs in the majority of people who have lost weight on virtually any type of treatment programme. It is regrettable that whilst for most diseases the patient receives an individualized prescription of treatment, the obese patient often has to fend for himself. The nurse should be aware that with each unsuccessful attempt at weight loss the overweight person's chance of successful weight reduction is theoretically reduced. Whoever is directing the weight reduction programme, the dietitian, nurse or doctor, should take the responsibility very seriously, motivating the individual and reinforcing the treatment at regular intervals in an attempt to achieve long-term success.

Weight reduction should be approached from three different angles:

1. Energy intake should be reduced by modifying the eating habits of the patient.
2. The patient should be motivated to adhere to the regimen through behaviour control.
3. There should be an increase of energy output, where possible, in the form of increased exercise.

Dietary history

As is essential with all forms of diet therapy, a detailed history should be taken before embarking on a suggested programme of treatment. Although superficially this may appear to be an extremely simple exercise, the accuracy of the information obtained depends to a large extent on the interviewer's handling of the situation. The following procedure may be helpful when interviewing an overweight patient.

Establish rapport with the patient as an indication that the relationship can be a sympathetic understanding one, and that he or she need not fear a dictatorial or derogatory lecture.

Enquire in detail as to what was consumed from the time of awakening until bedtime the previous day and whether this was representative of an average day's intake. As each meal or snack is discussed, assess quantities in terms of household measures and number of portions and note the time of day when it was consumed. Environmental stimuli are particularly relevant in pinpointing problem areas. For example, a patient who eats while cooking dinner, after frequent arguments with the spouse, or from boredom, will need help in directing his/her reactions along other channels. This is known as behaviour modification and is discussed in detail below.

As the 'night eating syndrome' is a well documented contributive factor in obesity, it should be established what food was consumed after the meal at night. Eating in bed, whilst studying, or in front of the television set, are all common problems of this kind.

Patients may not consciously consider the need to tell one about liquids consumed. Surprisingly, some people presume that energy ingested in the liquid state is less detrimental than solid food. Specific questions need to be asked about the intake of coffee and tea (with milk and sugar?), carbonated drinks, alcoholic beverages and water sweetened with fruit cordial. While the patient is recalling the previous day's intake it is essential that the interviewer should not show disapproval. If a patient is reprimanded about a particular food consumed he or she is understandably unlikely to disclose any other aberration and the interview may become biased.

Having ascertained the details of the previous day's intake, the nurse can use this as a basis for a modified diet in the future, bearing in mind the financial limitations indicated by the food eaten. Before discussing the recommended weight reduction plan it may be useful to look at a few of the major controversial regimens that have been proposed. Many overweight patients have unsuccessfully attempted a variety of programmes and the nurse will be questioned repeatedly about other methods of losing weight which appear to be simpler than dieting.

Popular weight-loss methods

The innumerable weight-reducing regimes which promise instant weight loss make up a huge financial empire surrounded by millions of gullible, dissatisfied people in their quest for thinness. These formula diets, appetite suppressants and gimmick regimens have become an enormous challenge to those of us involved in nutrition education. Misinformation and food faddism are often promoted by these programmes and it is often difficult to separate fact from fiction when reading the information provided by the astute marketing experts of many of the products. A few of the more popular regimens are discussed below.

Crash diets

The Mayo Clinic diet, the cheese and tomato diet, the liquid diet, the Scarsdale diet, the carbohydrate 'gram' diet — all have had their periods of popularity. There are several reasons why most of these are successful only for a short period. In the first place they do not get at the root cause of obesity, as they merely severely limit the foods allowed and stipulate meal components. Furthermore, they do not improve the eating habits which cause the condition.

Having adhered to the diet for a limited period of time, the choice confronting the dieter is two-fold; either to return to previous eating habits (thus returning to the previously excessive weight) or to go on a modified low-energy diet, which could have been used from the start. Diets in which the foods are limited to a few selected items (such as cheese and tomatoes) are usually deficient in several vitamins and minerals.

Recently there has been an upsurge of interest in the extremely low-carbohydrate diet or 'ketogenic' weight reduction regimen. This diet includes unrestricted amounts of fat and kilojoules and the proponents claim that such emphasis on fat consumption will result in more rapid weight loss than isocaloric diets of different composition. There is no scientific substantiation for these claims. In fact, such diets are potentially hazardous in that they promote the development of atherosclerosis and can increase the serum uric acid levels. They are not to be recommended.

Another controversial diet used for weight reduction includes grapefruit at each meal. Some claim that this fruit has a 'chemical' or 'catalytic' effect, and many people consume large quantities in order to increase energy expenditure. Although grapefruit contributes relatively few kilojoules to the diet and is an excellent source of vitamin C, it plays no active role in weight reduction.

The Beverly Hills diet is founded on the unscientific basis that correct food combinations are the key to successful weight reduction. It is suggested that combining carbohydrate and protein, for example, will promote deposition of fat, whereas if taken separately will not have the same effect. Calcium and protein intake are limited in this diet which includes predominantly fruit.

Drugs

APPETITE SUPPRESSANTS. There are two major modes of action of appetite-suppressing drugs. Some inhibit the feeling of hunger, whereas others influence the feeling of satiety, thus causing the individual to eat less at a meal. This approach is, of course, only effective in people where a fundamental predisposing factor to their overweight is an exaggerated sensation of hunger. These drugs often produce side-effects of irritability, drowsiness, depersonalization and depression. Addictive anorexic agents are dangerous, while others, although not habit-forming, may become a crutch without which the patient feels insecure. Furthermore, there is a wide range of variation in sensitivity to these drugs, probably related to differences in aetiology of the condition. In the long term, the individual must depend on his or her own self-discipline and the selection of foods for weight reduction, rather than omission of normal meals due to anorexia.

THYROID HORMONE. For many years the use of this drug for overweight has been controversial. In patients whose thyroid function has been shown to be inadequate, the administration of this drug is unquestionably useful. However, the routine treatment with this drug of overweight patients with normal thyroid function is seldom justified. Although a study has shown that in the short term there will probably be improved weight loss, serious side-effects may accompany this form of treatment. Both tachycardia and negative nitrogen balance may occur, the latter condition resulting from increased protein breakdown. This can be rectified if the protein content of the diet is increased but this measure is wasteful and, as the additional need is difficult to determine quantitatively, the energy content of the diet may be increased unnecessarily.

DIURETICS. These cause weight loss due to loss of fluid and not the reduction of adipose tissue which is the essential purpose of the weight-reduction regimen. They are contra-indicated in most cases. With the prescription of these drugs the doctor often consciously or unconsciously implies that they are an essential part of the weight reduction programme. Having taken a few of the pills the individual develops a false sense of success as she passes excessive amounts of urine and notices a loss in weight. Although this is usually a temporary phenomenon and the weight is rapidly regained, individuals may attribute a great measure of success to the diuretic.

There are two instances in which these drugs may be justified. Studies have shown that middle-aged overweight women tend to retain fluid, and should there be little weight loss in spite of adherence to a weight reduction regimen a trial of diuretic therapy may be effective. Patients should be told that an initial drop in weight is to be expected. If fluid retention is normal the weight will return to its previous level within a few days. However, in the event of the body retaining excessive amounts of fluid, administration of a diuretic will prompt a diuresis with more permanent effects. Premenstrual weight gain, attributable to hormonally induced fluid retention, can also be reduced by using a diuretic but the individual should realize that this weight loss bears no relation to loss of body fat.

Currently in vogue is a weight reduction programme in which patients are given a low-energy diet, a high fluid intake (up to 20 glasses of water per day) and daily diuretics. There appears to be no scientific basis for this regimen other than the high satiety value of this large volume of water.

METHYL CELLULOSE. Methyl cellulose preparations, particularly biscuits containing this product, have recently been sold extensively as a means of weight reduction. When ingested, this substance absorbs a considerable amount of water and it is claimed that individuals feel satisfied with a small quantity of food. To improve the taste of the substance, methyl cellulose may be combined with several other ingredients and if taken in the dosage prescribed these preparations may provide a considerable number of kilojoules. Other disadvantages are that the biscuits in particular are expensive and play no role in improving the basic unsatisfactory eating pattern which has caused the overweight.

Massage

Massage is a useful adjunct to the weight reduction diet for those who are unable to exercise. Massage stimulates the circulation to the extremities and increases muscle tone. However, it is of little use in increasing the energy output and patients should be discouraged from overemphasizing the importance of this form of therapy.

Sweating

Currently fashionable are a variety of 'treatments' consisting primarily of weight loss through excessive perspiration. Where physical activity (discussed below) is responsible these methods are valuable for healthy people. However, the use of non-porous underwear or tight bandaging of specific areas is an expensive and unnecessary pastime. Frequently these measures are accompanied by the instruction to follow a strict weight reduction diet, which is the all-important part.

Mechanical restriction of nutrient uptake

WIRING THE JAWS TOGETHER. This controversial procedure is still sometimes practised. The result is that the patient is unable to consume food other than that which can be made liquid enough to be sucked in through a straw. This technique is widely criticized because of the risk of aspirating vomit and also because it does nothing to improve the eating habits.

SURGICAL INTERVENTION. These relatively new operations are being widely undertaken today as a last-ditch stand against obesity. Patients should be only investigated prior to surgery and the operation undertaken when attempts to reduce on more conventional and less hazardous regimens have failed. Of particular relevance is a patient's attitude to the operation. It has been shown that it is seldom successful in salvaging a broken marriage: emotional stability is a prerequisite for success.

One procedure, the ileo-jejunal bypass, consists of creating an anastamosis between the jejunum and the ileum, causing the food to bypass approximately half a metre of gut. This reduces the absorption of the food eaten, and in successful cases satisfactory weight loss can be anticipated in spite of the ingestion of fairly large amounts of food. The adaptation period is one or two years, during which time long-term, foul-smelling, severe diarrhoea frequently occurs, often accompanied by abdominal pain. A variety of complications can occur, including electrolyte imbalance, deficiency of certain vitamins and liver damage. Approximately 30–40% of patients develop polyarthritis. During the period of adaptation extensive weight loss can be anticipated and this may be accompanied by a psychological reaction resulting from a changed body image.

Apart from the obvious advantage of weight loss and relative freedom from dieting, other advantages include a drop in serum cholesterol levels, improved cardiovascular and respiratory status and, often, improved mental outlook. However, severe metabolic disturbance and even death may result. A further disadvantage is that some patients fail to lose more than a small proportion of their excess weight. The operation may be reversed if the objectionable side-effects, in particular the diarrhoea, fail to subside. Interestingly, the arthritis also disappears if the bypass is reversed.

Another procedure used today restricts the reservoir capacity of the stomach. The use of staples to limit the size of the stomach to as little as 50 ml has been undertaken by some surgeons; however, as the staples sometimes become detached and the pouch can readily by expanded if excessive food is eaten, the results of this procedure are often disappointing. A third technique involving both the reduction of stomach size with stapling and a bypass anastomosis to the stomach is also being implemented with some success today.

Exercise

Jogging, organized gym classes and taped aerobic exercises have become a way of increasing energy expenditure for a large section of our society. Apart from dietary modification it is the most effective way of losing weight in the moderately overweight person. Strenuous exercise is both unpractical and hazardous for the obese but they, too, can usually benefit by at least undertaking more walking — unless cardiac involvement precludes it. Furthermore, regular moderate exercise is of value in weight maintenance for older people as the metabolic rate drops with ageing and increased activity elevates energy expenditure.

The belief that physical activity results in enhanced appetite and the consumption of an increased quantity of food has been shown to be incorrect. In fact, a recent animal study showed that rats that were exercising for one or two hours per day ate less than those who were not exercised at all.

Another aspect of importance is that it appears that obese people are generally less active than those of normal weight and thus tend more readily to put on weight. An interesting study done on children has further suggested that overweight children are not only less active than their slim counterparts but are more efficient in their movements, i.e. to execute the same activity, the overweight child uses less energy.

Also of importance is the fact that the benefits of exercise are of longer duration than originally thought. Following exercise the basal metabolic rate remains elevated for several hours, thus promoting additional effortless energy utilization. In fact, a study recently undertaken showed that subjects who doubled their exercise retained an elevated basal metabolic rate until the following day.

To be effective, exercise must be taken regularly. There may be a marginal weight gain at the commencement of an exercise programme, as the increase in muscle tissue, which is heavier than adipose tissue, may outweigh the loss of fat. This however is a slight and temporary effect.

There are several secondary effects which more than justify the inclusion of exercise in the weight reduction programme. In the first place, it is part of a regimen in which the individual is required to positively undertake a commitment which is frequently disliked. It is said that the extent to which an overweight individual adheres to an exercise programme can be directly correlated to his/her motivation to lose weight. Thus if a patient regularly finds excuses to miss out on exercise there will usually be an unsatisfactory weight loss due to lack of adherence to the diet as well. Secondly, the increase in muscle tone makes clothes fit better and gives the person an added sense of achievement. Furthermore, when participating in exercise, the overweight person is away from the temptation of the kitchen, and is being conditioned to have interests other than food.

THE COMPOSITION AND DISTRIBUTION OF THE DIET

The diet should supply between 4000 and 6000 kJ (approximately 950–1400 Cal) per day, depending on the activity and the age of the patient. This diet should result in a weight loss of 0.75–1.0 kg/week. Interestingly, it has been shown that weight loss is more successful in patients who take their diet as multiple meals than in those who take the same intake in one or two meals per day. The food should thus be divided into three meals, or if desired into six smaller snacks, per day. If possible the main meal should be taken at midday, or even at breakfast, as more energy is expended in digestion if the meal is followed by a reasonable amount of exercise than if it is followed by the relaxation which is probable after the evening meal.

The essentials of the successful weight reduction regimen are as follows:

1. It must supply *adequate protein*, not only to meet physiological requirements but also to ensure optimum satiety value after each meal. This will prevent early hunger and the need to nibble between meals (one of the major problem areas for overweight people).

2. Fat, the most concentrated source of energy in the diet, should be *severely restricted*. Food should be prepared by methods such as baking, stewing or steaming, as fried or creamed foods add enormously to the energy content of the diet.

3. *High-carbohydrate* foods selected for inclusion in the diet should be primarily those supplying starch in preference to sugar. Concentrated sweet foods provide a high proportion of 'empty kilojoules', i.e. energy from sources of poor nutritive value. This of course does not apply to fruits, which are good sources of vitamins, minerals and fibre. They also provide variety in the diet and two to four items of fruit are usually included per day.

4. *Fibrous* green and yellow *vegetables*, such as cabbage, sprouts and marrow, are valuable 'fillers'. They are primarily composed of fibre and water, and supply few kilojoules. They are normally allowed in unrestricted quantities as salads and cooked vegetables and in soups and stews.

5. Artificial *sweeteners, spices* and *herbs* are usually included to improve the flavour of foods and increase variety in the diet. Although sodium cyclamate has been incriminated as a hazardous food additive if taken in huge amounts, saccharine still appears to be permissible if consumed in reasonable quantities. The use of artificially sweetened drinks in excessive quantities is to be discouraged, as part of the treatment for obesity must involve adaptation to consuming moderate quanties of food and self-discipline in terms of intake.

CONSTRUCTING A MENU

The menu plan recommended below is based on several exchange lists which are modified to fit in with the life-style and eating pattern of the patient. Similar foods are listed together in portion sizes comparable in energy value enabling the patient to select preferred foods. The exchange lists used are as follows:

1. main course exchanges equivalent to a portion of meat or substitute at a main meal,
2. light meal exchanges equivalent to a portion of meat or substitute at a lunch or dinner,
3. starch exchanges, i.e. foods equivalent to one slice of bread,
4. fruit exchanges.

The patient is also informed about the unrestricted foods which may be used as fillers.

Main course exchanges

The patient should be aware that a 30 g slice of roast mutton contains as many kilojoules as two slices of bread and that 100 g of beef is equivalent to three to five slices of bread. It is thus not only essential that all visible fat should be removed from meat, but also that portions of lean meat are carefully controlled. The following list indicates equivalent portions. As most individuals usually have one meal a day at which large portions are consumed, the following exchanges have been measured specifically for the main meal. The weights given below are all cooked weights.

Beef	corned 100g
	roast 100g
	lean steak 120 g
Chicken	roast, skin removed 150 g
Ham	lean, boiled 100g
Kidney or liver	150 g
Mutton and lamb	lean chop, broiled/grilled 90 g
	leg of lamb 90 g
Pork	roast leg, all fat removed 90 g
Veal	roast leg 120 g

Fish	white fish (haddock, plaice, whiting, sole, monk fish, etc.) 200 g
	shellfish (e.g. lobster and prawns) 180 g
Eggs	two (large)
Vegetarian substitute	lentils, soya, dried beans or peas (cooked and drained) 250 ml (1 cup)

Lunch, breakfast and supper exchanges

At the remaining two meals of the day smaller portions of high-protein foods should be taken. The following equivalents will serve as a guide.

Bacon	lean, all fat removed, grilled crisp 2 strips
Beef	sliced corned 60 g
	steak mince 75 g
Cheese	cottage cheese 75 g
	processed cheese 1 wedge
	cheddar cheese 25 g (2 tablespoons grated cheese)
Chicken	75 g
Egg	one large
Fish	white fish 100 g
	canned pilchards 60 g
	salmon 40 g
Liver or kidney	60 g
Breakfast cereal	oatmeal porridge 200 g (cooked weight)
	weetabix 1 bar
	muesli 2 rounded tablespoons

Exchange list of starches

The following foods are interchangeable; each taken in the amount indicated can be regarded as one portion of starch.

| *Banana* | one small |

Beans, dried	cooked 3 tablespoons
Biscuits	2 cream crackers
	4 small round salty crackers
	3 strips of wholewheat crispbread
Bread	white, brown or wholewheat one slice, 1 cm thick (30 g)
Corn	one cob, 7–9 cm long, medium thickness
Macaroni, spaghetti, etc.	quarter cup, cooked
Parsnips	3 tablespoons cooked
Peas	3 tablespoons cooked
Porridge	⅓ cup, cooked
	2 tablespoons dry instant cereal
Potatoes	2 small
Rice	2 tablespoons cooked
Sweet potatoes	3 tablespoons cooked
Wine	one glass dry

Fruit exchanges

The following fruit portions are interchangeable and may be taken raw, stewed or baked without sugar.

Apple	1 medium
Apricot	3 small or 2 large
Fruit juice	1 small glass (125 ml)
Fruit salad	unsweetened, ⅔ cup (150 ml)
Grapefruit	half (large) or whole (medium)
Grapes	12
Melon, cantaloupe	quarter medium
Watermelon	⅓ of a round, 2 cm thick
Orange	1 medium
Peaches	2 medium or 1 large
Pear	1 small or half large
Pineapple	2 thin slices
Plums	2 or 3 small
Prunes	4–5 depending on size

Unrestricted foods

Although the following foods do contribute carbohydrate to the diet, this amount is relatively small and the foods can be taken in moderate amounts without regard to the kilojoule content. They act as fillers and provide variety, both essential aspects of a weight reduction diet.

asparagus	celery	horseradish	olives in brine
cabbage	cress	leeks	radishes
carrots	cucumber	marrow	rhubarb
cauliflower	green beans	mushrooms	spinach

clear soup   meat and yeast extract (Oxo, Marmite, etc)
soda water   black tea and coffee (not sweetened coffee
lemon juice   essence)
vinegar   artifically sweetened cool drinks
salt and pepper   Worcestershire sauce
    all spices and herbs
onions for flavouring and in cooking
unsweetened pickles and tomatoes

Sample menu (weight reduction)

The following diet provides 4600–5000 kJ (1100–1200 Cal) depending on the size of portions consumed and the amount of unrestricted foods taken.

Breakfast
    1 fruit exchange
    1 'light meal' protein exchange
    1 starch exchange
    unrestricted foods such as lemon juice, tomato, tea or coffee if
        desired, including skimmed milk from daily ration
Dinner (midday or evening)
    1 'main course' protein exchange
    vegetables and salads as desired from list of unrestricted foods
    1 fruit exchange
Supper or lunch
    1 'light meal' protein exchange
    vegetables or salads from list of unrestricted foods
    1 starch exchange
    1 fruit exchange
    tea or coffee with skimmed milk from daily ration
Daily ration: 300 ml (½ pint) skimmed milk + 1 teaspoon margarine or butter

Using the above as a framework for the diet, the patient can use foods which fit the family budget and eating pattern, provided they are cooked in the required way. The following menu plans illustrate this point.

Day 1

    Early morning tea or coffee
Breakfast
    orange juice (using 1 orange)
    1 scrambled egg
    1 slice wholewheat toast with 1 teaspoon butter and yeast
        extract
    tea or coffee with skimmed milk from ration
10 a.m.
    Tea or coffee with skimmed milk from ration
Lunch
    100 g grilled haddock with tomato
    2 small potatoes
    tossed salad
    1 apple
    tea or coffee
4 p.m.
    tea or coffee with skimmed milk from ration
Dinner
    1 plate of soup made from meat stock (all fat removed) and
        vegetables selected from unrestricted foods
    150 g roast chicken (skin removed)
    Brussels sprouts and carrots
    1 baked pear with cinnamon, sweetened with artificial sweet-
        ener
10 p.m.
    tea or coffee with skimmed milk from ration

Day 2

Breakfast
    5 dried stewed prunes
    ½ cup (125 ml) porridge with skimmed milk from allowance
    1 scrambled egg
    tea or coffee

10 a.m.
    tea or coffee with skimmed milk from ration
Lunch
    cheese on toast (1 slice of wholewheat toast topped with 1
        tablespoon grated cheese), 1 rasher of lean back bacon and a
        slice of tomato, grilled for 2 minutes
    lettuce and cucumber
    1 apple
4 p.m.
    tea or coffee with skimmed milk from ration
Dinner
    consommé
    100 g roast beef
    marrow, cabbage and green beans
    2 peaches stewed with artifical sweetener
10 p.m.
    tea or coffee with skimmed milk from ration

Complications

Mid-meal hunger is a frequent complaint of slimmers and patients
may be told to save their fruit or 'starch' portions for mid-meal
snacks.

    Constipation, due to both reduced food volume and minimal fat
intake, resulting in reduced lubrication of the gut, is a common
problem among those on a weight reduction diet. Adequate fluids
and large quantities of salads and cooked vegetables may be
beneficial but in some cases a routine intake of digestive bran may
be advisable. Increased fluid intake will then cause the bran to
swell and increase the contents of the digestive tract, usually
alleviating the constipation.

FOOD FALLACIES AND MISINFORMATION

Although misconceptions about food and nutritional value are
common in other aspects of feeding, the layman's lack of
knowledge in the field of weight control is particularly apparent.
Here the role of the dietitian and nurse as nutrition educator is
very important, not only to assist patients to develop a more
rational understanding of comparable foods, but also to take a

firm stand against the manipulative overweight individual. The following facts may be relevant to the nurse in this respect.

Both *bread* and *toast* have a similar energy content per slice and should be limited in the weight reduction diet. Ordinary baker's wholewheat bread, whilst contributing considerably more vitamin and mineral content to the diet, has approximately the same kilojoule content as white or brown bread. Home-made wholewheat bread which includes seeds, nuts, yoghurt, etc., will have a higher energy content.

Fats and *oils* are interchangeable with regard to their energy content per gram. Although oil is recommended in the treatment of coronary artery disease, its kilojoule content is no lower than that of butter or margarine.

Many patients misunderstand the role of *liquids* in the diet. Water, soda water, black tea and coffee and artifically sweetened cool drinks may be taken without restriction. However, alcohol, tea with condensed or fresh milk, synthetic cool drinks, fruit juice and soups contribute kiljoules to the diet. Many patients not only drink these in large quantities but fail to disclose the fact to the nurse.

Glucose, brown sugar and *honey* are, like *white sugar*, forbidden on the weight reduction diet. They all supply approximately 17 kJ/g (4 Cal/g).

'Dietetic' or *diabetic* foods may *not* be taken without restriction. Although 'diabetic' artifically sweetened cool drinks, fruit gums and chewing gum are virtually kilojoule-free, this is not the case with other products. The canned fruits and special jam, for instance, retain the fruit sugar even though the preparation includes only artifical sweeteners. These canned fruits should be used as exchanges and in the same quantity as the fresh product and the jam should be used in limited amounts. Chocolates and sweetened biscuits prepared for diabetics should be avoided due to the high fat content, and other ingredients used.

There is no basis for the routine advice to overweight people to avoid *salt*. Although for about the first fortnight the weight loss may be attributable to fluid loss (as discussed below), the misapprehension that salt intake and resultant fluid retention are the cause of overweight is unfounded in people with normal cardiac and renal function. Long-term abstinence from salt is unnecessary and can be hazardous in hot climates.

BEHAVIOUR MODIFICATION

Also known as behaviour therapy, this is a method of correcting the behaviour of individuals with psychological problems. Originally used in the treatment of alcoholism and certain phobias, behaviour modification is now being applied in the field of obesity. The purpose of behaviour therapy is to develop a permanent change in relevant behaviour in order to achieve weight loss, and thereafter permanent maintenance of ideal weight.

Initially, the problem is defined. Behaviour patterns which are directly responsible for the overweight are then modified as required. The patient should be made aware that obesity is a long-term — maybe a life-time — problem and requires a change in life-style to correct it. Because *self-management* is the key to weight reduction, it is an essential part of the therapy to furnish the patient with the understanding and skills to achieve the appropriate changes in behaviour.

The first step is to take a detailed dietary history, determining not only what and how much the person eats, but also emotional factors, which may be relevant. By instructing the patient to keep a record of food eaten for a week and the social, emotional and physical circumstances relating to its consumption, both the nurse and the patient usually gain valuable insight into the problem. During the course of the regimen which follows, positive reinforcement of essential changes in attitude are required and regular supportive therapy is essential for success. Some practical manoeuvres which are useful in implementing therapy are given below.

STIMULI. Establish the stimuli which prompt the patient to eat, and help channel this activity along other lines. For example, the individual who eats while watching television may replace food with knitting. The one who eats when depressed or lonely could perhaps be encouraged to work in the garden instead, and the teenager who eats from boredom could be encouraged to develop an interest in a hobby.

THE ACT OF EATING. To increase the emphasis on the eating of food a specific place setting may be used. A special glass and unusual cutlery will reinforce the stimulus of eating. Many overweight people are fast eaters and they should be encouraged to use only a fork to eat their meals, in order to slow down and thus reduce the quantity of food consumed. Other ways of emphasizing the procedure of eating are to hang a mirror directly opposite the overweight person's plate at table, to write down each food eaten, and to use a smaller plate for all their meals. All foods should be served in the kitchen — away from the place of eating — and problem foods such as chocolates and sweets should not be readily obtainable: these could be locked away and the key held by a supportive family member.

INITIAL WEIGHT LOSS. Using initial weight loss as incentive to further adherence to the regimen is often helpful. Children in particular benefit by the drawing of a graph, plotting weight loss on the vertical axis against 3-day intervals on the horizontal axis. However, the patient should understand from the start that initial weight loss may be considerably more than that which can be expected later. Commencement of a weight reduction regimen is followed by fluid loss as the individual starts depending on body fat reserves for energy needs. Loss of stomach contents accelerates this weight loss, which is gratifying initially but may result in despondence when the rate of weight loss returns to an average of 750–1000 g/week. Other dieters may lose satisfactorily for some weeks, after which their weight may remain constant in spite of continued adherence to the diet. Middle-aged overweight women are inclined to retain fluid after a weight loss of 8–10 kg, and this plateau effect is often the cause of their return to their previous unsatisfactory eating habits. Diuretics are often advisable for a short period at this stage, if only as a temporary morale booster.

REWARD. Rewarding people for weight lost is also an important part of treatment. Children may receive money and should be encouraged to put this away to a particular goal in preference to making a regular purchase of sweets, and housewives may accumulate the money previously spent on non-desirable foods for a particular item of clothing. Neither the amount of money nor the weight is important but rather the incentive that this self-reward provides. Another helpful hint is for the individual to buy an article of clothing which is a size too small and aim to fit it by a specific date.

People who need to lose weight need support and encouragement. Many find it helpful to diet as a group and gain from the encouragement and help of others with the same problem. Losing weight can be accompanied by a sense of deprivation and may be a lonely as well as a rewarding experience. It depends on the individual personality and the nature of the problem.

In conclusion, it is stressed that while the nurse may regard the above suggestions as juvenile and trivial, it has been shown that behaviour modification is in many cases all-important in the therapy of obesity.

NURSING MANAGEMENT HINTS

1. Positive reinforcement of the diet is very necessary. Regular weighing *on the same scale* helps maintain the patient's motivation, and the plotting of a graph (as discussed earlier) is a useful practice to commence in hospital. Routine, tactful checking of the contents of patients' lockers for foods brought in by visitors is relevant; patients should be aware that fruit is strictly restricted to that provided in the hospital diet. Sugar should never be offered to patients on a weight reduction diet by those serving tea and coffee in the ward. If a milk drink is served at night, these patients should either be offered an alternative, such as tea or a sugar-free cool drink, or this should be included as part of the patient's allowance. Whatever the situation, the practice should be constant and all should know the rule.

2. Constipation is a widespread complication among hospitalized patients on weight-reducing diets. Unless contraindicated, routine administration of approx. 2 tablespoons digestive bran and extra liquids are advisable from the outset in patients who tend to have this problem.

3. On discharge, routine follow-up of weight loss should be arranged. Whether the patient returns to see the dietitian in the out-patients department, visits his/her doctor or, if still housebound, is at least supervised by the community nurse, the interest of a health professional is helpful in retaining adherence to the diet.

BIBLIOGRAPHY

Ashwell, M. & Garrow, J.S. (1975) A survey of three slimming and weight control organizations in the UK. *Nutrition, 29(6)*, 347.

Bleicher, J.E., Cegielski, M. & Saporta, J.A. (1974) Intestinal by-pass operation for massive obesity. *Postgrad. Med., 55(4)*, 65.

Blonz, E. & Stern, J. (1981) Obesity and fad diets. In: Ellenbogen, L. (ed.). *Controversies in Nutrition*. London: Churchill Livingstone.

Blundell, J. (1975) Anorexic drugs, food intake and the study of obesity. *Nutrition, 29(1)*, 5.

Bradfield, R.D. (1973) Relative importance of SDA in weight reduction. *Lancet, 2*, 640.

Bray, G. (1982) 'Brown' tissue and metabolic obesity. *Nutr. Today, 17*, 23.

Bray, G.A. & Bethune, J.E. (1974) *Treatment and Management of Obesity*, London: Harper and Row.

Brightwell, D.R. (1974) Treating obesity with behaviour modification. *Postgrad. Med., 55(4)*, 52.

Bullen, B., Reed, R. & Mayer, J. (1964) Physical activity of obese and non-obese girls appraised by motion picture sample. *Am. J. Clin. Nutr., 14*, 211.

Council on Foods and Nutrition (1973) A critique of low carbohydrate ketogenic weight reduction regimens. A review of Dr. Atkin's diet revolution. *J. Am. Med. Ass., 224*, 1415.

Evans, E. & Miller, D.S. (1978) Slimming aids. *J. Hum. Nutr., 32*, 433.

Fabry, P., Fodor, J., Hejl, Z., Braun, T. & Zvolankova, K. (1964) *Lancet, 2*, 614.

Ferstl, R. (1976) Modifying behaviour in obesity. *J. Am. Med. Ass., 236(13)*, 1443.

Garrow, J.S. (1974) *Energy Balance and Obesity in Man*. London: North-Holland.

Garrow, J.S. (1983) Indices of adiposity. *Nutr. Abstr. Rev., 53*, 697.

Hawk, L.J. (1979) Influence of body fatness in childhood on fatness in adult life. *Br. Med. J., 1*, 151.

Himms-Hagen, J. (1983) Brown adipose tissue thermogenesis in obese animals. *Nutr. Rev., 41*, 261.

Hirsch, J. (1971) Adipose cellularity in relation to human obesity. *Adv. Internal Med., 17*, 289.

Holodinsky, C. (1982) The Beverly Hills diet: A critical review. *J. Can. Diet. Ass., 43*, 251.

James, W. (compiler) (1976) *Research on Obesity: A Report of the DHSS/MRC Group*, p. 94. London: HMSO.

Jeffrey, D.B. (1974) A comparison of the effects of external control and self-control on the modification and maintenance of weight. *J. Abnorm. Psychol., 83(4)*, 404.

Knittle, J.L. (1972) Obesity in childhood: a problem in adipose tissue cellular development. *J. Pediat., 81*, 1048.

Levitz, L.S. (1973) Behaviour therapy in treating obesity. *J. Am. Diet. Ass., 62*, 22.

Miffer, D.S. & Mumford, P. (1966) Obesity: physical activity and nutrition. *Proc. Nutr. Soc., 25*, 100.

Pi-Sunger, F.X. (1976) Jejunal bypass surgery for obesity. *Am. J. Clin. Nutr., 29(4)*, 409.

Stuart, R.B. & Davis, B. (1974) *Slim Chance in a Fat World*. Illinois: Research Press Co.

Vasselli, J., Clearly, M. & Van Itallie, T. (1983) Modern concepts of obesity. *Nutr. Rev. 41*, 361.

Watson, J. (1979) The vanishing nurse. *Nurs. Mirror, 12 July*, Suppl.

Wooley, O.W., Wooley, S.C. & Dunham, R.B. (1972) Can calories be perceived and do they affect hunger in obese and non-obese humans? *J. Comp. Physiol. Psychol., 80*, 250.

6   Underweight

Individuals whose weight falls to a level at which health is impaired and resistance to disease is lowered are regarded as underweight. This usually means a weight more than 10% below the accepted standard for age and sex. The lower the weight, the more serious the condition: at its most severe, underweight can threaten life.

AETIOLOGY

There are various causes for the condition, which can be classified as either physical or psychological.

Physical causes

There are three categories of physical disorders which may cause abnormal weight loss:

1. The intake may be inadequate for normal needs. This may be due to environmental causes (e.g. poverty, inadequate supplies on expeditions or deliberate starvation as in prisoner-of-war camps), or to anorexia, encountered in many illnesses.
2. Alternatively there may be an excessive demand for energy, resulting in a drain on the body energy stores with which the individual cannot keep pace by consuming normal quantities of food. This occurs frequently during puberty where accelerated growth often accompanied by excessive participation in sport may result in the gauntness and ultra-thinness sometimes seen in teenagers, particularly boys. Long-term strenuous exercise may have the same effect. Added to the vast energy expenditure of, for example, the long-distance runner, he or she frequently does not have the corresponding appetite or interest in eating. The concomitant anaemia that many runners develop tends to increase their anorexia.

    The excessive needs of patients with wasting disease such

as tuberculosis, cancer and AIDS result in long-term debilitation.

In hospitals postoperative weight loss is common. Appetite seldom keeps pace with the excessive energy needs for anabolism and, in patients where reserves are already depleted on admission to hospital the situation is even more likely to result in underweight (as discussed in Chapters 4 and 13). Chronic fevers have the same effect. Long-term nutritional demands to meet bacterial or viral invasion, and also to reduce body temperature to normal, deplete reserves and weight loss may result.

3. There may be abnormal loss of energy. With severe diarrhoea and vomiting there is a loss of unabsorbed nutrients. In extensive burns losses through the exudate will result in nutritional demands which will be extremely difficult to meet with food and/or parenteral feeding. Loss of glucose in the urine of uncontrolled diabetics and their inability to utilize and conserve the carbohydrate they eat effectively will also result in underweight, if the condition is not diagnosed and treated immediately.

Psychological causes: anorexia nervosa (Fig. 9)

In Western society today the wide variety of foods available, the impact of advertising and the symbolism of foods and eating (opulence, wealth, etc.), all make it extremely difficult for people to keep their weight within normal limits. On the other hand, the emphasis is on dieting and the correlation of extreme thinness with beauty further complicates the situation. Many young girls, developing an attitude of independence and adventure, enjoy cooking and tasting new and different foods and tend to become overweight; and the present early onset of puberty with its associated change in the fat distribution adds to the feeling of fatness. Many girls mature early in puberty, at least in physical terms. Prompted by the teasing of friends or a feeling of self-consciousness, a girl may voluntarily attempt to lose weight. In fact it has been suggested that a possible reason why this illness is seldom encountered in boys is the more gradual onset of puberty in males. Many workers have suggested that the condition develops as a result of a strong subconscious desire to return to the

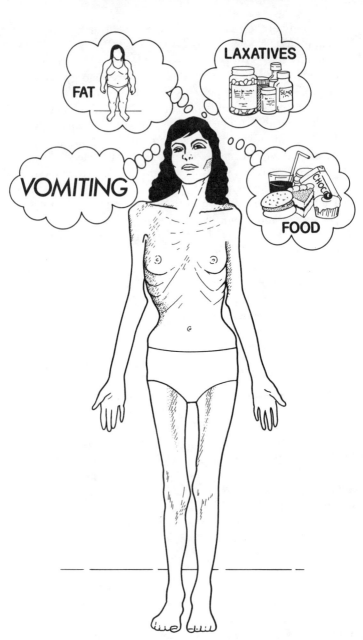

Fig. 9. *Psychological characteristics of anorexia nervosa.*

security of childhood and an aversion to approaching adulthood. The associated symptom of amenorrhoea which occurs with the illness is thus regarded as a solace by these patients.

Emotional disturbances and mental illness have a marked effect on eating habits. Some patients react by overeating whereas others develop an aversion to food. Rehabilitative nursing is perhaps of more importance with these patients than in those with any other dietary disorder. In most other conditions the patient is likely to be motivated to adhere to the necessary dietary instructions but this is seldom the case in patients where underlying psychological problems are the cause of their weight loss or gain.

Although generally regarded as a disorder of present-day living and stress, anorexia nervosa was first described by Gull in 1868. He initially called the condition *apepsia hysterica* but later renamed it *anorexia nervosa*. It occurs almost exclusively in girls from early teenage to mid-twenties. It is often preceded by domestic strife, over-dependence on parents, or a broken sexual relationship. A precipitating factor in many cases is the demand of sports teachers or dancing teachers on these individuals to lose weight in an attempt to excel in a particular activity. Anorexia nervosa is essentially a condition where a breakdown in communication with family or members of the peer group results in a poor self-image and a protest in terms of food rejection.

A feature of anorexia nervosa is a distorted body image: the girl who is marginally overweight continues to lose weight, prompted by the illusion that she is overweight, long after her weight has returned to normal.

Crisp (1976) undertook a large survey in England, comparing teenagers in comprehensive and independent (i.e. private, public and grant-aided) schools. He showed that social influence appeared to be important in that the condition was considerably more prevalent in the more affluent group. He concluded also that anorexia nervosa is a common condition and is probably becoming more widespread. The mortality rate can reach 20%.

Patients with anorexia nervosa tend to be similar in symptoms and temperament: they are frequently intelligent, active over-achievers. They are often depressed, introspective teenagers who delight in the preparing and serving of foods but eat minimal quantities themselves. Meals are accompanied by a feeling of guilt and often prompt vomiting afterwards. Some take large amounts of purgatives or secretly discard their food whenever possible. Invariably, they claim to be constipated.

The name 'anorexia' is in fact a misnomer as patients do not refuse food through lack of appetite but voluntarily starve themselves. Some develop the habit of binge-eating followed by vomiting (bulimia nervosa), or alternatively vomit the small amount of food they have been persuaded to eat.

Secondary metabolic abnormalities that accompany the disorder and have been described by Crisp (1970) are: endocrine abnormalities including amenorrhoea, sometimes hypogonadism, hypothyroidism and reduced adrenal function, major disturbances of carbohydrate and lipid metabolism, and electrolyte imbalance.

Recent research has raised the possibility of associated zinc deficiency playing a role in perpetuating the condition. It is suggested that the low zinc intake in the minimal food consumption of the anorectic may lead to the deficiency symptom of reduced taste sensitivity, which in turn may aggravate the poor intake by further reducing the desire for food (Bryce-Smith & Simpson, 1984).

Anorexia nervosa is essentially a psychiatric disorder and is the one diet-orientated condition in which the involvement of the dietitian (who represents to the patient an emphasis on food and eating) may in some cases do more harm than good. Certain workers suggest that food-forcing as a form of treatment often duplicates a causative home factor — food-preoccupied, over-forceful parents. It is essential that any nursing or paramedical worker who is responsible for the treatment of these patients understands the emotional problems, and although these patients need to be handled very carefully they should not be allowed to manipulate the situation, a common tendency in this condition. Behaviour modification, as applied in obesity, is seldom advisable, as the nutritional disorder is secondary to the psychological illness.

When binge-eating followed by deliberate vomiting, or *bulimia nervosa*, occurs it does not necessarily develop into overt anorexia nervosa; some women initiate this technique merely to maintain their weight at the desired level. It is, however, a hazardous habit, both because of the potential for advanced anorexia nervosa and because the teeth are adversely affected by the frequent contact with the strongly acid stomach contents. It is also a practice that can become progressively more difficult to control and can result in dehydration and hypotension. In a review article on the subject, Fairburn points out that the principal complaint of patients with bulimia nervosa is loss of control of eating. Often self-imposed dietary rules are broken by gross binge-eating but depression, loneliness or a morbid fear of getting fat can all precipitate this disorder or episodic binge-eating and vomiting.

These patients, not unlike many patients with anorexia nervosa, are frequently preoccupied with food, which they regard as 'fattening, forbidden' food or 'thin, permitted' food, becoming depressed and anxious if they 'lose control' of their intake.

Treatment

The treatment must to some extent be tailored to the severity of the illness. In severe cases, where hospitalization is necessary, therapy is appropriately more drastic. It is essential that the underlying psychological problem be treated, as merely attempting to change dietary attitudes will be of temporary benefit, if effective at all.

At the commencement of treatment, establishment of rapport between the patient and nurse, or patient and therapist, is essential. The patient is often resentful about the need for recovery and reluctant to accept treatment. She may minimize her weight loss and agree to stop vomiting her meals but will usually soon relapse unless closely supervised.

There is considerable controversy about the stated goals of treatment in grossly underweight patients. Some workers maintain that the precise weight gain required must be stipulated at the start of treatment. The appropriate diet is then commenced and aggressively reinforced until weight is within normal limits. Others feel that the patient's resistance to a target weight, which will be regarded as totally unrealistic by the patient, will hinder the effectiveness of treatment. It is understandable that a patient weighing 20 kg below her recommended body weight and still convinced that she is overweight will totally reject the suggestion that she should regain 20 kg. The patient will insist that a gain of more than a few kilograms will result in obesity. It is therefore suggested that the patient should rather approach the target weight gradually. A weight gain which is acceptable to the patient should be suggested, on the understanding that the situation will be reassessed when the objective has been reached. In this way the impact of rehabilitation is reduced.

Hospitalized patients are usually confined to bed for a large proportion of the day to reduce energy output by physical activity. They are encouraged to project their emotions to more positive actions than self-deprivation. Constant reassurance is necessary to make the patient realise that she will not become overweight by eating moderate quantities of food and that a maintenance regimen will be given when required. Firm handling is essential. The patient must be well supervised to ensure that meals are finished, that vomiting is not induced, and that purgatives are not smuggled into the ward. Supplementary tube feeding at night is sometimes necessary.

Patients will often try to manipulate the staff into replacing a high-energy item with a less suitable food and no omissions or substitutions in the served diet should be tolerated. It is sometimes necessary to allow these patients to use only a commode so that the nurse may observe whether vomiting or purging is taking place. On admission to hospital such patients generally have a lower weight than patients treated as out-patients, and an initial weight gain of 0.91–1.8 kg/week is recommended. However, rehabilitation may be associated with an unpredictable weight gain at times and patients, as well as staff, should be aware that no precise weight gain should be anticipated each week.

In less severe cases and where the condition is not associated with domestic conflict or, as in bulimia nervosa, weight is within acceptable limits, treatment may be attempted at home, on the understanding that inability to achieve the goal weight in a particular period (e.g. 1 kg in a fortnight) will necessitate immediate hospitalization. These patients often respond by exercising vigorously to increase energy utilization, unless directly forbidden to do so. They should also not have access to a scale as they tend to weigh themselves repeatedly. Twice weekly supervised weighing to reassure them that they will not suddenly become obese is a reasonable routine.

During the course of the illness patients usually choose exclusively protein foods, avoiding fats and carbohydrates as 'fattening'. From the commencement of treatment the diet should be adapted to be as near to a normal diet as possible.

For patients who are unmotivated and obstructive about

treatment this varied diet is sometimes preceded by a diet consisting solely of milk. From 6 a.m. to 10 p.m. the patient is fed one glass of milk every hour, on the hour, for three days. An exclusive milk regimen has a relatively high energy value and is tolerated and digested well in the majority of cases. It is said that after this period the patient is usually more easily won over to commence a more normal diet. Lactose intolerance precludes a milk diet.

DIETARY MANAGEMENT OF UNDERWEIGHT PATIENTS

It is of particular importance that the nurse takes cognizance of the emotional, pathological, social and financial difficulties confronting the patient and related to the aetiology of this condition. It is essential to identify and treat the underlying cause of weight loss. Where underweight results from psychological causes the patient may be reluctant to co-operate. The nursing skills in managing this problem are described in detail by Jack Lyttle.

The first decision to make is the form of feeding, i.e. whether nutrients should be taken orally, parenterally or enterally. The latter two methods of rehabilitation are discussed elsewhere. Initially the patient's capacity, and hence the intake, may be small and supplementary feeding may be necessary per tube. Progressive increments of approximately 850 kJ (200 Cal) per day should be made.

Nutrient requirements

Inclusion of good quality *protein* at each of six snacks per day will assist in replenishing body muscle stores. Carbohydrate is also required for its protein-sparing effect and should play an important role. Concentrated *sugars*, such as candy and chocolate, are most useful concentrated foods but they will usually be rejected by an underweight patient resisting treatment as being 'too rich' or causing nausea. *Fat* is particularly useful in the diet as a concentrated source of energy. Mineral and vitamin deficits may occur with excessive weight loss and so these, too, are required in larger amounts: supplements are usually advisable. Energy intake should gradually be increased to approximately 12 000 kJ (2900 Cal).

A recipe for an appropriate high-energy milk drink useful for mid-meal snacks is given below but caution must be exercised as debilitated patients occasionally suffer from lactase deficiency.

750 ml milk
150 g milk powder
2 eggs
synthetic colouring (e.g. cochineal)
flavouring
sugar or Caloreen (a glucose polymer discussed in Chapter 16)

Whisk together these ingredients and serve chilled as a milkshake.

The following sample menu is given as a guide.

Sample menu

Breakfast
  muesli with bananas and creamy milk
  2 scrambled eggs (mixed with cream prior to cooking)
  a slice of toast, well buttered while hot
  a glass of milk
Mid-morning
  3 biscuits liberally spread with butter and cheese
  a glass of milk
Dinner
  roast chicken — a thigh and a leg — with 2 small roast potatoes,
    peas and roast marrow
  175 ml of fruit yoghurt or baked pudding and custard
Mid-afternoon
  high-energy milk drink (recipe given above)
Supper
  a medium helping of fried fish and chips
  beetroot salad
  a small helping of coleslaw mixed with mayonnaise
  cheese and biscuits
9 p.m.
  high-energy milk drink

NURSING MANAGEMENT HINTS

1. Six small meals must be daily routine for these patients. Unless contra-indicated (e.g. in patients with lactose intolerance), milk should play an important role in supplementary feeding. It is rapidly absorbed and if the patient misses the serving of morning or afternoon tea — due to medical procedures or visits to other departments — a glass of milk or a milk drink at the earliest opportunity will help meet the deficit and not remove their appetite for the next meal.

2. Routine weighing of these patients is necessary wherever possible. In physically debilitated patients it encourages a realism that their efforts are helpful and motivates them to continue to persevere to eat — a difficult challenge to those with little appetite. Where no weight gain is observed in spite of a voluntary attempt to compensate for increased needs, and there is no obvious cause such as diarrhoea, burns or other causes discussed earlier in this chapter, a hidden reason such as cancer or hyperthyroidism may need to be sought.

   In the patient with anorexia nervosa, regular weighing reassures her that her weight is controllable, i.e. that she will not, in a few days, put on an excessive amount of weight and become obese as many of these patients fear.

3. The bowel habits of underweight patients should be carefully observed. Diarrhoea due either to organic disease or laxative abuse may play an important role in their weight loss.

BIBLIOGRAPHY

Anon (1983) The enigma of anorexia nervosa. *Nutr. Rev., 41*, 121.
Armstrong-Esther, C. (1977) Anorexia nervosa: aspects of care and treatment. *J. Adv. Nurs., 2*, 127.
Bryce-Smith, D. & Simpson, R. (1984) Case of anorexia nervosa responding to zinc sulphate. *Lancet, 2*, 350.
Crisp, A. (1970) Anorexia nervosa: 'feeding disorder', 'nervous malnutrition' or 'weight phobia'? *World Rev. Nutr. Diet., 12*, 452.
Crisp, A., Palmer, R. & Kalucy, R. (1976) How common is anorexia nervosa? A prevalence study. *Br. J. Psychol., 128*, 549.
Day, S. (1974) Dietary management of anorexia nervosa. *Nutrition, 28*, 289.
Fairburn, C. (1983) Bulimia nervosa. *S. Afr. J. Hosp. Med., 9*, 145.
Goodsitt, A. (1974) Anorexia nervosa. *J. Am. Med. Ass., 229*, 372.
Groen, J.J. (1973) Psychocultural influences of nutrition behaviour. *Nutrition, 27*, 393.
Gull, W.W. (1868) The address in medicine delivered before the annual meeting of

APPLIED NUTRITION AND DIETETICS

the British Medical Association at Oxford. *Lancet, 2*, 171.

Huse, D. & Lucas, A. (1983) Dietary treatment of anorexia nervosa. *J. Am. Diet. Ass.*, 687.

Lacey, H. (1976) Anorexia nervosa. *Nurs. Times, 72*, 407.

Lyttle, J. (1986) *Psychiatric Nursing.* London: Baillière Tindall. (In preparation).

Marshall, M.H. (1978) Anorexia nervosa: dietary treatment and re-establishment of body weight in 20 cases studied on a metabolic unit. *J. Hum. Nutr., 32*, 349.

Spector, S., Wolpe, J. & Bouch, H. (1975) Behaviour therapy in anorexia nervosa. *J. Am. Med. Ass., 233*, 317.

7 Diabetes mellitus

Diabetes mellitus is a condition of chronic hyperglycaemia. Glucose is a normal intermediary product in the digestion of food and in the provision of energy from sources within the body. Carbohydrates — sugars, starches and glycogen — are broken down to glucose, and so to some extent are proteins (especially when inadequate amounts of carbohydrates are consumed) and fat.

Glucose is formed by the action of various enzymes on foods, as discussed in Chapter 8. The immediate effect of glucose entering the blood stream from the digestive tract is restoration of low blood sugar (glucose) to normal levels, if required. Glucose is transported to muscle tissue for energy needs as required and also to a lesser extent, to be stored as glycogen for later use. However, the liver is the main depot for reserve glucose in the form of glycogen. The conversion of glucose to glycogen can occur only through the action of *insulin*, the hormone which also plays an essential role in allowing sugar to enter cells and be used as fuel. In the absence of adequate sources of insulin, glucose will accumulate in the blood stream resulting in hyperglycaemia. When the concentration rises above approximately 9.5 mmol/litre of blood — the normal *renal threshold* — glucose is excreted in the urine (glycosuria), and can be detected by 'Stix' or other specific tests. A fasting blood glucose level of over 5.6 mmol/litre is indicative of diabetes. In certain conditions (e.g. late pregnancy or immediately following injury or a coronary thrombosis) this condition can occur transiently due to acute metabolic stress. Furthermore, a low renal threshold may cause glycosuria in a non-diabetic person, just as a high renal threshold may prevent hyperglycaemia inducing glycosuria in a person with inadequate supplies of insulin.

What then is the physiological basis for this inadequacy of insulin? The condition may result from impairment of insulin synthesis and/or release by the beta-cells of the pancreas. It can also result from the presence of 'anti-insulins' in the blood of an individual who, while able to produce normal amounts of insulin, is unable to overcome resistance to its action at the cellular level.

Diabetes is an inherited disease, usually preceded by a symptom-less stage characterized by certain abnormalities such as increased urinary output of insulin, multiple miscarriages, large babies (over 4.5 kg) and vascular changes. This stage is known as *pre-diabetes*. In the presence of other diabetogenic factors such as obesity, growth and possibly virus infection, pre-diabetes may develop into overt diabetes.

JUVENILE-ONSET DIABETES

Juvenile-onset diabetes, sometimes called insulin-dependent dia-betes, usually occurs in children and teenagers and often follows a period of growth. It is often encountered in individuals with a positive family history of diabetes.

These patients have a reduced number of beta-cells, resulting in an inadequate output of insulin. Consequently, the sugar content of the blood increases and spills over into the urine. Fat depots are depleted for energy purposes, and ketones, which are intermedi-ary products of fat metabolism, accumulate due to the absence of carbohydrate, which is essential for the complete breakdown of fat. The onset of the condition is acute, but is usually preceded by a short period of weight loss and the three classical signs, increased thirst (polydipsia), increased urination (polyuria) and increased hunger (polyphagia). The patient may present initially with severe vomiting and weakness or coma, the last resulting from the toxic effects of ketones. The nurse should be aware that the onset of diabetes in children is an emergency for which immediate medical help is required.

Management

Patients with juvenile-onset diabetes present a unique problem to the team responsible for treatment and management. The nurse, doctor, dietitian and social worker play an essential role of reassuring, guiding and helping the patient and his family adapt to the necessary regimen. Parents may have feelings of shock, guilt and anxiety which may be accentuated by the memory of their child's recent diabetic crisis. The child is often depressed and apprehensive at the prospect of daily injections and the need for a permanent dietary regimen.

Motivation is the keyword of treatment, and regular appointments should be arranged with the dietitian at the out-patients' clinic to maintain adherence to the diet and restimulate interest in the regimen. Regular reassessment of the diet is necessary for growing children to ensure that it is adequate for optimum development. Diabetic children — and their parents — sometimes develop an overconfident and ultra-casual approach to diabetes and regular remotivation is of the greatest importance. Teenagers often go through a stage when they react to the discipline that is vital in the diabetic regimen and demonstrate their independence by non-compliance. Authoritative but tactful handling is essential to satisfactory management.

These patients require insulin supplementation, achieved by the administration of an injection once or twice daily. Various types of insulin are available and these are used either singly or in combination, depending on several factors including the severity of the condition, the patient's activity and the distribution of meals. When the disorder is diagnosed, treatment is initiated with soluble insulin. This is a short-acting compound (the action lasts 1–8 h) and is administered before each meal. When the patient's blood sugar level has been stabilized, a combination of soluble with longer-acting insulin is usually introduced to reduce the number of injections required daily. Alternatively, a single injection of an insulin with a relatively quick onset and a medium action may be used. The insulin preparations Isophane and protamine zinc insulin (PZI) fall into this class. Lente and ultra-lente insulin have a long-acting effect and require a substantial bedtime snack to counteract the hypoglycaemic effect during the hours of sleep. In children long-acting insulins are seldom advisable, because children go early to bed and may thus have a hypoglycaemic attack in the early hours of the morning.

A recent development in this field is the development of monocomponent insulins. These are highly purified porcine compounds and cause less cutaneous reaction and fat atrophy at the injection site. They are also thought to reduce the incidence of long-term complications such as retinopathy and atherosclerosis. Short-acting and long-acting forms are available in this type of insulin (e.g. Actrapid, Monotard).

Insulin was previously widely available in concentrations of 40 or 80 units/ml and soluble insulin was also obtainable in a concentration of 20 units/ml. Today most countries, including the UK, have standardized the concentration to 100 units/ml in an attempt to prevent errors of measurement and incorrect dosage.

It is essential that food be taken 20–30 min after the insulin injection. Both parents and patients should be aware that the daily food intake must be distributed to allow for snacks between meals and before bedtime to counteract the hypoglycaemic effect of the insulin.

All diabetics, but particularly those with newly diagnosed juvenile diabetes, should understand the complication of *hypoglycaemia* and be advised always to carry glucose tablets or a wrapped sugar cube. Sweets, of course, are equally effective, but the temptation to eat them unnecessarily if far greater for a youngster, particularly if the child feels deprived anyway. In Britain, newly diagnosed patients are often given a supervised attack of hypoglycaemia so that they can be aware of the symptoms and will know how to treat them. Hypoglycaemia may be caused by strenuous or long-term activity which has not been preceded by the consumption of an appropriate snack, or by illness, particularly when accompanied by vomiting. Diabetic youngesters also often have inherently labile blood sugar levels which may drop or rise spontaneously at times. Although lack of control of blood sugar levels within normal limits is *usually* the result of dietary aberrations, a punitive attitude by those in authority is not always fair, nor will it result in rapport and adherence. Patients should be encouraged to join the British Diabetic Association, 10 Queen Anne Street, London W1M 0BD. The association provides advice and information and runs camps for diabetic children.

Dietary requirements

In the pre-insulin era, extreme rigidity of diet was essential and many young patients were virtually starved during their short lives. Today, however, dietary deprivation is not regarded as a prequisite for optimum control. The current choice is, roughly, between a 'free' diet or a controlled and regularly monitored diet in which the carbohydrate intake is based on a specific number of exchanges from which interchangeable portions can be selected for variety. Few people today recommend an unrestricted diet for juvenile diabetics. Proponents of the free diet usually restrict only concentrated sweetened foods such as sweets and cakes (although occasionally even these are allowed), and specify the distribution of meals throughout the day. They maintain that this attitude causes less psychological trauma and rebellion than a restrictive regimen. However, as these patients often require several daily injections of insulin and are thought to develop more complications in later life, this liberal diet is seldom recommended. Furthermore, as juveniles often have a more brittle, labile type of diabetes, they cannot afford the lack of control and the fluctuations in blood sugar level which are precipitated by a free diet.

MATURITY-ONSET DIABETES

When onset occurs in adulthood, diabetes is usually less serious, manifesting itself in a less dramatic way, and often related to the recent onset of obesity. It is usually more stable and milder than the juvenile-onset type and is caused either by suboptimal output of insulin or by resistance to insulin utilization. Oral agents (particularly sulphonylureas and biguanides) which stimulate increased production or promote more efficient action of insulin in the body are used very effectively in this group, but diet is an essential part of treatment. Diabetes occurs particularly in people over the age of 40 with a family history of the condition. In its mild form it is often largely reversible in the overweight patient if the required weight loss occurs.

Management

Many maturity-onset diabetics are overweight and their prime need is a controlled low-energy diet. A low-carbohydrate, low-fat diet is recommended in the hope that with weight reduction improved control of blood sugar levels will be achieved, and the long-term use of oral hypoglycaemic agents will be avoided.

The maturity-onset diabetic whose weight is within normal limits is usually merely given instructions to omit concentrated sugars, to distribute the intake of fat throughout the day and to modify the fat intake as discussed below (under General principles of diet).

COMPLICATIONS OF DIABETES

Although not a disabling disease in itself, particularly the maturity-onset type, diabetes can cause extremely severe complications. Atherosclerosis resulting in coronary heart disease, gangrene due to affected peripheral arteries, and retinopathy resulting from lesions in the ocular capillaries, with blindness in severe cases, all occur frequently in patients with long-standing diabetes. A variety of renal complications can occur, including toxaemia in pregnancy and glomerulonephritis. Meticulous control of the diabetes, i.e. retaining the blood sugar level within normal limits with the necessary drugs, diet and exercise, is generally thought markedly to reduce the possibility of complications. Self-discipline, the ability to give a relatively constant insulin injection and the probable effect of a controlled diet on most complications all contribute to an improved outlook for the patient. It should also be noted that there is a higher prevalence of complications in the obese patient and *the importance of weight reduction cannot be overemphasized.*

GENERAL PRINCIPLES OF DIET

When, centuries ago, diabetes was first identified, patients were fed on large quantities of carbohydrate to replace that lost in the urine. Later, diabetics were given a virtually carbohydrate-free diet. More recently patients have been told to omit sugar from their diet and to eat complex carbohydrates (such as potatoes, rice and bread) preferentially. This is the advice that is still given today but with the recent work done on the 'glycaemic index' of various foods, there has been a change of emphasis.

The glycaemic index compares the blood sugar response of various foods with an equivalent amount of glucose. Taking the two-hour blood response of glucose as 100%, it is clearly advantageous to emphasize foods with a lesser and more prolonged effect on the blood sugar level in the diabetic diet (i.e. a lower glycaemic index).

Jenkins *et al* report many studies indicating surprising results when a wide range of foods are compared to glucose on this basis. For example, potatoes provoked a greater response (i.e. had a higher glycaemic index) than the equivalent amount of rice and bread had a higher index than spaghetti. On testing, fructose also gave an unpredictable response, having a lower glycaemic index than anticipated. Several factors, including the presence of fibre, appear to influence the glycaemic index but the problem is complex.

The dilemma is expressed in the recent recommendation of the British Diabetic Association: 'A general increase in the fibre content of the diabetic diet is a useful therapeutic measure. More effective normalization of postprandial glycaemia may be achieved by a more selective approach to dietary carbohydrates and by consideration of the glycaemic effects of foods and meals in their entirety rather than on the basis of sucrose or total carbohydrate alone. More research is urgently needed to unravel this complicated but fundamental aspect of dietary advice.'

Thus, at this stage, the implications are still unclear except to indicate the following.

1. Legumes are to be encouraged in the diabetic diet (in controlled quantities and distributed as indicated below).
2. The total carbohydrate should not be as restricted as in the past. In fact, the general recommendation today is that the carbohydrate intake should contribute 40–50% of the total daily kilojoule requirement.
3. Fibre should be liberally included in the diet as this slows down the release of available carbohydrate taken concurrently and hence lowers the glycaemic index.
4. The role and quantity of fat and protein in the diabetic diet remain the same.

Modifying his daily intake according to changes in activity or occupation will ultimately be the patient's responsibility and it is imperative not only that the diet is tailored to his individual needs, but that the patient fully comprehends the principles of the regimen. A summary of these principles follows.

Energy

The controlled diabetic requires the same energy intake as the normal individual of the same weight and activity (see Table 1). Overweight patients should adhere to a weight reduction regimen and those who are underweight (especially the recently diagnosed juvenile diabetic who has undergone a period of debilitation) should take a high-protein, high-energy diet.

Protein

The protein requirement of the controlled diabetic is also similar to that of the non-diabetic. The standard recommended amount — approximately 0.75–1 g/kg body weight for adults, which in practice is readily attained with a diet of 60–90 g protein/day — covers the needs of controlled diabetics. However, it should be remembered that most high-protein foods also contain relatively large amounts of fat, and meat in particular should be considered with regard to its saturated fat content (see below).

During the early stages of juvenile diabetes, which often results in considerable wasting of tissue, a high-protein diet is recommended to restore depleted resources. A diet providing up to 120 g protein/day may be advisable for the newly diagnosed teenager. However, the carbohydrate intake should remain as controlled as is practical, because of the difficulties of insulin regulation at this stage. Initially, large quantities of meat, cheese and milk may be required, but when the necessary weight has been regained these foods will be reduced to normal limits because of their high fat content. However, milk is also a source of carbohydrate (lactose); 300 ml (½ pint) contributes 15 g of carbohydrate to the diet, which should be included in dietary calculations.

Carbohydrates

Cane sugar (sucrose) or glucose has a dramatic elevating effect on the blood sugar concentration and is also a source of 'empty' kilojoules; it is thus omitted from diabetic diets. Fruit is included in controlled amounts, as the sugar present in fruits is more slowly absorbed than sucrose (partly because of the accompanying fibre and partly because of the inherent metabolic effects of fructose) and because of the added advantage that fruit contains other nutrients. Although a wide range of stipulations regarding carbohydrates may be recommended, the usual regimen provides 200–280 g carbohydrate/day. This includes sugar (in fruit) and starch (in bread, rice, potatoes, etc.). Overweight patients should take less than 120 g carbohydrate/day and very active teenagers may take more than 280 g/day: this is a diet relatively high in carbohydrates and an appropriately lower fat intake may be required.

The carbohydrate requirement of children may be determined in various ways. The following rule is easy to remember and apply: multiply the child's age in years by ten and add 100 or 110. Thus an 8-year-old child is given 180–190 g of carbohydrate, divided into 10 g portions, throughout the day.

Fat

Diabetics are more prone than others to develop hyperlipidaemia, atherosclerosis and coronary heart disease. Unlike women in the general population, diabetic women are as likely to suffer from these conditions as men.

Epidemiologically, it appears that a diet low in saturated fat and cholesterol protects against the elevation of serum cholesterol and retards the deposition of atheroma in susceptible individuals (see Chapter 9). For this reason the diabetic is advised to replace the saturated (animal) fats such as butter, lard, suet, etc., with polyunsaturated (vegetable) oils. Foods high in cholesterol should also be limited. Having established the energy, protein and carbohydrate requirements of the patient, the dietitian or nurse may ascertain his fat requirements by difference. This may be done as follows, although in practice strict limitation of fat is seldom necessary, except for the overweight diabetic.

Example

A patient requires 8000 kJ (approx. 1900 Cal), 80 g of protein and 220 g of carbohydrates.
1 g of protein or carbohydrate gives 17 kJ (4 Cal) of energy
 80 × 17 = 1360 kJ (320 Cal) energy from protein
220 × 17 = 3740 kJ (880 Cal) energy from carbohydrate
         5100 kJ (1200) Cal
8000 — 5100 = 2900 kJ more energy required
This balance is divided by 38 (because 1 g fat yields 38 kJ), giving the patient a daily requirement of approximately 76 g fat.

Fibre

Following the widespread research undertaken to ascertain the role of fibre in the maintenance of good diabetic control, current practice is to include large amounts in the diabetic diet. Some of the studies indicated that the consumption of water-soluble gums and pectins results in improved blood glucose levels, possibly because they form gels and delay gastric emptying. In particular pulses (legumes), with a low glycaemic index — possibly due to reduced digestibility — should be liberally used, as also salads, fibrous fruit and wheat bran, within the framework of the diabetic diet.

In conclusion, the recommended diabetic diet must be tailored to the patient's income, way of life and family circumstances. The goals of the regimen are the same for the juvenile-onset and the maturity-onset diabetic:

1. to retain the blood sugar (i.e. glucose) concentration within normal limits, avoiding both glycosuria and hypoglycaemia;
2. to supply adequate amounts of nutrients;
3. to maintain or restore health and keep the weight at a normal level;
4. to modify fat intake so that the levels of serum cholesterol and lipids will reduce the likelihood of atherosclerosis;
5. to be adaptable to changes in life-style of the patient.

It is vital that the diabetic understands both the need for his diet and the basis on which it has been compiled.

Distribution of the diet

The nutritional demands of the juvenile- and maturity-onset diabetic differ, as discussed earlier.

The *maturity-onset* patient is often overweight and is advised to adhere to a weight reduction regimen with or without oral agents to lower blood sugar. Those being treated by diet alone should take three meals a day, in the first place because regular small meals cause more manageable demands on the pancreas and, secondly, because 'skipping' meals often results in the consumption of high-carbohydrate snacks. Furthermore, those on short-term hypoglycaemic agents (e.g. tolbutamide) also need food to compensate for the blood sugar lowering effect of these drugs taken at meal-times.

Juvenile diabetics, however, and those on once-daily hypogly-caemic oral agents, should have three meals and three mid-meal snacks per day to counteract the effect of their single daily long-acting drug or insulin injection, whether long-acting or soluble insulin is being used. The comparative effect of three large meals as opposed to six smaller ones in this situation is graphically depicted in Fig. 10. It is obvious that the dramatic preprandial (before meals) drop in the blood sugar and the postprandial (after meals) elevation beyond normal limits is not indicative of satisfactory control. Distribution of the diet over six smaller snacks causes less impact on the blood sugar level. Smaller intervals between food intake result in a smaller drop in blood sugar concentration.

As can be seen from Fig. 10, the blood sugar lowering effect of soluble insulin taken at, say, 7 a.m. commences almost immediately but is soon counteracted by breakfast. (*After any injection containing soluble insulin, food must be taken within half an hour.*) Later in the day, should an interval of more than about 2½–3 hours be allowed to elapse between food intakes, the blood sugar level will drop below normal limits; hence the great importance of mid-meal snacks. Long-acting insulin exerts its hypoglycaemic effect for up to 24 hours and it can thus be seen that the late evening snack is of particular importance. When small meals are taken more frequently, there is also less chance that hyperglycaemic peaks, as indicated on the graph, will occur.

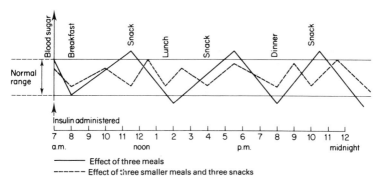

Fig. 10. *The effect of blood sugar levels of food intake after an insulin injection.*

PRACTICAL DIETARY MANAGEMENT

It is understandable that patients are sometimes upset or depressed when the diagnosis of diabetes is made. To be confronted with a negative attitude and a prohibitive, complex diet will not cheer the unhappy patient. It is thus strongly advised that patients be given a diet based on a carbohydrate exchange system, which can be modified to the individual's way of life. A nurse with a cheerful, positive attitude rather than a restrictive approach will greatly help the patient, bewildered by a regimen which encroaches on his life-style.

Initially, it is advisable to weigh out certain foods like bread, potatoes, etc., or to use appropriate food models to indicate food portion sizes to patients. In a short period of time the patient's familiarity with the regimen will help him to be more adept at estimating quantities. However, regular reinforcement is necessary as an over-casual attitude to the diet often develops after some time and this is to the detriment of the patient's blood sugar control.

Interchangeable portions of 10 g of carbohydrate are the cornerstone of the diet. Although both the fruit and 'starch' portions given below are similar in carbohydrate content, they are classified separately to encourage inclusion of both in the diet. However, where finances prevent the inclusion of a wide variety of foods, a bigger proportion of carbohydrates may be taken as starch. Furthermore, although milk is included below as a source of carbohydrate, it should be used as an interchangeable item only in exceptional circumstances: generally, it should be included routinely due to its high nutritional content.

Patients in hospital are usually given 400–800 kJ (100–200 Cal) less than on their return home to greater activity. This should be made clear to patients, i.e. that they increase their intake in relation to their increase in activity.

Exchange list

STARCHES. The following foods taken in the amount mentioned are interchangeable. Each provides 10 g of carbohydrate. Cooked weights are given for all foods.

Potato	1 medium (60 g)
Porridge	½ teacup
Vegetables	beetroot, parsnips, peas, dried or broad beans, or sweet potatoes 2 tablespoons
Bread	1 slice, 1 cm thick (20 g)

Rice	2 tablespoons cooked
Breakfast cereal	cornflakes or rice crispies 3 tablespoons
Pasta	macaroni or spaghetti 2 tablespoons
Biscuits	2 cream cracker biscuits, water biscuits or similar crackers
Milk	200 ml
Yoghurt	1 small carton
Ovaltine etc.	2 teaspoonsful Ovaltine, Horlicks or similar drink
Potato crisps	1 packet
Other pulses	soya beans ½ teacup

FRUIT. The following fruit portions are interchangeable and may be taken raw, stewed or baked. The weights are 'as purchased'.

Apple	1 (approx. 100 g)
Apricots	2 medium
Banana	1 small banana
Grapes	8
Melon	1 large slice
Peach	1 medium
Pear	1 medium
Pineapple	½ cup, diced
Plums	3 large
Orange	1 medium
Strawberries	⅔ cup
Fresh fruit juice	1 small glass

Although clearly defined limits must be set for the diabetic, the inclusion of certain foods in unrestricted amounts can be a tremendous morale booster. Giving the patient a list of foods which may be taken as desired increases rapport and helps ensure co-operation. The following foods have relatively little carbohydrate and a low energy content and are therefore considered to be 'free foods'. However, many of these foods do still contain some carbohydrate albeit in small amounts. This means that the excessive amounts that the occasional voracious patient consumes (e.g. a bunch of carrots or half a cauliflower) will contribute considerable carbohydrate and patients should be made to realize that this is not recommended.

asparagus	cress	runner beans	rhubarb
broccoli	marrow	cauliflower	sprouts

cabbage	celery	cucumber	turnips
carrots	onions	radishes	peppers
lettuce	swedes	tomatoes	spinach

Seasoning: all herbs and spices, horseradish, unsweetened pickles, curry

Liquids: clear soup, tea, coffee (not sweetened essence), meat and vegetable extract (Marmite etc.), lemon juice

Sample menu

Breakfast
  2 carbohydrate portions, e.g.:
    1 portion of fruit and a slice of toast
    or a bowl of porridge with milk from ration
    or baked beans on toast
  1 slice poached haddock
  7g (1 teaspoon) of polyunsaturated margarine
  tea with milk from ration

Mid-morning
  2 cracker biscuits or a thin slice of toast
  1 teaspoon polyunsaturated margarine
  coffee or tea with milk from ration

Lunch
  2 thin slices of bread or 2 other carbohydrate exchanges
  2 teaspoons of polyunsaturated margarine
  2–3 tablespoons of cheese (preferably low-fat cheese)
  1 fruit
  salad (tomato, lettuce, carrots, cucumber)

Mid-afternoon
  same as mid-morning

Dinner
  fat-free broth made with unrestricted vegetables
  chicken fried in oil
  either 1 potato and 1 portion of fruit for dessert
  or 2 other carbohydrate exchanges, e.g. peas, spaghetti
  cabbage and marrow

Bedtime
  1 fruit or 2 plain biscuits
  tea or coffee with milk from ration

Daily milk ration: 200 ml (⅓ pint) preferably skimmed

Note: Patients on long-acting therapy may need a more substantial snack at bedtime; additional cheese, milk or nuts may be recommended. It may be advisable to withhold some food from the previous meal if there is concern about overweight.

DIABETIC INVALID'S DIET

The diabetic who is debilitated (e.g. after surgery) or anorexic may at times prefer lighter foods to the hearty menu given above. These patients may be given 10 g carbohydrate exchanges as follows:

Fruit juice	1 small glass
Porridge	½ cup strained oats
Skimmed milk	200 ml
Jelly	2 dessertspoons
Soup	½ cup, cream of vegetable
Ginger ale	½ cup

The following diet is suggested as a short-term emergency replacement for patients receiving their usual dose of insulin or oral hypoglycaemic agent who are unable to eat their normal diet.

Sample menu

The following menu contains approx. 190 g of carbohydrate. The ingredients should be evenly divided between six meals.

Oatmeal	1 teacup, cooked measure
Milk	1 pint (600 ml)
Eggs	1
Orange juice	1 pint (600 ml)
Bread/biscuits	6 slices of toast (or 12 cream crackers), spread with 30 g of butter
Banana	1 large (or 2 small)
Soup	1 cup, cream of mushroom

The questions patients ask

How does a vegetarian diabetic manage?

Ovolactovegetarians have less of a problem than vegans. The

former should replace two or three of their carbohydrate exchanges with milk and their meat and fish portions should be replaced with cheese, cottage cheese, yoghurt and eggs. Soya, peas, beans, lentils and chickpeas should also play a prominent role in the vegetarian diabetic's diet — particularly the limited diet of the vegan: 50 g cooked peas, beans and lentils, 100 g cooked soya beans and 35 g cashew nuts are each equivalent to one portion of starch plus the protein portion for that meal. Similarly, 3 tablespoons of peanut butter are equivalent to one carbohydrate and one protein portion. However, cashew nuts and peanuts have a higher fat content than legumes and therefore contribute a considerably greater amount of energy.

A major problem with vegetarians is that they frequently eat a large amount of rice and potatoes. For example, Hindus traditionally enjoy a plate of vegetable curry or vegetable breyani (hot spiced stewed vegetables) with rice. The need to control their carbohydrate intake should be stressed to these patients.

What about artificial sweeteners?

Although theoretically it may be preferable for diabetics to try and lose the taste for sugar completely, studies have shown that many diabetics find that the use of artificial sweeteners increases the variety and palatability of the diet. Horwitz reports the findings of Court who ascertained that 72% of the mothers interviewed used artificial sweeteners for their diabetic children. Mehnert, too, found that only 17% of the diabetics in his study could do without sweets.

The question, then, is which sweetener to use? This has for some years been a highly controversial question. The three main sweeteners and their attributes are as follows:

1. Cyclamate is a compound approximately 450 times as sweet as sugar, which has recently lost favour due to reported carcinogenicity when taken in large quantity. It was previously widely used both domestically and in the processing industry, its main advantages being a true sweet flavour with little after-taste and stability at high temperatures.
2. Saccharin, which has a similar sweetening strength, has more recently come under scrutiny regarding toxicity. It is less

expensive than most other sweeteners but is of limited use because of its instability at cooking temperatures.

3. Aspartame. Unlike the two above which are non-nutritive compounds, this is regarded as a nutritive sweetener. It enters normal metabolic pathways, and is broken down to the amino acids phenylalanine and aspartic acid. It is approximately 180–200 times as sweet as sugar and has a true sweet flavour but loses this at cooking temperatures. This is most suitable for sweetening beverages such as tea and coffee.

What about other sugars?

Both fructose and sorbitol are sometimes advised for diabetics. These sugars have a much less dramatic elevating effect on the blood sugar concentration and do not require insulin for metabolism, while containing the same energy per gram as sucrose. They have the advantage over cane sugar of being sweeter so that smaller quantities are required. Small amounts may be taken by diabetics who are not overweight, but some patients cannot tolerate even limited quantities of sorbitol, because of its purgative effect.

Which 'diabetic' or 'dietetic' foods are acceptable?

Fruit canned *'without sugar'* (i.e. the water-packed product or that sweetened with artificial sweetener) still contains fruit sugar and should be taken in the same quantity as fresh fruit. Artificially sweetened *fruit gums* and *chewing gum* are suitable for diabetics. *Diabetic chocolate* has a high saturated fat content and consequently a high energy value and thus large amounts are inadvisable. *Sweets, blancmanges, biscuits* and *cakes*, while not being sweetened with sugar, are still often made with many other ingredients unsuitable for diabetics. *Fruit cordials* contain a small amount of carbohydrate derived from the base and so each glass of the made-up drink contains about as much energy as a quarter of a slice of bread. Similarly, dietetic *cola drinks* should not be taken in enormous amounts, not because of any carbohydrate content but because of the caffeine present. The practice of drinking more than a litre of such drinks per day, occasionally encountered in diabetics, is not to be encouraged. *Diabetic jams* retain the sugar present in the fruit, but as they are seldom eaten in any quantity due to their high cost, they may provide a welcome change occasionally. The sorbitol present may prompt diarrhoea if taken in large amounts.

What about the effect of exercise on food intake?

Physical activity is to be encouraged in diabetics except in exceptional circumstances. It stimulates the blood circulation, increases energy expenditure and lowers blood sugar levels. This latter aspect is of particular importance if the satisfactory control achieved in hospital is lost when the patient returns home and resumes his former activities. The diet must often be increased to allow for additional exercise. For this reason the patient who is admitted to hospital for purposes of control should be encouraged to undertake at least mild exercise as soon as this is possible. Exercise helps to maintain good control and the insulin requirement is often reduced. The diabetic should take an extra one or two 10 g portions of carbohydrate, as well as additional protein or fat for prolonged sustenance, prior to participating in physical activity. If the exercise is strenuous or extended, an additional carbohydrate portion should be taken afterwards as well. On such occasions controlled amounts of sweetened foods are justified, as the sugar has an early effect on the blood sugar level. Examples of sweetened foods containing 10 g carbohydrate include:

50 g of vanilla ice-cream or sorbet
2 sponge finger biscuits
1 crumpet
1 chocolate wholemeal biscuit
20 ml (1 level tablespoon) of full-cream sweetened condensed milk
60 g (2 dessertspoons) of ordinary canned fruit with juice
125 ml (1 small glass) of cola or other carbonated beverage

NURSING CONSIDERATIONS

Constant balance between insulin injections and food intake is essential. Regarding insulin-dependent diabetics:

1. When patients feel too ill to eat the required meal, give them an alternative source of carbohydrate (see Diabetic invalid diet).
2. If they need to fast prior to a procedure, check with the doctor before administering insulin. A much lower dose will normally be given; small dosages will sometimes be omitted altogether until later.
3. If the patient will be absent from the ward during the time that a meal or snack would normally be consumed, ensure that a cheese or peanut butter sandwich is taken along with instructions to eat it only at the usual time.

Regarding non-insulin diabetics:

1. These invariably overweight patients should be regularly monitored to ensure weight loss.
2. Patients should understand that the hypoglycaemic effect of the oral agents must be counteracted with food and that at least three regular meals providing a small amount of complex carbohydrate are essential for maintaining normal blood sugar levels.

Regarding *all* diabetics:

1. Check the bedside locker for food brought in by visitors and confirm that both day and night staff are aware that the patient should not be offered sugar with beverages served, nor fruit cordials (e.g. lemon squash) or sweetened drinks (e.g. drinking chocolate).
2. When therapy starts, patients should be made aware of the symptoms of hypoglycaemia. Should a patient have a hypoglycaemic attack, ascertain the next insulin dosage from the doctor, as less will be required. Standard practice is usually to give half the usual dose of insulin for the 24 hour period following the hypoglycaemic attack.

BIBLIOGRAPHY

Bantle, J., Laine, D., Castle, G., Thomas, J., Hoogwerf, B. & Goetz, F. (1983) Postprandial glucose and insulin responses to meals containing different carbohydrates in normal and diabetic subjects. *N. Eng. J. Med., 309*, 7.
British Medical Journal (1970) Diets for diabetics. *Br. Med. J., 2*, 66.

Court, J.M. (1972) *Your Child has Diabetes*. London: William Heinemann Medical Books.

Craig, O. (1977) *Childhood Diabetes and its Management*. London: Butterworth.

Creak, S. (1978) Observations on juvenile diabetics in a metabolic ward. *J. Hum. Nutr., 32*, 289.

Horwitz, D. (1983) Can Aspartame meet our expectations? *J. Am. Diet. Ass., 83*, 142.

Jackson, W.P.V. & Vinik, A.I. (1977) *Diabetes Mellitus, Clinical and Metabolic: A Shorter Textbook*. Cape Town: Juta.

Jenkins, D. (1982) Lente carbohydrate: a newer approach to diabetes mellitus. *Diabetes Care, 5*, 634.

Jenkins, D., Taylor, R. & Wolever, T. (1982) The diabetic diet, dietary carbohydrate and differences in digestibility. *Diabetologia, 23*, 477.

Nutrition Subcommittee of the British Diabetic Association's Medical Advisory Committee (1981) Dietary recommendations for diabetes for the 1980s. Final Draft, July 1981.

Nuttall, F. (1983) Diet and the diabetic patient. *Diabetes Care, 6*, 197.

Oakley, W.G., Pyke, D.A. & Taylor, K.W. (1975) *Diabetes and its Management*, 2nd edn. Oxford: Blackwell Scientific.

Ostman, J. (ed.) (1969) *Diabetes: Proceedings of 6th Congress of the International Diabetic Federation*. Amsterdam: Excerpta Medica.

Paxinos, R. & Ferguson, R. (1978) Juvenile diabetes — a team approach. *J. Hum. Nutr., 32*, 294.

Ricketts, H.T. (1976) Fiber and diabetes. *J. Am. Med. Ass., 236(20)*, 2321.

Soskin, S. (1941) The blood sugar: its origin, regulation and utilization. *Physiol. Rev., 21*, 140.

Tredger, J. & Ransley, J. (1978) Guar gum — its acceptability to diabetic patients when incorporated into baked food products. *J. Hum. Nutr., 32*, 427.

Tunbridge, R. & Wetherill, J.H. (1970) Reliability and cost of diabetic diets. *Br. Med. J., 2*, 78.

Williams, R.H. (ed.) (1965) *Diabetes*. New York: Harper and Row.

8   Digestive tract disorders

The digestive tract is a highly complex organ nearly 9 m in length, the functions of which are to convey ingested food from the mouth to the rectum by a series of peristaltic movements, and to convert the food, through the actions of numerous specific enzymes, into substances which can be utilized and absorbed by the body. More than any other organ, it reflects the physiological and psychological status of the individual. The nurse will notice repeatedly that in disorders of the digestive tract it is the patient and not the gut which must be the prime target of treatment. This aspect will be elaborated on where appropriate in this chapter.

PHYSIOLOGY

In various areas throughout the digestive tract there are a variety of enzymes, each of which plays a specific role in the digestion of food. These enzymes are catalytic agents produced by the cells in the mucosal lining. They are produced in clearly defined areas and each is responsible for the splitting of an individual food component into simpler substances.

Digestion (Fig. 11) commences in the mouth. The food is masticated into small particles and mixes with the saliva which moistens the food, making it more manageable and helping with its transport through the digestive tract. Saliva contains the enzyme *amylase* which hydrolyses *starch* to *dextrins*. On being swallowed the food is conveyed to the stomach by oesophageal peristalsis, which is assisted by gravity when the patient is upright. The food is allowed to enter the stomach by a relaxation of the *gastro-oesophageal sphincter* at the lower end of the oesophagus, which then constricts again to retain the stomach contents. The food now makes contact with the gastric juices which contain weak *hydrochloric acid* and the enzyme *pepsin*, and forms what we call *chyme*, the partially digested food mixture.

Several factors influence the secretion of hydrochloric acid. In the first place, sensory stimuli such as the thought, appearance, aroma and taste of food increase gastric acid output, whereas tension or 'unappetizing' stimuli decrease the output. Certain foods also have a specific effect on gastric acid secretion. Alcohol and meat extracts increase secretion, whereas fat and protein have inhibitory effects. One useful effect of this is that foods that are predominantly protein or fat take longer to be digested and therefore have a greater satiety effect.

Food leaves the stomach by way of the *pyloric canal* after a ariable length of time in the stomach that depends on both the texture and the composition of the food. Under normal circumstances, liquids leave the stomach within half an hour, carbohydrates take a little longer, and proteins and fats may remain up to six hours in the stomach, undergoing partial digestion during this period.

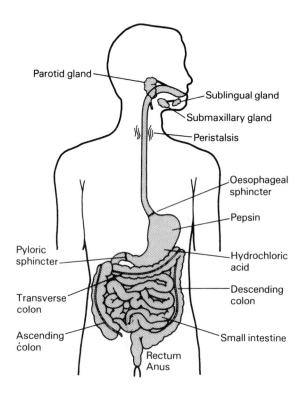

Fig. 11. *Normal digestion.*

The small intestine

The major digestion of all nutrients occurs predominantly in the *duodenum* and *upper jejunum* and to a lesser extent in the *lower jejunum* and *ileum* (Fig. 12). The *terminal ileum* is the site for absorption of *bile acids* and *vitamin B_{12}* and in diseases of this part of the small intestine (e.g. Crohn's disease) inadequate absorption of these substances occurs. A variety of enzymes are secreted by the mucosal glands and digestion is aided by the entry into the digestive tract of *bile*, the secretion of which is stimulated by the presence of food in the duodenum. Furthermore, the acid chyme stimulates the output of a hormone, *secretin*, which stimulates the secretion of pancreatic juice into the small intestine. This raises the pH of the chyme which becomes alkaline — a conversion necessary for the action of the intestinal enzymes. The pancreatic

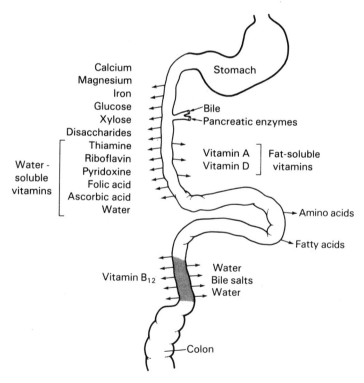

Fig. 12. *Areas of nutrient absorption in the digestive tract.*

juice transports the pancreatic enzymes to the chyme to help with digestion.

Carbohydrates are converted to disaccharides by *pancreatic amylase* and then further reduced to glucose by the action of *lactase, maltase* and *sucrase* (see Chapter 1). *Proteins* are converted to simpler compounds by *trypsin* enzymes and then reduced to amino acids by the *peptidases. Fats* are emulsified by bile and reduced by *lipases* to fatty acids. Vitamins and minerals are released and made available, and intestinal bacteria degrade the cellulose.

The wall of the small intestine is covered with *villi*. There are four or five million of these small, finger-like projections or tufts, which are rich in capillaries. Absorption of nutrients into the blood stream occurs through these villi, assisted by peristaltic movement.

The fibre in food is unaffected by the enzymes in the human digestive tract (unlike the situation in animals which are equipped to utilize it for energy purposes). Fibre is necessary to form bulk in the stool and promote peristalsis and evacuation.

The large intestine

The primary function of the large intestine is to concentrate the remaining digestive mass. Peristalsis promotes contact between the liquid chyme and the absorptive surface of the intestinal wall which results in the absorption of water and considerable reduction in the volume of stool. Speed of passage through the large bowel is largely dependent on the proportion of fibre present in the chyme — a low-fibre diet provides little stimulus for peristaltic contractions and emptying time is prolonged (as discussed under Constipation.)

DISORDERS OF THE UPPER DIGESTIVE TRACT

Numerous abnormalities can occur at different sites in the digestive tract. Organic changes of the mucosal wall, variation in peristaltic movements, and inhibition of enzyme output are all abnormalities which may result in symptoms.

Oesophagitis

Oesophagitis is caused by reflux of gastric contents precipitated by decreased gastro-oesophageal sphincter pressure. This results in the characteristic symptom of heartburn which is probably the most common gastrointestinal symptom encountered today. Nebel suggests that 36% of normal people suffer from heartburn at least once a month, with a considerably higher incidence in pregnant women. In people with suboptimal sphincter competency, oesophagitis can be precipitated by the ingestion of specific foods. The mechanism of these food intolerances is not completely understood but it appears that fatty foods, alcohol and chocolate reduce the constriction of the gastro-oesophageal sphincter. Other food items such as strongly spiced dishes, orange juice, and carbonated beverages and coffee cause heartburn by direct irritation of the mucosal lining of the oesophagus; smoking has the same effect. Patients should be advised to avoid irritating foods and also to eat small meals to reduce gastric reflux. The overweight patient will often have more frequent symptoms owing to the pressure of adiposity. The condition is alleviated by slow drinking of buffering liquid such as milk to wash out the oesophagus. Most patients are told to remain upright for 1– 1½ hours after meals to prevent symptoms by minimizing reflux.

Acute oesophagitis caused by the ingestion of caustic or corrosive compounds must be treated with great caution as ingestion of coarse foods can result in perforation. Initially, parenteral feeding may be necessary to allow healing, but less severely affected individuals are fed from the start with a bland semi-solid diet. With improvement of the oesophageal wall the texture of the diet is liberalized.

Hiatus hernia

A hiatus hernia is a protrusion of a loop of the stomach through a gap in the diaphragm. It is a common condition, particularly in women, and particularly with advancing age. Burkitt and James suggest that the prevalence of the condition in Western communities may be related to our low-residue diet and subsequent exaggerated bowel contractions which result in increased intraluminal pressure. The condition may run an asymptomatic course. However, some patients may experience symptoms ranging from discomfort to severe chest pain (often confused with cardiac pain), especially if the hernia is complicated by oesophagitis (which occurs commonly) or by stricture. Heartburn, regurgitation, epigastric pain, vomiting and even bleeding may occur. Swallowing may cause pain and if the stricture is severe the patient may not be able to swallow solids.

Surgical treatment is occasionally necessary but generally medical treatment is effective. The basic aim of such therapy is to reduce oesophageal reflux. The patient is advised to sleep with his head well elevated, to avoid wearing constricting belts and not to go to bed soon after a large meal. Antacids will help neutralize the stomach contents so that should reflux occur there will be less damage to the oesophageal lining. The main dietary modification is weight reduction where necessary, as the reduction in abdominal pressure is extremely effective in alleviating symptoms. Other dietary changes which are helpful are avoidance of foods causing oesophagitis (discussed above) and reduction of foods with a high content of coarse fibre; pips, fruit skins and coarse fibrous vegetables such as cabbage and onions readily cause the production of gas with subsequent distension of the stomach. The recommendations made in Appendix A (The low-fibre diet) are often helpful. Should stricture occur, the semi-solid diet discussed in Chapter 16 is appropriate.

Gastritis

Gastritis is inflammation of the gastric lining. It is characterized by nausea, vomiting, epigastric pain and bleeding. It can occur as a single acute episode or chronically and may be due to alcohol, smoking, infections or ingestion of toxins and irritating substances. It may initially be necessary to feed the patient intravenously, but as soon as vomiting stops small quantities of easy digestible fluids such as milk, sweetened tea and jellies are given. Milk is particularly useful because of its acid-buffering reaction and its inhibitory effect on gastric acid secretion: the consumption of a glass of milk can cause the pH of the stomach contents to rise from about 2 to over 5. Within a few days, a bland diet can be introduced with continued emphasis on frequent small meals. Foods can be selected from those included in Appendix A. This modified diet may be necessary for one or two weeks, after which the patient may return to a normal regimen. Naturally the cornerstone of treatment of the condition is removal of the cause (e.g. alcohol or orally ingested drugs) to prevent recurrence of the inflammatory state.

The peptic ulcer

A peptic ulcer is a lesion in the mucous membrane of the stomach (*gastric ulcer*) or duodenum (*duodenal ulcer*). It occurs when for some reason the mucosal lining loses its inherent resistance to the digestive juices, which then erode an area in the membrane. This mechanism is not well understood.

Aetiology

Peptic ulcer is a commonly encountered condition. It has been estimated that 5–10% of the population of the UK suffer from it. There is no evidence that diet plays a role in the aetiology of ulcer formation, but a variety of other environmental factors have been correlated to increased risk. Stress, seasonal changes and analgesics have all been implicated. Although the pathogenesis of the disease remains unclear, it appears to be less frequent in the UK than it was in the 1960s and although previously it was encountered largely in higher-income groups, today it is seen more commonly in poorer people. A recent editorial in the *Lancet* comments: 'if the cause of ulcer remains poorly understood, the logical basis of treatment totally escapes us'.

Diet

Early this century, when Sippy introduced his regimen of frequent small feedings of milk and cream, milk played a prominent role in the ulcer diet. The Sippy diet was based on the understanding that the fat would inhibit gastric juice secretion and that the acid-buffering effect of the milk would be protective to the stomach lining and assist in the healing of the ulcer. Some years later the diet was modified by Meulengracht, who introduced a more liberal regimen — the bland diet which was used as the basis of diet therapy for many years afterwards. It was based on the principle of omitting foods that were mechanically, chemically or thermally irritating.

It is only during the last 10–15 years that these principles have been seriously challenged. It became clear that the restrictions of the 'ulcer diet' were largely traditional, and scientific understanding questioned the concepts on which the diet was based. From studies which compared the effect of the traditional ulcer diet on patients with gastric ulcers with the effect of an unrestricted diet on a similar group, it emerged that there was no difference in response between the two groups. Fried foods, spicy foods and those with a high fibre content appeared to have no detrimental effect on the healing of the ulcer or its symptoms of pain and discomfort, and milky diets appeared to be no more effective in terms of positive improvement, nor did they have any particularly 'soothing' effect on the stomach lining. Furthermore, it appeared that the bland diet might even be harmful in that it was extremely difficult to include all necessary nutrients in such a restricted diet. This diet, based primarily on milk, is also inadvisable for those with a tendency to hypercholesterolaemia, or lactose intolerance.

However, there are a few rules which are still considered useful, particularly for patients with a gastric rather than a duodenal ulcer. Such patients suffer more from food-induced symptoms and are also at risk of developing carcinoma, a complication not seen with a duodenal ulcer. These rules are as follows:

1. *Small frequent feedings* are of major importance in reducing acidity and alleviating symptoms. Patients should be advised to take five small meals each day in preference to three large ones. Late evening snacks stimulate nocturnal acid secretion and patients should be discouraged from eating immediately before retiring.
2. *Alcohol* causes excessive secretion of stomach juices. Patients are thus advised to drink in moderation and then only if the alcohol is buffered by a meal. Smoking is usually only allowed immediately after meals, if at all. *Caffeine* has the same effect, and so strong *tea, coffee* and *cola* beverages should not be taken in large amounts.
3. Certain *spices* have been shown to cause gastric irritation. These include *chilli powder, black pepper* and *mustard seed*, and avoidance of these and other strong spicy foods is thus generally recommended to reduce symptoms.
4. Patients should be advised to *eat slowly* and masticate their food properly. This is also important from a psychological

aspect, as *relaxation* and *reduction of tension* are cornerstones of the management of ulcer patients.

5. There is no evidence that coarse, fibrous foods are badly tolerated by these patients, if well chewed, but individuals without teeth, or with ill-fitting false ones, should possibly limit their intake of excessively fibrous foods.

It must be stressed that considerable controversy remains about the subject of what constitutes a good diet for an ulcer patient. There are still some conservative practitioners who maintain that the low-residue diet plays an important role in the therapy of ulcers, and there are patients who have less discomfort on a restricted dietary regimen. Furthermore, psychological factors are of enormous importance in digestive tract disorders. Active participation in a trusted form of management is often of great psychological value to these patients. They should, at all times, feel that they are involved with the management of their disease and should be advised to avoid any foods which they do not tolerate well. Most patients will find that they are free of symptoms on a normal diet, omitting only a few selected items, and well distributed throughout the day; a few may find that the low-fibre diet (see Appendix A) is more suitable.

Bleeding ulcer

A peptic ulcer may haemorrhage, causing haematemesis and melaena with associated symptoms of nausea and vomiting. In the case of massive bleeding, shock and even loss of consciousness can occur. In severe cases surgical intervention is necessary; in others conservative medical treatment is effective.

In the past, the patient with a bleeding ulcer was starved for the first few days in order to 'rest the stomach'. Chips of ice were given to keep the mouth moist with a limited fluid intake, but all other foods were withheld. However, current therapy is more liberal, as it has been found that regular small feedings help to reduce acidity and inhibit gastric acid output. Initially, parenteral feeding or limitation to clear fluids may be necessary, but within a few days, when vomiting has subsided, feeding commences with frequent small meals of light, bland foods. Large quantities of food and fibre must be avoided to prevent distension: feeding usually starts with milk, jelly, custard, sweetened tea and milk soups, in quantities of approximately 150 ml every one or two hours. Within a few days the patient may be given larger quantities less frequently, and after seven to ten days the low-fibre diet discussed in Appendix A will be appropriate.

DISORDERS OF THE SMALL INTESTINE

In this part of the digestive tract, food components are broken down and absorbed and thus malabsorption states, with associated symptoms, will occur if there is inadequate enzyme activity or organic changes preventing normal absorptive processes.

Coeliac disease (gluten enteropathy)

Coeliac disease, also known as gluten enteropathy, is a congenital malabsorption disorder precipitated by exposure of the gut lining to gluten, the protein compound found in wheat, barley and rye. Atrophy of villi occurs, but this can be reversed by withdrawing the offending substance from the diet. The condition occurs in 1 in 1500 people and may be diagnosed both in children and in adults. It is generally regarded as a permanent disability: although there can be a remission of symptoms in teenagers and young adults there is often a return to the overt condition in later life.

In children, where it is more readily recognized, patients usually present with diarrhoea, with characteristic frothy, foul-smelling stools, a distended abdomen, irritability and weight loss. Symptoms occur after the introduction of mixed feeding, including foods containing flour. Adults may suffer from long-term ill-health, weight loss, diarrhoea, anaemia and oedema before the diagnosis of coeliac disease is established.

Aetiology

Gluten is composed of two compounds, *gliadin* and *glutenin*. It has been proposed that gliadin causes a biochemical defect in sensitive individuals. Although the mechanism is not well understood, it is thought that gliadin may either have a direct allergic effect or, alternatively, cause vulnerability of the villi and subsequent atrophy due to the toxic effect of partially metabolized gluten.

Diagnosis is usually confirmed by a jejunal biopsy.

Absorption of other nutrients is adversely affected, hence the frequent intolerance of fats. *Anaemia* is also a common complication, due to impaired iron and folic acid absorption; and degeneration of bone, with tetany and osteomalacia, can result from reduced absorption of calcium and vitamin D. Deficiencies of electrolytes and vitamins can result from excessive losses in diarrhoea.

Dietary management

Although the diet may at first glance appear to be a relatively easy one to follow — merely omitting bread, cake and biscuits from the normal diet — there are associated problems which make the application of the gluten-free diet rather complicated in practice:

1. There is controversy as to whether wheat, oats, barley and rye are the only foods to be avoided by these patients. Some workers exclude buckwheat from the diet.
2. Secondary lactose and sucrose intolerance may be present initially, and temporary adherence to a lactose-free or sucrose-free diet is often necessary to relieve symptoms.
3. The widespread use of flour and gluten-containing products in processed foods presents problems. Pudding powders, processed meat, stock cubes and packet soups frequently contain gluten. Even coffee from vending machines may have to be avoided for this reason. Food additives such as stabilizers, fillers, emulsifiers and cereal thickeners frequently contain wheat. Processed cheese, malted products and combination foods of unknown composition must all be omitted from the diet.
4. There may be psychological problems. Children's parties and school lunches can be traumatic experiences for the young coeliac, and the refusal of Communion bread may result in embarrassment for adults.
5. Although gluten-free flour and other products are available with an EC 10 form from Welfare Foods, Stockport (address: 63/65 Higher Hillgate, Stockport, Cheshire SK1 3HE), these are sometimes difficult to use as gluten is the fraction which causes elasticity in dough mixtures, resulting in retention of air and the rising of products made with flour (the word

'gluten' comes from the Latin word meaning glue). This effect is thus largely absent in gluten-free products and perseverance may be necessary to master the technique of producing acceptable gluten-free products.

It is of the greatest importance that the nurse take a positive attitude in assisting these patients to adapt to the dietary regimen. They should be strongly advised to join the Coeliac Society (address: PO Box 181, London NW2 2Q7), which has up-to-date lists of permitted processed foods, recipes and other helpful literature. Cookery demonstrations are also sometimes organized for groups of coeliac patients. Patients should be advised to emphasize fresh products in their diet rather than processed foods which can give rise to symptoms. A list of suppliers of various gluten-free products is given in Appendix D. The following foods may be included in a gluten-free diet:

all fruit and vegetables — fresh, frozen, dried, plain or canned, also fruit juices
all varieties of meat and fish (including smoked) (*except* sausages, mince dishes with flour or breadcrumbs, or processed meat such as corned beef and luncheon loaves)
milk of all types
eggs and cheese (*except* processed spreads)
maize (including cornflour, custard powder and cornflakes)
rice (including rice crispies, puffed rice and 'baby rice')
soya flour and tapioca
butter, margarine, oil
herbs, spices, Marmite, Bovril and similar extracts
tea, coffee and cocoa
sugar, jam and honey
products made from gluten-free flour, arrowroot, potato and rice flours
plain sweets and chocolates (*excluded* are liquorice, filled chocolates and other combination sweets such as Smarties, Kit Kat, etc.)

It is emphasized that this is essentially a brief summary of appropriate foods and that a comprehensive list of foods should be obtained by the patient either from the local dietitian or directly from the Coeliac Society.

Disaccharide intolerance

Under normal circumstances carbohydrates are first broken down to disaccharides in the gut. These are then acted upon by disaccharidase enzymes (lactase, maltase and sucrase) in the brush border of the small intestine to produce monosaccharides. When there is enzyme deficiency, the sugars are used by intestinal bacteria which cause fermentative diarrhoea, resulting in losses of not only sugar but also other nutrients due to accelerated peristalsis. Abdominal cramps, distension and irritability may also be present. The condition may occur either as a congenital primary abnormality or secondary to a disease process in the intestinal wall. The latter situation may be transient, and reversible by withdrawal of the offending sugars until the intestinal function has returned to normal. Causes of secondary disaccharide intolerance include gastrointestinal infection, gastrointestinal surgery, malnutrition, drug-induced inhibition of lactase output, and radiotherapy for cancer.

Lactase deficiency

Lactase deficiency can occur as a relative or an absolute deficiency and may be either permanent or temporary. This defect occurs widely as a congenital abnormality in Asian and Negro people: in a recent study in American school children it was found that 40% of the black children who refused the subsidized milk programme did so as a result of a relative lactose intolerance. Figures of incidence vary, but it has been suggested that up to 90% of Asians and Negroes are affected. A recent study in Israel also demonstrated an extremely high incidence.

It appears that lactase activity is directly related to the lactose content of the diet. If dietary lactose is drastically reduced when the infant is weaned there is a greater possibility of rapid decline in lactase activity. It can also occur as part of the normal process of ageing. Acquired lactose intolerance can result from mucosal damage, which may be caused by:

1. disease states such as acute gastroenteritis (especially in infants), coeliac disease,
2. surgery to the gastrointestinal tract,
3. administration of certain drugs,
4. debilitation resulting from kwashiorkor.

Diet therapy

Milk and all foods containing milk must be avoided. This includes processed foods which contain milk solids or whey (such as most margarines and confectionery), many drugs, in which lactose is used as a filler, and all foods of which the components are unknown. All medicines should be checked before use for even a small amount can have a detrimental effect on these patients. However, butter, cottage cheese and yoghurt are often well tolerated because of the breakdown of most of the lactose to lactic acid during the manufacture of these products. Initially, both cottage cheese and yoghurt should be administered cautiously to those with an absolute deficiency of lactase. This is because the action of microorganisms in commercially produced yoghurt is often stopped when the product reaches the required pH and it is possible that a small proportion of lactose remains intact. With regard to cottage cheese, a small amount of unconverted lactose may be present in the whey of smooth soft cheeses; thus the drier the cottage cheese, the less likelihood of lactose in the product. Permitted margarines include Tomor Kosher Margarine, Outline low-fat spread and also low-fat spreads made by Safeways and Sainsbury.

Sucrase-isomaltase deficiency

Although not commonly encountered, sucrase deficiency is occasionally seen in infants, or secondary to diffuse mucosal damage of the small intestine. Chronic diarrhoea is the predominant symptom, resulting in dehydration and malnutrition.

Diet therapy

Sugar must be avoided. This includes cane, beet and maple sugar, and also molasses and pineapple, which contain sucrose. Starch intolerance is seldom a problem as only negligible amounts of maltose are consumed, being present in malted products, barley and honey.

PANCREATITIS

Pancreatitis is an inflammatory disease of the pancreas, characterized by reduced secretion of digestive enzymes from the pancreas, affecting the absorption of protein, fat and carbohydrate. It is accompanied by nausea, vomiting and severe epigastric pain and can occur as a single isolated attack (acute pancreatitis) or recurrently (chronic pancreatitis). It is most commonly caused by excessive alcohol consumption or by cholelithiasis. Type V hyperlipidaemia can also precipitate the condition (see Chapter 9).

Chronic pancreatitis is often accompanied by steatorrhoea (due to fat malabsorption) and weight loss (due to nutrient losses in the stool, and the malnutrition usually accompanying alcoholism).

For the first three to five days until the acute episode subsides, patients are treated with parenteral feeding to replace fluid and electrolyte losses resulting from profuse vomiting. Thereafter, the patient is given small, easily digestible meals frequently throughout the day, both to prevent distension and to reduce the digestive load on the pancreas. The patient with chronic pancreatic insufficiency should continue with this regimen indefinitely. Preparations of pancreatic enzymes are often administered to assist with digestion.

Fat absorption is affected by impairment of pancreatic lipase secretion, but the high reserve potential of the digestive tract will promote absorption of a large proportion of the fat intake in many patients. However, those with steatorrhoea or Type V hyperlipidaemia are advised to reduce their fat intake to the minimum. Medium-chain triglycerides, which are absorbed in the absence of lipase, are often recommended as a source of supplementary kilojoules and to provide variety in the diet.

Carbohydrate absorption is impaired in most patients with acute pancreatitis but this problem usually resolves itself rapidly and insulin administration is seldom necessary. However, there is a high incidence of diabetes in patients with chronic pancreatitis and, should this occur, the dietary principles appropriate to diabetes will be applicable.

Protein will be digested largely through other compensatory mechanisms and thus, although pancreatic trypsin secretion may be minimal, patients are advised to have a high-protein diet.

CYSTIC FIBROSIS OF THE PANCREAS

This is a congenital disorder seen in children, causing degeneration of active cells into fibrous tissue and cysts, resulting in diminished output of pancreatic juices. Food is thus less efficiently digested and pronounced steatorrhoea occurs. Malfunctioning of mucus-producing glands in the bronchial tree results in chronic respiratory disease, and impairment of function of the sweat glands results in the secretion of sweat with a very high sodium and chloride content.

Diet therapy

These children absorb only about 50% of the food consumed, the balance being lost in the stool. Pancreatic enzymes such as Pancrex and Cotazyn are given orally with each meal to compensate for deficiency of natural enzymes and the patient is given a very high-kilojoule diet to make up for losses. Six smaller meals per day are preferable to three large ones.

Fat digestion is impaired owing to the reduced output of pancreatic lipase. Previously a severely reduced fat intake was recommended because of the increased excretion of fat seen in the stool. However, it has recently been shown that although fat excretion is increased when fat intake is increased, fat absorption is correspondingly improved. Today, fat intake is usually adjusted to individual tolerance and many patients need merely a moderate reduction in fat. Affected adolescents who have extremely high energy requirement may benefit from the inclusion of MCT oil to maintain an adequate energy intake.

Starch absorption may occasionally be impaired due to the steatorrhoea but sugars and starches should be emphasized, both for their protein-sparing effect and as a source of much-needed kilojoules.

Protein is well tolerated and should be prominent in the diet. Generous vitamin and mineral supplements are given to ensure adequate absorption.

DISORDERS OF THE LARGE INTESTINE

As mentioned earlier, the enzymatic breakdown of foods occurs predominantly in the small intestine. The function of the large intestine is primarily absorption and concentration of the faecal mass.

Ulcerative colitis

Ulcerative colitis is a chronic condition of ulceration of the mucosal lining of the colon, characterized by diffuse diarrhoea containing blood and mucus. Psychogenic factors play a prominent predisposing role and the condition is potentially malignant. It occurs predominantly in young adults. The diarrhoea can be accompanied by considerable losses of blood, of protein in the exudate from the raw surface and of other nutrients. Weight loss, anorexia, anaemia, dehydration and malnutrition result.

Diet therapy

A high-protein, high-energy intake with adequate vitamins and minerals forms the basis of dietary management. Coarse fibrous foods are avoided to prevent irritation of the colon and food is given throughout the day to ensure a satisfactory intake. A trial of milk withdrawal is advisable as milk intolerance is sometimes encountered in these patients. However, as milk is such a highly adaptable, nutritious food it should be introduced as soon as lactose intolerance is excluded, although the patient must be observed for the occurrence of aggravated diarrhoea.

These patients need supportive management and encouragement to participate in their treatment. Meals should be appetizing and nutritious, with emphasis on preferred foods. In some hospitals these patients are routinely supplied with snacks throughout the day and the nurses are instructed to repeatedly encourage the patient to eat these, not only to ensure an adequate intake but also as a form of supportive therapy and attention to the patient. Personality traits of tension, anxiety, insecurity, frustration and stress are commonly encountered in these patients who require emotional help possibly to a greater extent than others with gastrointestinal disease. The following sample menu is suggested once tolerance of milk is confirmed.

Sample menu (ulcerative colitis)

Breakfast
    fruit juice
    cereal (refined) with milk and sugar

2 eggs, scrambled, served with savoury mince
white toast, butter and smooth jam
milky tea with sugar

Mid-morning

peanut butter sandwiches and milk

Dinner

large helpings of roast chicken and rice, boiled potato, carrots
baked milk pudding and cream

Mid-afternoon

crackers, butter and cheese with Milo or a similar beverage

Supper

large helping of baked fish in cheese sauce, mash, avocado pear
stewed apple and custard

Bedtime

Ovaltine or similar beverage, chopped egg on toast

Additional daily ration

1 litre of high-energy milk (see Chapter 6)

Diverticulitis

Diverticular disease of the colon is characterized by the protrusion
of the inner lining of the large bowel through the muscular layer,
resulting in flask-like sacs forming outside the wall (diverticulosis:
Fig. 13).

These sacs most commonly occur in the sigmoid colon but every
part of the colon may be involved. Inflammation of these sacs (or
diverticula) is known as diverticulitis.

Diverticulosis is very common in the elderly and it is currently
thought possibly to result from the long-term consumption of a
low-residue diet. It appears that patients with diverticular disease
have a lower crude fibre intake than healthy controls: the
condition occurs less frequently in vegetarians than non-
vegetarians who consume significantly less fibre. Interestingly, the
rise in death rate from diverticular disease in Britain was halted
during the war and post-war years when white bread was not
available and sugar was rationed. In a recent editorial in the
Lancet it was stated that 'since the dietary fibre boom the number
of operations done for uncomplicated diverticular disease has
fallen impressively'.

The need for adequate fibre in the diet as a preventative

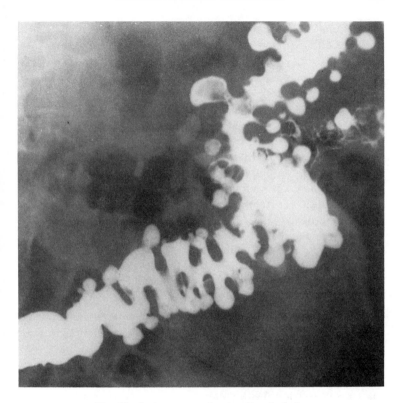

Fig. 13. *Barium enema showing diverticulosis.*

measure is thus stressed. Cereal fibre, in particular, is of great importance, as it is poorly digested by colonic bacteria and causes the greatest increase in stool weight and decrease in transit time. Whenever possible, patients, particularly older ones, should be encouraged to consume wholewheat bread, fruit and vegetables in an attempt to avoid diverticulosis or to reduce the inflammatory condition if the disorder is already present. This may in practice be difficult for many elderly people, both from financial considerations and because of the difficulties of carrying home quantities of perishable foods. Bran is an inexpensive and relatively light product and is a useful alternative: the daily use of one to three tablespoons of bran mixed with cereal or salad is a practical measure which most elderly people could employ. Adequate fluid (approximately eight glasses per day) is essential to combine with the fibre and cause an increase of faecal mass.

Diet therapy

Acute episodes are initially treated with low-residue foods and liquids (usually tea, jelly, fruit juices, etc.) to reduce irritation of the intestine, with progression in texture as soon as is practical. When they can be tolerated, bran and foods with a high cellulose content should be emphasized in the diet, although sometimes coarse fibrous items such as fruit pips and skins and hard particles such as cauliflower stalks cause discomfort and pain, in which case they should be avoided. The reader is referred to Appendix B for the high-residue diet.

Spastic colon (irritable colon)

'Spastic colon' is one of the most common digestive tract disorders. Known by several names, including irritable bowel syndrome and mucous colitis, it occurs more widely among women than men and is seen particularly in patients between the ages of 20 and 40. It is characterized by abnormal contractions of the colon causing abdominal pain and distension and constipation or diarrhoea associated with cramps. As with several other digestive tract disorders psychogenic factors play a prominent role in the aetiology of this condition and it is frequently seen in people who over-react to the stresses of every day living. The repeated lack of response to the urge for defecation, which is a common characteristic of people living rushed, irregular lives, has also been implicated as a causatory factor. Lack of exercise and a dietary pattern of hurried meals consisting predominantly of refined carbohydrates are also regarded as important contributory causes.

Education in improved habits of hygiene is an important part of treatment. The patient must understand the importance of regularity in eating, evacuation, relaxation and exercise.

Diet therapy

A high-fibre diet (see Appendix B) is recommended, with the inclusion of eight to ten glasses of liquid per day. Patients often react adversely to specific foods, especially coarse fibrous ones, which should be omitted from the diet. Patients should initially increase their fibre intake slowly as there may be aggravation of symptoms if a high-fibre diet is introduced too rapidly.

The patient with a spastic colon and diarrhoea presents a special problem. Many are unable to tolerate even normal amounts of fibre and for them a low-fibre diet (Appendix A) is necessary until the diarrhoea subsides, after which the diet should contain the maximum amount of fibre which can be tolerated without discomfort.

Constipation

Constipation is a disorder in which the evacuation of faeces occurs irregularly and with difficulty.

Many people have a regular bowel action daily, whereas others defecate less frequently. Constipation is thus a condition which is relative to normal regularity. Physical causes can be similar to those discussed above, i.e. repeatedly omitting to respond to the urge to defecate, lack of exercise and a hurried pattern of living, with poor eating habits. The major dietary causative factor is lack of adequate fibre and it has been shown repeatedly that the high-fibre diet produces an accelerated transit time in the gut, much larger stool weights and more frequent bowel actions. Interestingly, a study by Beyer *et al* showed that in addition to these effects, a high-fibre diet resulted in faecal losses of protein, fat, carbohydrate and energy which were more than double those of people on a similar diet with low fibre. Perhaps the common combination of people on a highly refined high-kilojoule diet being both obese and constipated is a self-perpetuating situation due to the increased efficiency of absorption of nutrients caused by a low-fibre diet.

Another factor which contributes to constipation is the consumption of insufficient fluid to combine with the fibre in the bowel. As mentioned in Chapter 2, wheat bran can absorb up to 200 times its weight in water and it is thus imperative that consumption of larger quantities of bran is accompanied by the drinking of additional beverages. The constipated individual should drink eight to ten glasses of liquid per day and consume adequate bran, fibrous fruit and vegetables (see Appendix B).

Dried prunes contain a fraction known as *diphenylisatin*, which prompts a gastrocolic reflex. Patients should thus be advised to take about six prunes daily, not only for the effect of the fibre in the gut but also because of this compound.

It is strongly recommended that the above simple dietary modifications should be attempted before resorting to potentially harmful purgatives. Should laxatives become necessary they should be used only intermittently to prevent dependence and loss of efficacy of the bowel.

Diarrhoea

Diarrhoea occurs when impaired absorption of fluids from the gut results in frequent discharge of liquid faeces. The condition can result from accelerated peristalsis due to infection, toxic substances (induced by drugs, bacteria, etc.), defective enzyme output (e.g. lactose intolerance) or organic disease. It is essential to diagnose the cause of the disorder as soon as possible rather than treat the patient symptomatically. For example, diarrhoea caused by pathogenic bacteria will be treated with antibiotics, and that due to lactose intolerance by milk withdrawal. Ulcerative colitis will be treated systemically. Severe diarrhoea, particularly in children, can rapidly result in dehydration and death if not treated quickly, and it is of the utmost importance that urgent attention is given to these patients. Diarrhoea in infants is discussed in Chapter 2.

Diet therapy

Fluid replacement is of paramount importance and the patient should drink — or be given intravenously if necessary — fluids adequate to replenish losses. The more profuse the diarrhoea, the greater the need for fluid. Potassium, sodium and chlorides are also required in increased amounts to replace losses, and these should be given in either drug or dietary form. In severe acute cases, clear fluids are usually given for 24 hours to rest the gut. Stock cubes or extracts such as Marmite and Bovril, dissolved in hot water, supply much-needed electrolytes and should be given several times a day. Weak tea, fruit juices (which are excellent sources of potassium) and 'degassed' carbonated beverages can also be included. Patients with severe diarrhoea who are weak and dehydrated are fed parenterally until depleted stores of fluids and electrolytes are replenished.

The treatment of milder cases, after the first 24 hours, is a subject of controversy. Most practitioners today recommend that the diet be rapidly liberalized to a low-fibre diet (Appendix A), whatever the state of the stools. More conservative treatment emphasizes the continued administration of very light bland foods such as gruels, thickened with refined starch (e.g. cornflour) or, more commonly in paediatric care, Nestargel, Arobon (which is a mixture of carob bean powder, starch and cocoa) or pectin (as grated apple or as a pharmaceutical product). These are bulk-producers and will reduce the discomfort and improve the consistency of the stools of many patients. However, until the bowel has fully recovered, fluids and electrolytes are of paramount importance in dietary management.

Crohn's disease

'Crohn's disease' is a term used to refer to chronic regional enteritis involving all or any area of the digestive tract, although seen principally in the distal ileum and colon. The area is chronically inflamed, with deep ulceration. The disease is usually progressive, but can go through periods of remission. The predominant feature is diarrhoea accompanied by rectal losses of mucus and blood. Fever, abdominal discomfort, generally poor health and intestinal obstruction are other common symptoms, and perianal fissures commonly occur.

Diet therapy

Patients are frequently malnourished due to losses in the stool and impaired absorption. A high-protein, high-energy intake to replenish depleted body stores is thus of primary importance. Patients are encouraged to take a high-kilojoule diet in the form of three meals a day with three additional snacks of high-protein foods. Potassium may be lost in copious quantities in the diarrhoea and emphasis on foods high in potassium is recommended practice. Vitamin supplements are often prescribed due to losses and reduced absorption. Medium-chain triglycerides are often included to allow increased absorption of fat. Only those foods which are low in residue are included because they have no irritating effect and a slow transit rate through the gut. As patients may be lactose intolerant, a trial of milk withdrawal is usually advisable. In practice, the recommended diet is similar to that given to the patient with ulcerative colitis. If bowel obstruction occurs the patient is temporarily given a fluid diet.

It is advisable that supplementary nutrition in the form of liquid nutrient concentrates be considered for these patients. A. Harries *et al*, in a recent study, demonstrated the efficacy of such supplementation which when taken in addition to the regular diet resulted in improved nutritional status, including increased weight and skinfold thickness, and higher serum protein levels.

NURSING CONSIDERATIONS

Profuse foul-smelling diarrhoea and excessive flatulence are embarrassing and unpleasant features of several digestive-tract disorders. Whenever practical, retain a bedpan or commode, a toilet roll and an aerosol air-freshener at the patient's bedside for immediate use as required. Furthermore, satisfactory hand-washing facilities are an integral part of the nursing of these patients. If the exclusion of specific food components (e.g. gluten, lactose) is required, ensure that the patient as well as the staff understand the implications. The attitude of 'just a small amount (of milk in tea, for example) couldn't hurt' is both erroneous and hazardous to the patient.

Monitor the intake of fluids by constipated patients. The consumption of large quantities of fibre is less effective if inadequate liquid is taken.

Keep a small plate of sandwiches with 'high-protein' fillings constantly at the bedside of patients with ulcerative colitis and suggest that passing ward staff encourage the patient to eat them. Apart from the obvious benefits of the additional protein and energy, these patients, who are often tense and highly concerned about themselves, usually react positively to this supportive interest. They also learn that they play some role in their own treatment.

The state and regularity of the patient's stools should be accurately charted if at all abnormal. This would usually reflect progress of a gastrointestinal illness or indicate increased morbidity. Patients with a bleeding ulcer will have black stools and medical staff must be immediately alerted to the situation as a blood transfusion may be required.

The frothy, foul-smelling steatorrhoea resulting from malabsorption should return to normal within a few days of exclusion of the offending nutrient. The routine avoidance of both gluten and milk products as an initial precautionary measure in the treatment of coeliac disease is usually wise as such a high proportion of these patients have secondary lactose intolerance. After a few weeks, challenge with milk will confirm the diagnosis.

Each stool of the patient with ulcerative colitis should be observed and noted. Repeated losses of small amounts of blood can cause anaemia.

Severe diarrhoea can be a life-threatening condition, particularly in infants and children. Whether the child requests a drink or not, fluid replacement is an integral part of the treatment.

Infants with cystic fibrosis may pass undigested food particles through the digestive tract; thus the colour of the stool may vary according to the colour of the recently consumed food.

Whilst constipation is a widespread problem in hospital patients, laxative addiction is also a common phenomenon of our time, especially in women. Before responding to a patient's request for routine administration of laxatives, ensure that this is in fact necessary.

BIBLIOGRAPHY

Allan, J. Mason, A. & Moss, A. (1973) Nutritional supplementation in treatment of cystic fibrosis of the pancreas. *Am. J. Dis. Childh.*, *126*, 22.

American Academy of Pediatrics, Committee on Nutrition (1974) Should milk-drinking by children be discouraged? *Pediatrics, Springfield, 53*, 576.

American Dietetic Association (1971) Position paper on bland diet in the treatment of chronic duodenal disease. *J. Am. Diet Ass., 59*, 244.

Anderson, C. & Goodchild, M. (1976) *Cystic Fibrosis.* Oxford: Blackwell Scientific.

Anon (1978) Operations for diverticular disease. *Lancet, 2*, 25.

Arthur, A., Clayton, B., Coltom, D., Seakins, J. & Platt, J. (1966) Importance of disaccharide intolerance in the treatment of coeliac disease. *Lancet, 1*, 172.

Aylett, S. (1971) Cancer and ulcerative colitis. *Br. Med. J., 2*, 203.

Bennett, J. (1980) Biochemical abnormalities and nutritional control in inflammatory bowel disease. In: Brooke, B. & Wilkinson, A. (eds.) *Inflammatory Disease of the Bowel*. Bath: Pitman Medical.

Beyer, P. & Flynn, M. (1978) Effect of high and low fibre diets on human faeces. *J. Am. Diet. Ass., 72*, 271.

Bingham, S. (1979) Low residue diets: a reappraisal of their meaning and content. *J. Hum. Nutr., 33*, 5.

British Medical Journal (1977) Sucrose malabsorption. *Br. Med. J., 1*, 1558.

Burkitt, D. & James, P. (1973) Low residue diets and hiatus hernia. *Lancet, 2*, 128.

Cunningham, K. (1973) Coeliacs and the people who help them. *Nutr. Lond., 27*, 23.

Dodge, J. (1975) Dietary treatment in cystic fibrosis. *Health Magazine, Lond., (Chest Heart Ass.), 12(2)*, 3.

Gear, J., Ware, A., Fursdon, P., Mann, J., Nolen, D., Brodribb, A. & Vessey, M. (1979) Symptomless diverticular disease and intake of dietary fibre. *Lancet, 1*, 511.

Harries, A.D., Davis, V. & Heatley, R. (1983) Controlled trial of supplemented oral nutrition in Crohn's disease. *Lancet, 1*, 887.

Harries, J., Muller, D., McCollum, J., Lipson, A., Roma, E. & Norman, A. (1979) Intestinal bile salts in cystic fibrosis. *Archs. Dis. Childh., 54*, 19.

Kilby, A., Burgess, E., Wigglesworth, S. & Walker-Smith, J. (1978) Sucrase-isomaltase deficiency. A follow-up report. *Archs. Dis. Childh., 53*, 677.

Lancet (1975) Why does peptic ulcer happen? *Lancet,1*, 1076.

Nebel, O., Forbes, M. & Castell, D. (1976) Symptomatic gastro-esophageal reflux: incidence and precipitating factors. *Am. J. Dig. Dis., 21*, 953.

Odell, A. (1971) Ulcer dietotherapy — past and present. *J. Am. Diet. Ass., 58*, 447.

Painter, N. & Burkitt, D. (1971) Diverticular disease: a deficiency disease of Western civilisation. *Br. Med. J., 2*, 450.

Price, S., Smithson, K. & Castell, D. (1978) Food sensitivity in reflux esophagitis. *Gastroenterology, 75*, 241.

Shatz, B., Bane, A., Wessler, A. & Avidi, L. (1970) Medical and surgical aspects of hiatus hernia. *J. Am. Med. Ass., 214*, 125.

Singleton, J.W. (1974) Crohn's disease. In: Conn, H.F. (ed.) *Current Therapy*. London: W.B. Saunders.

Townley, R. (1966) Disaccharidase deficiency in infancy and childhood. *Pediatrics, Springfield, 38*, 127.

Walker-Smith, J.A. (1979) Coeliac disease: a life-long problem. *Mod. Med. S. Afr., 4(3)*, 13.

Weijers, H. & Van de Kamer, J. (1962) Diarrhoea caused by deficiency of sugar splitting enzymes. *Acta Paediat. Belg., 51*, 371.

9 The heart and circulatory system

Cardiovascular disease is the most important cause of death in the Western world. In spite of the vast incidence and massive research programmes in many parts of the world the exact aetiology is still obscure. There are many risk factors involved and a variety of inter-related conditions. In this chapter the two major disorders will be discussed (atherosclerosis and cardiac failure) with particular emphasis on contributory factors that are dietary related.

ATHEROSCLEROSIS

This is the most common form of hardening of the arteries deriving its name from the Greek *atheros*, meaning porridge and *sclerosis*, meaning scarring. The accumulation of soft lipid-rich plaque in the intima lining of the artery walls affects particularly the larger arteries and may result in progressively more narrowing of the lumen and restricted blood flow. Should a blockage occur owing to the occlusion of the artery by a clot of blood or plaque, the area being served by these arteries will be deprived of nutrients and oxygen. If this happens in the arteries leading to or situated in the brain the individual will suffer from a stroke or cerebrovascular accident; in the feet gangrene will occur. Should an artery in the legs be affected the individual will have pain when additional demands of oxygen are made, the condition being known as *claudication*. However, it is particularly the arteries feeding the heart that are of vital importance. This atherosclerotic progression, known as coronary heart disease (CHD), results in these arteries becoming blocked and part of the heart muscle will die, i.e. the patient will have a myocardial infarct or a 'heart attack'. When a large area is affected premature death can result.

Although previously diet was thought to be the all-important risk factor, it is now known that numerous other influences can affect the pathogenesis of atherosclerosis. These include the following:

SMOKING. CHD occurs three times more frequently in cigarette smokers than in non-smokers. This is probably the most important risk factor for if the individual with established atherosclerosis stops smoking his risk of progression of the disease is reduced. Mortality in non-inhaling cigar and pipe smokers and former smokers is about the same as in non-smokers.

SEX. Men suffer from about eight times the rate of CHD as premenopausal women. However, after the menopause the incidence in women rapidly increases and is about the same in both sexes.

HYPERTENSION. This is a major risk factor for CHD and (as discussed below) the dietary implications of restricting salt, as well as reducing obesity, make this risk factor at least in part dependent on patient compliance.

HEREDITY. This is extremely relevant in CHD. According to McLaren the hereditability of raised serum cholesterol levels has been calculated at 35–40%. Overweight people frequently have raised levels of both cholesterol and triglyceride. Added to this the raised blood pressure they often develop makes them likelier candidates for CHD.

DIABETES. Individuals with diabetes are also more prone to CHD because of impaired carbohydrate tolerance as well as raised serum cholesterol levels being an integral part of the diabetic disease process.

COFFEE-DRINKING. This has for a long time attracted attention as a possible risk factor in CHD. In a recent Norwegian study involving nearly 15 000 participants it was found that serum levels of both cholesterol and triglyceride were adversely affected in those with a high coffee consumption. The association was statistically significant even after adjustment was made for other covariates. The fact that 60% of the subjects drank five or more cups of coffee per day, that it was generally the boiled type that was consumed, and that the coffee was predominantly taken black may possibly affect the result.

DIETARY FATS. CHD occurs widely in populations taking a diet high in saturated fats, and serum lipids drop when appropriate dietary manipulations are made. It appears that, while reduction of total fat is relevant, the proportion of polyunsaturated fats and oils to saturated fats (known as the *p/s* ratio) is of major importance. (For further explanation of these terms, see Chapter 1.) Saturated fats have a formative role in the production of cholesterol in the serum, whereas research indicates that polyunsaturated fats not only do not have this deleterious effect, but that they assist in the clearance of cholesterol from the body.

Serum lipids

There are several fats normally present in the serum but the two fractions most closely related to diet are cholesterol and the triglycerides.

Cholesterol

Cholesterol is manufactured in the liver and it is also absorbed from dietary sources by the digestive tract. It occurs in all tissues. Serum levels are influenced by age and sex, but the normal range is approximately 3.8–7.2 mmol/litre. The optimum value for health, up until middle-age, is less than 5.6 mmol/litre. Saturated fats and cholesterol in the diet appear to have some effect on serum levels, as strict reduction of these fats in the diet of patients with certain types of hyperlipidaemia results in a drop in serum cholesterol. The degree of risk of myocardial infarct has been correlated to the elevation of serum cholesterol. Some workers have suggested that for every 1% drop in serum cholesterol there is a 3% reduction in the risk of developing coronary heart disease in predisposed individuals. Regrettably, most hypercholesterolaemic patients are unaware that their level of cholesterol is abnormal until they have a myocardial infarct. It is thus strongly recommended that, where the nurse is aware of a strong family history or the presence of several predisposing factors in an individual, especially a middle-aged male, since this group is particularly prone to this condition, she advise him to have a serum cholesterol examination. Patients often exhibit xanthomata, which are white or yellowish nodules of lipid material, particularly around the eyes, on the elbows and on the feet, and the nurse may be alerted to the disorder in this way.

Triglycerides

These fats, like cholesterol, are found in the blood not in the free form but bound to specific proteins. Elevated serum triglyceride levels are encountered in diseases of abnormal fat or carbohydrate metabolism (such as diabetes mellitus); also, some individuals who respond to an excessive intake of carbohydrate in this way. People who either consume large quantities of alcohol or who demonstrate increased sensitivity to moderate quantities frequently also have raised triglyceride levels. Hypertriglyceridaemia appears to increase the risk of ischaemic heart disease, but its role is less well documented than hypercholesterolaemia. Some workers suggest that elevated triglyceride levels are an independent risk factor, whereas others hold the view that this factor is supplementary to that of hypercholesterolaemia. Normal triglyceride levels are 0.3–1.7 mmol/litre but in affected individuals can rise to five times this amount, or even higher.

Lipoproteins

Lipoproteins are the major transport forms of lipids in the blood. They are identified according to their specific composition. Today, the classification of hyperlipoproteinaemia set out by Frederickson *et al* and based on quantitative electrophoresis is the most generally accepted. Frederickson categorized inherited forms of hyperlipidaemia, manifested in elevated lipoprotein levels, in five major classes. Each type of hyperlipidaemia tends to respond to a specific form of therapy. As hyperlipidaemia of all categories may be familial, it is usually advisable for close family members to be examined if an abnormally elevated lipoprotein level is found. In secondary hyperlipidaemia, where a primary disease is the cause of the hyperlipidaemia, treatment of the primary condition is a prerequisite for lowered lipid levels.

TYPE I is rare and is encountered exclusively in children. It is generally caused by lipoprotein lipase (enzyme) deficiency preventing normal utilization of fats. Eruptive xanthomata may be evident on the skin (Fig. 14) and the patient complains frequently of severe abdominal pain. These young patients cannot handle fats normally and strict dietary restriction of fat intake to less than 30 g/day is usually recommended. The relative proportion of satu-

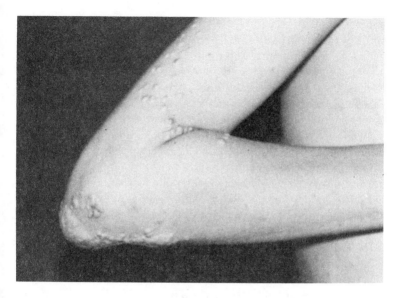

Fig. 14. *Eruptive xanthomata caused by lipoprotein lipase deficiency.*

rated and polyunsaturated fats is unimportant. Medium-chain triglycerides (MCT), which bypass the usual absorption pathways, are sometimes used to increase the energy intake of these patients. They must be introduced slowly into the diet as MCT can cause osmotic diarrhoea if large quantities are introduced too rapidly. A high-protein, high-carbohydrate diet is given. Dietary cholesterol plays no role in the causation or therapy of this condition, but will be low in a diet severely restricted in fat. The diet is particularly difficult to apply because children wish to attend parties, consume school dinners and eat the same foods as their families. The psychological effects of the application of a stringent diet from an early age may be detrimental to the normal development of the child. The use of MCT oil for frying, the inclusion of herbs and seasoning for enhanced palatability and emphasis on fruit-based or farinaceous desserts to increase the energy intake and add variety will all help to make this diet acceptable to the child.

TYPE II is the most commonly encountered hyperlipo-proteinaemia. Cholesterol levels are elevated due to congenital causes, environmental factors or certain diseases. Triglyceride levels are normal in patients with Type IIA hyperlipoproteinaemia but raised in those with Type IIB. The restriction of cholesterol and saturated fats will effect a drop in cholesterol of 15–25% in many of these patients. Saturated fats should be replaced where practical with polyunsaturated fats: there is considerable evidence to suggest that polyunsaturated fats do not elevate serum cholesterol levels but in fact actively reduce them and promote the excretion of cholesterol. Thus many workers suggest the daily inclusion in the diet of a few tablespoons of a highly polyunsaturated oil (e.g. sunflower seed oil) as part of the treatment of this condition. However, others consider that the routine consumption of this amount of oil each day will readily lead to obesity and that the disadvantages of the added energy intake outweigh the other advantages: weight reduction is an important aspect of treatment, particularly if the triglyceride level is elevated. In such cases carbohydrates, particularly refined sugars, should be drastically reduced and alcoholic drinks should also be severely restricted.

TYPE III is a rare familial disease where the patient has both elevated cholesterol and elevated triglyceride levels. It is accompanied by an increased incidence of coronary thrombosis and peripheral vascular disease in young subjects. The triglyceride levels are sensitive to carbohydrate intake and demonstrate an exaggerated response to carbohydrate loads. Weight reduction will usually form an essential part of the management. A diet low in refined carbohydrate is recommended and restrictions of saturated fat and cholesterol are generally prescribed to reduce the hypercholesterolaemia.

TYPE IV, carbohydrate-induced hyperlipidaemia, is often manifested by a moderate to markedly elevated triglyceride level. It is frequently associated with diabetes and may be compounded by obesity. Serum cholesterol levels may be within normal limits and thus require no dietary modification. The patient is told to avoid alcohol, which can directly affect triglyceride levels, and reduce the amount of fat and sucrose in his diet as part of the essential weight loss programme. Weight reduction may result in normal triglyceride levels and is an essential part of treatment.

In *TYPE V*, as in Type I, the triglyceride levels may become extremely high. When plasma from these patients is allowed to stand for 24 hours, the excess triglyceride may form a characteristic greasy layer on the surface. The condition can be secondary to pancreatitis, alcoholism and certain other disorders. Type V is encountered infrequently and symptoms are similar to those of Type I. Weight reduction is of primary importance in this condition. Total fat restriction is essential and consumption of alcohol is restricted.

In addition to the above classification recent research has indicated that two other fat carriers are of great importance in the aetiology of atherosclerosis. Low-density lipoproteins (LDL) contain approximately 50% cholesterol and, in fact, transport about 70% of the body's total cholesterol. These carriers are therefore specific indicators of the amount of circulating cholesterol and raised levels will thus indicate CHD.

However, this positive correlation appears to be less important than the negative association between high-density lipoproteins (HDL) and CHD, as these fat carriers have a markedly protective effect on the individual.

As the above blood fractions are fat carriers and both HDL and LDL are affected by very low total fat intakes or very high intakes of polyunsaturated fat, patients should be advised merely to modify their diets in the manner discussed below and not over-react.

Table 13 summarizes the dietary management of hyperlipoproteinaemia.

Dietary management of hypercholesterolaemia

The lowering of elevated serum lipid levels by diet and other environmental modifications such as an increase in exercise and a reduction in smoking is usually attempted before drugs are used, unless levels are exceptionally high and the patient at major risk, i.e. having angina attacks or severely hypertensive. As indicated above, the diet prescribed for hypercholesterolaemia is low in saturated fats, which are mainly encountered in animal and dairy fats. Thus lard, suet, butter, cream and similar fats must be omitted from the diet. *Fish oils* (from sardines, pilchards, tuna, etc.) and *vegetable oils* (from sunflower, avocado and most nuts) are unsaturated and should be used as a replacement. Coconut is an exception to the rule in that coconut fat is saturated. The acceptability of specific *margarines* depends on the method of production. In order to convert vegetable oil into the solid state required for margarine, oils undergo *hydrogenation* which satu-

Table 13. Dietary management of hyperlipoproteinaemia.

Type	Fat	Cholesterol	Kilojoules	Carbohydrate	Alcohol
I	Reduce to 30 g/day Type of fat not important	Minimal in this restricted fat diet	Unrestricted	Predominates in diet due to fat restriction	None allowed
II A	Low saturated fat High polyunsaturated fat, approx. 30% of kJ intake	Less than 250–300 mg/day	Restricted if patient overweight	Unrestricted	1–2 glasses wine per day recommended
II B III	Low saturated fat, high polyunsaturated fat	Less than 250–300 mg cholesterol/day	Weight reduction major aspect of regimen for overweight patients	Complex carbohydrates preferable to concentrated sweet foods	Restricted; in weight reduction regimens, alcoholic drinks forbidden
IV	Low saturated fat and high polyunsaturated fat, if serum cholesterol elevated	Less than 250–300 mg cholesterol/day	Weight reduction imperative if overweight	Complex carbohydrates preferable to concentrated sweets	Forbidden
V	Type of fat unimportant; reduce to 30 g/day, all types	Less important; reduced to approx. 500 mg/day	Weight reduction essential aspect of dietary regimen	Diet high in complex carbohydrates; omit sweetened foods if overweight	Forbidden

rates, at least in part, the fat molecules present. Margarines which are only partially hydrogenated are sold in plastic tubs to prevent leaking and are sometimes labelled as containing more than 40% or 50% polyunsaturated fats. These highly polyunsaturated margarines (e.g. Flora) should be used exclusively when a spreading fat is required, although liquid oil is obviously more unsaturated and should take preference for cooking purposes. Lean beef has approximately 10–12% fat, and mutton, too, has a high fat content. All visible fat on meat should be removed before cooking. Chicken (without the skin) and veal are preferable to other meats.

As discussed above, implementation of these dietary rules should still include a small amount of both saturated and unsaturated fat. The recommended allowance is an intake of approximately 30 g/day, being equal quantities of both types of fat. This is referred to as the *p/s* ratio which, with equal quantities of each type of fat, is 1:1.

Only *low-fat dairy products* should be used, with skimmed milk and skimmed milk cheese replacing the full-fat products. Non-dairy coffee creamers usually contain coconut oil and should not be used. Boiled and jellied sweets should be taken in preference to chocolates and toffees.

Egg yolks should be restricted to one per week as each one contains 240–275 mg of cholesterol. However, *egg whites* are unrestricted and can be used to replace whole eggs in cookery. Two egg whites plus a teaspoonful of oil are approximately equivalent to one whole egg in many recipes. An acceptable omelette substitue may be made by lightly whisking together two egg whites, a teaspoon of oil, a little skimmed milk, seasoning and a drop of synthetic egg-yellow colouring and frying in a little oil.

Alcohol is allowed in moderate amounts to people with atherosclerosis but should not be taken in excess. (Immediately after a coronary thrombosis alcohol must be strictly forbidden as such patients are prone to arrhythmias at this stage and these occur more readily following the consumption of alcohol.) The daily diet should be divided into three meals per day: patients should be discouraged from táking one large meal at the end of the day, as so many working people do. More numerous, smaller meals cause less strain on the heart and circulatory system than one large one.

Monounsaturated fatty acids are consumed mainly in the form of oleic acid which is present in olives, poultry and various nuts, including peanuts, cashew nuts, almonds and pecan nuts. These fatty acids have little effect on serum cholesterol. However, nuts are an extremely concentrated source of energy, and overweight patients should be discouraged from eating these in more than small quantities.

Lecithin is a phospholipid which plays a role in the intermediary metabolism of fats and decreases the uptake of cholesterol by the cells. Although found in certain foods, particularly egg yolk and organ meats, it is also synthesized by the body. The role of dietary lecithin does not appear to be related to the serum cholesterol level. The current fad — encouraged by health store assistants and nature cure enthusiasts — of consuming lecithin capsules or spreads on bread is unlikely to have any beneficial value: it appears that ingested lecithin is degraded in the intestine. In a recent study in which lecithin was administered by injection a more favourable effect was noted, but this research is still at the experimental stage.

The following sample menu is recommended for the patient with hypercholesterolaemia. Should the condition be compounded by obesity or hypertriglyceridaemia, the menu will need to be modified accordingly.

Sample menu (hypercholesterolaemia)

Breakfast
   orange juice
   muesli and skimmed milk
   wholewheat toast, polyunsaturated margarine and marmalade
Lunch
   cottage cheese, peanut butter or fish paste sandwiches
   salad
   fresh fruit
Dinner
   fried fish
   chips and vegetables
   jelly and custard (made with skimmed milk and custard
      powder, which is merely coloured and flavoured cornflour)

Note: The above menu is merely a recommendation of how to modify fat intake. Naturally the overweight individual should apply the guidelines in Chapter 5, i.e. omitting sweetened foods and replacing the fried fish with a grilled or baked fish dish. The hypertensive patient should include minimal salt as discussed later in this chapter.

In conclusion, it is emphasized that studies have shown that even strict implementation of the low saturated fat, high polyunsaturated fat diet will result in a drop of only approximately 10% in serum cholesterol levels in free-living individuals.

In reviewing the situation, Oliver concludes: 'There is good enough circumstantial evidence to give some advice and it is this. Reduce total energy, reduce energy from fat to below 35% of the total, reduce energy from saturated fat to about 10% (thereby increasing the *p/s* ratio) and reduce salt. But there is much more to arterial disease and CHD than diet alone.'

Dietary management of hypertriglyceridaemia

As in the case with hypercholesterolaemia, the diet for these patients is open to some degree of controversy. However, until there is conclusive evidence, it seems reasonable to apply the knowledge we now have, especially as the modifications involved impose little inconvenience on the patient and his family.

The role of *alcohol* is particularly important. Patients with a predisposition to the disorder improve their triglyceride levels when alcohol is reduced; some patients, who show particular sensitivity to a small amount of alcohol, will have to avoid it altogether.

Secondly, *weight loss* is to be strongly recommended to the overweight patient as this will usually help to normalize elevated levels of serum triglycerides. The overweight individual frequently handles a glucose load abnormally and elevated triglyceride levels are regarded as being a secondary symptom of disorders of carbohydrate metabolism. As discussed in Chapter 7, overweight is of prime importance in the aetiology of maturity-onset diabetes mellitus.

The third modification suggested for this condition is less precise in application. It is known that carbohydrate influences triglyceride levels, at least temporarily. Thus, sugars appear to be contra-indicated and patients are usually told to reduce their sucrose intake to the minimum. Unrefined cereals seem to have an advantageous effect and complex carbohydrates, including fibre (e.g. baked potatoes in their jackets) are thus preferable.

To sum up: on consideration of the available evidence the following dietary recommendations are advisable:

1. Reduce weight, if necessary, to within normal limits.
2. Reduce alcohol intake, and avoid it completely for a trial period, if strict adherence to other suggested dietary manoeuvres does not cause a satisfactory drop in serum triglyceride levels.
3. Avoid sugar if overweight and replace with artificial sweeteners if desired.
4. Starches should be limited to complex carbohydrates and wholegrain cereals wherever possible.

To test the efficacy of these rules, the author recently conducted a study on hypertriglyceridaemic patients attending the out-patient department of a large teaching hospital. When patients were following the appropriate dietary rules, there was a significant drop in triglycerides, amounting to a drop of 50% or more in the triglyceride levels in 28% of the experimental group.

Research on hyperlipidaemia

Finally, discussion on the subject of hyperlipidaemia would be incomplete without reference to the role of two other relevant dietary factors.

DIETARY FIBRE. Several studies have shown that fibre exerts a protective effect on serum cholesterol levels. Even when large quantities of butter had been consumed to raise the serum cholesterol levels there was a reduction in levels when crude fibre was ingested. It is suggested that the mechanism for this effect is a decreased reabsorption of bile salts and an increase in faecal excretion of cholesterol. Although the evidence to date is largely circumstantial it seems prudent to advise hypercholesterolaemic patients to emphasize foods with a high fibre content within the framework of their other dietary modifications.

OMEGA-3 OILS. More recently the role of omega-3 (ω–3) fatty acids on the development of vascular disease has been studied. These fatty acids are so named because of the position of the first double bond on the chemical chain. They are taken in large quantities by Eskimos, who have a low incidence of atherosclerosis, low serum cholesterol and triglyceride levels and high serum levels of these ω–3 fatty acids, the latter being found predominantly in marine oils.

Although patients have for many years been advised to take fish in preference to meat, the recommendation specifically to include salmon and pilchard oils and other marine oils high in ω–3 fatty acids may, in years to come, become a specific directive in the diet for individuals with atherosclerosis.

HYPERTENSION, CARDIAC FAILURE AND OEDEMA

Hypertension is a condition of sustained abnormally high blood pressure, which has a potentially detrimental effect on the heart, kidneys, eyes, brain and peripheral circulation. The increased force exerted by the blood in the peripheral arteries causes damage at these vital sites. In some cases, hypertension can be due to renal or endocrine causes, but in many instances the aetiology is not well understood and the condition is known as 'essential hypertension'. Aggravating factors are stress, obesity and, probably, long-term salt intake. Treatment involves:

1. eradication of the cause, if possible. This is not always successful as irreversible renal damage may perpetuate the hypertension, creating a vicious circle.
2. specific drugs, which are available for the control of elevated blood pressure; in particular, diuretics are often prescribed for mild hypertension.
3. diet therapy directed especially at weight reduction (where necessary) and sodium restriction.

Sodium and hypertension

Over 35 years ago, Kempner recommended a diet for hypertension which consisted primarily of rice. This very monotonous regimen was found to be highly effective, and the observation that it was primarily the low salt intake which was responsible for the drop in blood pressure prompted research workers to study the relationship between the sodium content of the diet and hypertensive disease. For over a quarter of a century, Dahl and other workers have investigated the effect of varying levels of sodium intake on experimental animals and in epidemiological studies. It appears that in areas where much salt is consumed the population is at much greater risk of developing hypertension than are groups in areas with a low salt intake. Furthermore, reduction of sodium in the diet of hypertensives usually ameliorates the condition. Today, when highly effective diuretics are widely used in the treatment of hypertension and urinary fluid loss is accompanied by increased sodium loss, severe sodium restriction is no longer the all-important form of treatment except where patients manifest an individual resistance to the action of diuretics.

Some years ago there was considerable discussion about the relevance of salted bottled infant foods to the later development of hypertension. It was said that compared with adult consumption on the basis of relative kilojoule consumption, infants on a high-milk diet supplemented with bottled baby foods would have a higher salt intake. However, Lowe pointed out that, given adult body weight as compared with the weight of an infant, the proportionate sodium intake of the infant is considerably less. Nonetheless, action has recently been taken in Great Britain to reduce the sodium content of baby foods.

The average intake of sodium in a Western-type diet is 3–6 g/day. Most of it is consumed in the form of sodium chloride which contains 40% sodium: this means that the average salt intake is 7.5–15 g/day. In other areas, particularly in Japan where there is a high incidence of hypertension, salt intake has been found to be considerably higher.

Hypertensives who are responding favourably to diuretic therapy are usually advised merely to reduce their sodium intake by avoiding foods which are heavily salted. These include bacon, ham, corned beef, cheese, potato crisps, anchovies, tinned fish, sausage rolls, etc. However, more specific instructions are frequently necessary to ensure a more restricted consumption. The following rules reduce the sodium intake to 1 g/day, i.e. 2.5 g of salt.

1. Omit foods cooked or tinned with salt (baked beans, meat and fish products, sweetcorn, etc.), with monosodium

glutamate (soups, sauces), or baked with baking powder. Restrict high-sodium foods and emphasize fruit, vegetables, cereals (oat porridge, rice, barley, etc.), all prepared without salt.

2. Restrict milk intake to 250 ml/day or 3 tablespoons (50 g) of plain cottage cheese.
3. Restrict bread intake to 100 g/day, which means four thin (25 g) slices of baker's white, brown or wholewheat bread.
4. Include a total of 25 g butter on the above slices of bread.
5. Each day include two medium (120 g) portions of meat and/or fish. One egg may be taken daily but only if atherosclerosis is not a consideration.

Should it be necessary to restrict the sodium intake further, the omission of commercially processed bread and salted butter will reduce the sodium intake to approximately 350 mg (equivalent to 900 mg of salt). Further reduction of sodium intake to 200 mg (500 mg salt) can be made by replacing the milk with special low-sodium milk. Such drastic limitation of sodium intake, accompanied by diuretic therapy, may necessitate regular monitoring of serum electrolytes to confirm that serum levels do not drop too low. This diet is also unpalatable and is used only as a last resort.

Cardiac failure

In the event of the heart failing to meet the demand imposed upon it due to an underlying cardiac condition, cardiac failure can occur. This results in fluid retention, which can manifest itself as pulmonary or hepatic congestion, venous engorgement or oedema. Oedema is caused mainly by increased hydrostatic pressure at the venous end of the capillary network, but output of the hormone aldosterone and its effect on sodium retention are also precipitating factors.

Other causes of oedema

There are other important mechanisms involved in the development of oedema, the most important of which is lowered osmotic pressure due to hypoalbuminaemia. This may result from: (1) decreased protein intake such as occurs in malnutrition; (2) decreased protein absorption, as in malabsorption states; (3) decreased protein formation, as in chronic liver disease; or (4) increased protein loss, as occurs via the kidneys in the nephrotic syndrome or via the gastrointestinal tract in protein-losing enteropathies. In such cases sodium restriction is of secondary importance, increased protein intake being far more important. These aspects are discussed in the appropriate chapters.

Venous obstruction is another mechanism of oedema but here too sodium restriction is clearly inappropriate.

THE LOW-SODIUM DIET IN PRACTICE

Initially, patients may find it difficult to tolerate the low-salt diet as they find it tasteless and unpalatable. However, it is surprising how quickly they adapt. Here are some suggestions on how the food may be made more acceptable.

1. Salt substitutes may be used. These are compounds of potassium instead of sodium and may usually be used in moderate amounts unless there is severe kidney damage in which case these potassium salts may be contra-indicated.
2. Home-made unsalted mayonnaise or salad dressing and unsalted soups add flavour and variety to the diet.
3. Recipes using yeast as rising agents should be used in preference to those incorporating baking powder or soda. Sodium-free baking powder may be made up by mixing together 40 g of potassium carbonate, 30 g of cornflour and 8 g of tartaric acid. One and a half teaspoons of this mixture may be used in recipes to replace a teaspoon of baking powder.
4. Recipes including large amounts of eggs or milk should be avoided and salted butter in made-up dishes should be replaced with either salt-free butter or oil.

RELATED DIETARY ASPECTS

A *weight reduction* regimen in overweight hypertensive patients is of vital importance. A drop in blood pressure usually accompanies weight loss and there is also evidence that weight gain causes increased blood pressure. Whyte suggests that with each increase in body weight of 28 lb (12.6 kg) a rise of 10 mmHg in systolic and 7 mmHg in diastolic pressure can be anticipated. The weight reduction diet discussed in Chapter 5 will usually be effective, although the salt content may need to be modified.

Apart from the effect of sodium in cardiac failure, certain other ingested substances play a role in the efficient functioning of the heart muscle.

As discussed in Chapter 1, *thiamine deficiency* can result in cardiac failure with enlarged heart and marked fluid retention, so-called 'wet beri beri'.

Iron deficiency can give rise to anaemia with resultant dyspnoea and palpitations. However these instances are usually academic for the nurse as they are encountered infrequently.

Serum potassium is depleted by many diuretics and this is replaced either with the use of potassium supplements or, commonly, merely by an emphasis on high-potassium foods in the diet; these include bananas, oranges, pineapple juice, fish, meat and meat extracts, including gravies and soups. However, in the presence of renal complications or during the use of potassium-sparing diuretics such as spironolactone, a high intake of potassium must be avoided. Both high and low serum potassium levels can result in cardiac arrhythmias and regular monitoring of this electrolyte may be necessary.

In conclusion, the recent recommendations by the Joint National Committee on Detection, Evaluation and Treatment of High Blood Pressure summarize the current role of diet in this condition:

1. weight reduction for all obese persons;
2. moderate sodium restriction, coupled with blood pressure monitoring to ascertain individual sensitivity to sodium restriction;
3. moderation of alcohol intake;
4. reduction in abnormal levels of blood cholesterol.

NURSING CONSIDERATIONS

1. Rationale of nutritional principles and practical management of these patients has been discussed in depth in this chapter. In summary these cover;

(a) reducing total fat in the diet and increasing the proportion of polyunsaturated fats;
(b) implementation of a weight reduction diet for overweight patients;
(c) restricting salt intake, particularly if the patient is hypertensive.

2. Patients at risk for CHD should stop smoking immediately as this will reduce the risk to almost that of a non-smoker. Furthermore, women who take contraceptive pills and who also smoke heavily markedly increase their risk of CHD.

3. Many patients find cholestyramine, widely prescribed for clearing cholesterol from the body, extremely constipating. The consumption of 2–3 tablespoons of digestive or crude bran and an adequate fluid intake may relieve this. The powder is more palatable in orange juice or yoghurt or 'chased down' with skimmed milk.

4. Stress is a major risk factor and although CHD is undeniably a serious condition, the patient should be reassured and helped to cope with his anxieties.

5. Whilst the role of excessive coffee drinking in the development of atherosclerosis is still controversial there is no doubt that cardiac arrhythmias can be aggravated by smoking or the consumption of coffee, tea or alcoholic drinks, all of which should be avoided by affected patients.

BIBLIOGRAPHY

Borushek, A. & Borushek, J. (1981) *The Complete Australian Heart Disease Prevention Manual.* Perth: Family Health Publications.
Council on Foods and Nutrition (1972) Diet and coronary heart disease. *J. Am. Med. Ass., 222,* 1647.
Dahl, L.K. (1954) Evidence for relationship between sodium chloride and essential hypertension. *Archs. Intn. Med., 94,* 525.
Dahl, L.K. (1972) Salt and hypertension. *Am. J. Clin. Nutr., 25,* 231.
Dawber, T.R., Kannel, W. & Gordon, T. (1974) Coffee and cardiovascular disease. *N. Engl. J. Med., 291,* 871.
Dyerberg, J., Bang, H. & Stoffersen, E. (1978) Eicosapentaenoic acid and prevention of thrombosis and atherosclerosis. *Lancet, 2,* 117.
Evans, D., Turner, S. & Ghosh, P. (1972) Feasibility of long-term plasma-cholesterol reduction by diet. *Lancet, 1,* 172.
Fredrickson, D. (1975) It's time to be practical. *Circulation, 51,* 209.
Fredrickson, D. & Lees, R.S. (1965) A system for phenotyping hyperlipoproteinaemia. *Circulation, 31,* 321.
Goodnight, S., Harris, W. & Connor, W. (1981) The effects of dietary ω–3 fatty

acids on platelet composition and function in Man; A prospective controlled study. *Blood*, *58*, 880.

Housel, E.L. (1961) Diet and anti-hypertensive therapy. In: Brest, A. & Moyer, J. (eds.) *Hypertension Recent Advances*. Philadelphia: Lea & Febiger.

Huskisson, J.M. (1978) Effectiveness of dietetic consultation at the Lipid Clinic, Groote Schuur Hospital. *J. Diet. Home Econ. (S.A.)*, *6(3)*, 87.

Joint National Committee on Detection, Evaluation and Treatment of High Blood Pressure (1984) The 1984 report of the Joint National Committee on Detection, Evaluation and Treatment of High Blood Pressure. *Archs. Intn. Med.*, *144*, 1045.

Kannel, W. (1977) Preventive cardiology: what should the clinician be doing about it? *Postgrad. Med.*, *61*, 74.

Kannel, W., Castelli, W & Gordon, T. (1979) Cholesterol in the prediction of atherosclerotic disease. *Ann. Intn. Med.*, *90*, 85.

Keys, A. (1979) The diet/heart controversy. *Lancet*, *2*, 844.

Lewis, B. (1976) *The Hyperlipidaemias*. London: Blackwell Scientific.

Mann, J.I. (1979) A prudent diet for the nation. *J. Hum. Nutr.*, *33*, 57.

Margolis, S. & Elfert, G. (1984) Dietary modification of plasma lipid and lipoprotein levels. In: *Nutritional Management: The Johns Hopkins Handbook*. London: W.B. Saunders.

Oliver, M. (1982) Diet and coronary heart disease. *Hum. Nutr.*, *36*, 413.

Parijs, J., Joossens, J., Van der Linden, L., Versteken, G. & Amery, A. (1973) Moderate sodium restriction and diuretics in the treatment of hypertension. *Am. Heart J.*, *85*, 22.

Richards, A.M., Nicholls, M.G., Espiner, E.A., Ikram, H., Maslowski, H., Hamilton, E. & Wells, J.J. (1984) Blood pressure response to moderate sodium restriction and to potassium supplementation in mild essential hypertension. *Lancet*, *1*, 757.

Richardson, C. (1978) Regional project for the prevention of coronary heart disease. *J. Hum. Nutr.*, *32*, 373.

Shaper, A.G. (1976) Primary and secondary prevention trials in coronary heart disease. *Postgrad. Med. J.*, *52*, 464.

Stein, E., Mendelsohn, D., Fleming, M., Barnard, G., Carter, K., du Toit, P.S., Hansen, J. & Bersohn, I. (1975) Lowering of plasma cholesterol levels in free-living adolescent males; use of natural and synthetic polyunsaturated foods to provide balanced fat diets. *Am. J. Clin. Nutr.*, *28*, 1204.

Thele, D., Arnesen, D. & Forde, O. (1983) The Tromso Heart Study: Does coffee raise serum cholesterol? *N. Eng. J. Med.*, *308*, 1454.

Trowell, H. (1972) Ischaemic heart disease and dietary fibre. *Am. J. Clin. Nutr.*, *25*, 926.

Trowell, H., Painter, N. & Burkitt, D. (1974) Aspects of the epidemiology of diverticular disease and ischaemic heart disease. *Am. J. Dig. Dis.*, *19*, 864.

Truswell, A.S. (1976) Diet in the pathogenesis of ischaemic heart disease. *Postgrad. Med. J.*, *52*, 424.

Walser, M., Imbembo, A., Margolis, S. & Elfert, G. (1984) *Nutritional Management: The Johns Hopkins Handbook*. London: W.B. Saunders.

Watermeyer, G., Mann, J., Truswell, A.S. & Levy, I. (1975) Type IIIa hyperlipidaemia: an evaluation of four therapeutic regimes. *S. Afr. Med. J.*, *49*, 631.

Whyte, H.M. (1959) Blood pressure and obesity. *Circulation*, *19*, 511.

World Health Organization (1982) *Prevention of Coronary Heart Disease*. Geneva: WHO.

Yudkin, J. (1971) Sugar consumption and myocardial infarction. *Lancet*, *1*, 296.

10   Haematological disorders

Blood is the life-line to other stationary cells in the body. It is vitally important that the internal environment of tissues and organs remains constant and homeostasis is largely dependent on the highly specialized functions of the blood system. Blood transports nutrients from the digestive tract and oxygen from the lungs to the cells. It distributes hormones from various endocrine glands throughout the body to organs where they are required, as well as antibodies to counteract infection. Blood prevents the accumulation of waste products by removing them to the excretory organs and also helps maintain a constant body temperature.

Disorders of the circulatory system can therefore have far-reaching effects throughout the body. Although a wide range of abnormalities can obviously affect the many components and functions of blood, this chapter is specifically directed at conditions that are affected by dietary components. Diseases unrelated to diet (such as sickle-cell anaemia) are only included where relevant for explanatory purposes.

ERYTHROCYTE DISORDERS

Anaemia

The most widely encountered blood disorder is *anaemia* — a condition in which there is a reduced number of erythrocytes (red blood cells), a decrease in haemoglobin, or both. Incidence of the condition is variable, ranging from over 90% in some parts of the world where hookworm with resultant blood loss is endemic, to very low levels in communities of people who are well educated and have a high standard of living.

Symptoms of the condition result largely from reduced oxygenation of the tissues due to inadequate haemoglobin, the oxygen carrier of the blood. Patients are usually listless, weak and generally lacking in energy and motivation. They are pale, this pallor being particularly evident when reflecting the lower eyelid where the healthy reddish-pink colour is absent. Anaemic patients often have palpitations and headaches.

Causes of anaemia can be classified as follows:

Blood loss

The commonest cause of blood loss is the occult (or hidden) loss occurring from the digestive tract. Ulceration, ulcerative colitis, hookworm and other parasites and tumours of the digestive tract can all cause long-term losses of small quantities of blood, unrecognized over a long period of time.

A major cause of anaemia in women is blood loss due to constant heavy periods (menorrhagia) and the situation can be aggravated by the consumption of an unbalanced or inadequate diet. As with occult loss the situation can develop insidiously and often goes undiagnosed for long periods of time. Large quantities of blood can also be lost following extensive surgery or trauma and is seen in the vitamin K deficient infant (haemorrhagic disease of the newborn — see below). Blood loss can also occur via the pulmonary or renal tract (rarely) in diseases where these organs are affected.

Haemolysis

This is the destruction of an abnormally large number of red blood cells. The average 120 day life-cycle of the red blood cells involves the regular breakdown and replacement of erythrocytes. However, if this breakdown happens at a much quicker rate due to some abnormality, the body cannot replace the cells fast enough and the individual becomes anaemic. Certain drugs, burns and some diseases, such as malaria and infections by *Clostridium welchii* (which can occur with septic abortions) can also cause haemolysis. More rarely, genetic disorders, such as favism which is discussed in Chapter 15, can result in haemolysis. In some congenital abnormalities the shape and content of the red cell is affected. In conditions such as sickle-cell anaemia and thalassaemia and in spherocytosis the spleen reacts to these abnormal cells by breaking them down and causing haemolysis.

Furthermore, the mechanical breakdown of erythrocytes can occur with certain heart-valve abnormalities where the physical destruction results from the crushing valve movement. This type of mechanical destruction is also thought to contribute greatly to the anaemia often encountered in runners. It is thought that continual pressure of the feet against hard surfaces results in loss of free haemoglobin into the blood, which is then excreted in the urine. The condition is called March haemoglobinuria.

Reduced haemopoiesis (impaired blood formation)

There are two main causes of this disorder:

1. *Functionally impaired blood-forming sites.* This is seen in diseased or affected bone marrow or spleen or if these organs are damaged, for example by radiotherapy, or secondary to severe liver or renal damage.
2. *Nutritional anaemia.* Deficiences of several nutrients will cause anaemia, the type of resultant abnormalities of the blood cells being dependent on the stage at which the particular deficient nutrient is involved in haemopoiesis.

Iron is the most important nutrient involved in the production of haemoglobin and most of the body's iron is found here. Inadequate supplies will result in a condition known as microcytic hypochromic anaemia which refers to the fact that the cells are smaller and reduced (hypo) in colour (chromic). Iron deficiency anaemia is the most frequent form of anaemia in children and in some surveys 5–25% of children have been found to be iron deficient (Schneider *et al*). The body is unable to get rid of excess iron so the uptake is normally geared to the need of the individual. Approximately 10–30% of iron consumed is absorbed by the body. The recommended dietary requirement is small: 10 mg/day for males and 18 mg/day for females of child-bearing age to compensate for monthly menstrual losses. In fact the body requires considerably more, but 90% of the daily need is met by the reclycling of old worn-out blood cells. The body also stores iron in the liver, spleen and bone marrow.

Treatment of the iron-deficient individual includes the administration of optimal quantities of iron as well as attention to other factors which promote its absorption and utilization. For example, as iron is absorbed only in an acid medium, conditions which result in a deficient output of hydrochloric acid in the stomach (such as after a gastrectomy) will impair iron absorption and promote anaemia. Absorption will also be impaired in patients with diarrhoea or steatorrhoea and who consume abnormally large quantities of organic salts such as phytate (which is found in wholewheat products) and oxalate (found in spinach, rhubarb, etc.). The consumption of large quantities of tea concurrently with iron-containing food also has an adverse effect on absorption.

Ascorbic acid intake is of great importance to create a favourable environment for the absorption of iron. Anaemia can be precipitated by reduced serum iron levels secondary to scurvy. In a study by Gilooly *et al* the enhancing effect of vitamin C intake with a food source of iron was demonstrated.

Copper is essential for the formation of haemoglobin in that it is part of the enzyme necessary to convert ferric iron, the dietary form, to ferrous iron, the form in which it is transported.

Folic acid is another nutrient which forms an integral part of the mature erythrocyte. With inadequate intake red cell production is arrested in the bone marrow and large rudimentary cells (megaloblasts) which mature into large cells (macrocytes) are produced. Anaemia resulting from folic acid deficiency is seen particularly at times of exceptional physiological need such as during pregnancy and in prematurity, or with limited intake particularly in alcoholics or deprived children. Excessive utilization can also be secondary to other disorders. Such anaemia is seen in people with sprue, Crohn's disease and coeliac disease or in times of excessive demands of haemopoiesis, such as in haemolytic anaemia.

Vitamin B_{12} deficiency is seen in vegans with no food intake of animal origin. More frequently, pernicious anaemia occurs as a result of impaired vitamin B_{12} absorption due to the absence of Intrinsic Factor. This compound is found in normal, healthy gastric mucosa and is essential for the absorption of vitamin B_{12}. Atrophy (due to ageing) or removal of part of the necessary mucosa (as in a gastrectomy or with ileal resection) will result in reduced vitamin B_{12} uptake. The red blood cells seen in this type of anaemia are indistinguishable from those seen with folic acid deficiency.

Protein deficiency is frequently characterized by anaemia — not surprisingly — as haemoglobin is itself a protein. The aggravating effects of malaria, hookworm and other nutritional deficiencies have a marked effect on erythrocyte integrity but low protein intake *per se* may well have a significant effect as well.

Vitamin B_6 (pyridoxine) deficiency results in anaemia and microcytic hypochromic, normoblastic and megaloblastic types have all been described. This is of little practical relevance to the nurse who is unlikely to see a deficiency of this vitamin in the course of her duties. However, vitamin B_6 deficiency is occasionally seen secondary to the antagonistic effect of certain drugs (see Chapter 18).

Vitamin A deficiency has recently been incriminated as an anaemia-causative nutrient. In a recent study by Mejia and Arroyave it was shown that vitamin A fortification had a favourable effect on iron metabolism and nutritional status. Their data was obtained from Guatemalan children receiving vitamin A fortified sugar in a national supplementation programme. This interesting result requires further study.

Vitamin E after many years of controversy is now also considered to play a major role in erythrocyte formation. In a review of the subject, Drake and Fitch emphasized that improved erythropoiesis with administration of vitamin E has been observed in controlled studies with patients suffering from protein energy malnutrition and state that 'vitamin E should be viewed as a potential erythropoietic factor for humans and it should receive further carefully controlled therapeutic trials in patients with anaemia of obscure etiology'. However in practice this deficiency is hardly seen except in the neonatal period (i.e. haemolytic anaemia) and in states of chronic fat malabsorption (e.g. in cystic fibrosis).

Vitamin K is of indirect but significant relevance in anaemia. In the absence of adequate blood clotting (the prime function of vitamin K in the body), haemorrhagic disease of the newborn can occur resulting in blood loss. (Also, clotting cannot effectively proceed if the liver is not functioning adequately to produce sufficient prothrombin, see Chapter 11). Anticoagulant therapy counteracting the function of vitamin K can result in anaemia caused by blood loss.

Iron accumulation

The implications of nutritional anaemia as discussed relate largely to reduced iron uptake and utilization. There are, however, two rather rarer conditions where the opposite effect is seen, i.e. the pathological absorption and deposition of iron in the body.

Haemochromatosis

This disorder occurs predominantly in males, causing tissue damage particularly in the pancreas (destroying the insulin-producing cells and causing diabetes) and in the liver. Patients develop a characteristic bronze discolouration of the skin. This is usually treated by the routine 'tapping off' of the iron-rich blood; chelating agents which bind the iron are also used. As a dietary measure, the concomitant use of tea can be used to help block the excessive iron absorption. Vitamin C with iron overload can cause a toxic myocarditis and should be restricted in the diet.

Haemosiderosis

This is a condition in which iron is deposited in several organs and in particular in excessive amounts in the liver. It can occur for two reasons: in the first place as a result of abnormal blood destruction and the subsequent release of large quantities of iron or, secondly, due to excessive intake by mouth or from numerous blood transfusions. In Africa where iron pots are widely used for cooking, as well as for the production of alcoholic brews with a low pH in which the iron is more readily dissolved, a much greater incidence of the condition is seen than in other countries. The use of iron pots is hazardous and should be emphatically discouraged.

Dietary manipulation is of little significance in the above conditions which are essentially metabolic disorders related to excessive absorption. Patients are generally informed about foods having a high iron content and advised to limit these to moderate levels. Interestingly, it was the concern for people with haemochromatosis that led the US Food and Drug Administration to recommend against an increase in the amount of iron added to breads and cereals in the American enrichment programme.

LEUKOCYTE DISORDERS

This chapter would not be complete without some brief reference to leukocyte (white blood cell) diseases, such as multiple myeloma and leukaemia. There is little of specific relevance to these cancers, and dietary modification and manipulation is similar to that for patients with other types of cancer (see Chapter 14). An interesting aspect of therapy is the use of a folic acid antagonist in leukaemia. This temporarily blocks the rapid production of cells in malignant disease due to its inhibitory action on folic acid which plays an essential part in this process.

NURSING CONSIDERATIONS

1. 'Spoon-shaped' nails, i.e. nails which are concave instead of being convex with longitudinal ridges, are often seen in patients with long-term iron deficiency. If this characteristic is noted the patient's diet should immediately come under scrutiny. Other common symptoms of this condition relate to the tongue and mouth. Glossitis (inflammation of the tongue), atrophy of the papillary surface of the tongue and soreness of the mouth and tongue are all features of iron deficiency anaemia.

2. Night nurses should be alerted to note any colour change in urine. The diagnosis of a condition known as paroxysmal nocturnal haemoglobinuria, caused by a change in pH in the blood during sleep and resulting in anaemia, can be missed unless an observant nurse reports of the discoloured urine.

3. Check the diet of anaemic patients, not just for iron but also for stores of folic acid, vitamin B_{12}, ascorbic acid and general adequacy regarding all other nutrients. This can be done rapidly with reference to the basic four food groups as discussed in Chapter 1. The adult presenting with folate deficiency is most often addicted to alcohol.

4. Many patients become constipated when iron pills are administered for iron deficiency anaemia. Unsupervised laxatives taken to counteract this effect can result in diarrhoea, hence bowel activity should be well supervised in these patients.

5. Liver is the most highly recommended food for patients with a nutritional anaemia as it provides iron, copper, folic acid and vitamin B_{12} as well as protein and vitamin A. Pork liver is highest in iron; chicken liver while not quite so outstanding is advisable too, particularly for the many individuals who reject other types of liver. However in practice the consumption of large quantities of liver is usually less effective than giving the appropriate nutrients in concentrated form as a drug.

BIBLIOGRAPHY

Anon. (1980) *Am. J. Clin. Nutr., 33*, 2386.
Drake, J. & Fitch, C. (1980) Status of vitamin E as an erythropoietic factor.
Dubovsky, D. (1984) Anaemia — an aid to diagnosis. *J. Cont. Med. Ed.*
Gilooly, M. *et al* (1984) Factors affecting iron absorption from cereals. *Br. J. Nutr., 51*, 37.
McLaren, D. & Burman, D. (1976) *Textbook of Paediatric Nutrition.* London: Churchill Livingstone.
Mejia, L. & Arroyave, G. (1982) The effect of vitamin A fortification of sugar on iron metabolism in pre-school children. *Am. J. Clin. Nutr., 36*, 87.
Oppenheimer, S. & Hendrikse, R. (1983) The clinical effects of iron deficiency and iron supplementation. *Nutr. Abstr. Rev., 53*, 588.
Schneider, H., Anderson, C. & Cousin, D. (1977) *Nutritional Support of Medical Practice.* London: Harper and Row.
Wenck, D. & Baren, M. (1983) *Nutrition*, 2nd edn. Boston: Prentice Hall.
Williams, S. (1977) *Nutrition and Diet Therapy*, 3rd edn. St. Louis: C.V. Mosby.

11   The liver and biliary system

The liver, the largest organ in the body, is the site of a variety of metabolic activities and the storage depot for many reserve nutrients. It may be regarded as the watershed of the digestive process. Among its many complex functions are:

1. the conversion and modification of a number of nutrients,
2. the detoxification of various drugs (including alcohol) and food additives,
3. the destruction of various pathogenic organisms.

Although they are discussed in more detail in other parts of this book, a summary of the major dietary functions of the liver is relevant at this point. These are:

1. the conversion of ingested *amino acids* to *plasma proteins* and *urea*;
2. the production of *lipoproteins* (including *cholesterol*), various *plasma fats* (such as *phospholipids*) and *bile acids (salts)* during fat metabolism;
3. modification of ingested *carbohydrates* in various ways, including the conversion of *fructose* and *galactose* to *glucose* and the *production of glycogen* from glucose. Glycogen is stored in the liver and used as required for energy purposes, thus making the liver largely responsible for maintaining the blood sugar level within normal limits. *Gluconeogenesis* (i.e. the formation of glucose from fatty acids and amino acids) also occurs here, as well as some production of energy by the conversion of glucose to carbon dioxide and water;
4. The liver also plays a major role in *vitamin metabolism*. The fat-soluble vitamins A and D are mainly stored here. Vitamin D is metabolized in the liver and converted to $25\text{-}OH\text{-}D_3$. It is also inactivated in the liver for excretion in the bile. The liver is the site of the production of prothrombin, a process in which vitamin K plays an essential role. Large reserves of vitamin B complex, especially vitamin B_{12} and folic acid, are also stored here.

5. Various *minerals*, in particular iron and copper, are stored in the liver.

A word of caution: there has always been a strong emotional link between the liver and a feeling of well-being. Because of the complexity of the functions of the liver this is understandable, but there is no basis for the assumption that a vague feeling of nausea or malaise is the result of 'liverishness'. A diversity of dietary modifications commonly suggested by the layman, such as the omission of coffee, alcohol, fats, reduction of fibre and consumption of glucose, often bear no relationship to physiological requirements and are based purely on the mystique associated with this organ.

JAUNDICE

This is a discolouration of the skin caused by elevated blood levels of bilirubin, a pigment produced by the reticulo-endothelial system in the breakdown of haemoglobin. The body produces about 200–250 mg of bilirubin per day. Normally, this is cleared from plasma by the liver, where it is conjugated or modified in composition, rendering it soluble in bile, in which it is excreted. There are various possible causes for the accumulation of bilirubin in the blood, namely:

1. *Haemolytic jaundice*, caused by an increased load of haemoglobin due to excessive haemolysis of the red blood cells. The inability of the liver cells to handle the increased quantity of bilirubin results in the accumulation of unconjugated pigment.
2. *Hepatocellular jaundice*, due to hepatitis, usually resulting from infection or alcohol. This results in an accumulation of both unconjugated and conjugated bilirubin in the blood. The plasma level of unconjugated bilirubin is increased because of reduction in the capacity of the liver cells to remove bilirubin from plasma. Conjugated bilirubin increases due to a defect of the excretory mechanism of the liver cells.
3. *Obstructive jaundice* occurs in conditions such as gall-stones, carcinoma of the gall-bladder or strictures of the bile duct, preventing the normal output of bile necessary for the excretion of the bilirubin.

In all cases it is the underlying condition that requires treatment and not the symptom of jaundice, although the depth of colour usually reflects the severity of the condition.

HEPATITIS

This is an inflammatory condition which can be caused by chronic over-indulgence in alcohol, by certain viruses, or by drugs and toxins such as carbon tetrachloride. It is usually accompanied by accumulation of bilirubin in the blood resulting in the classical jaundiced appearance of the patient. Hepatitis can be a precursor to cirrhosis, particularly in the patient who continues to consume alcohol. The patient should take adequate protein and a high-carbohydrate diet to promote regeneration of the cellular mass. Furthermore, carbohydrate is valuable for replenishing glycogen deposits which become depleted during the early stages of this illness, to prevent the marked weight loss which usually occurs early in the illness, and for its protein-sparing effect. This last function means that carbohydrates will be used to meet the body's demands for energy, allowing the protein to be utilized for tissue repair.

Anorexia is a feature of this disease and thus meals should be attractive and emphasize preferred foods. If the patient feels nauseated by fats, these should be temporarily excluded from the diet. However, individuals who wish to consume fats in their meals should be encouraged to do so. Although only minimal quantities will be absorbed, the presence of fat invariably improves the palatability and variety of the menu and will probably encourage the patient to eat more, thus increasing the intake of other nutrients. As in gall-bladder disease, discussed below, short-chain fats are usually tolerated best. The following sample menu can be regarded as a guide. Of course, strict abstinence from alcohol is essential for all patients with this illness and for 6–12 months thereafter. Where over-indulgence is the cause of hepatitis, patients should be encouraged to refrain permanently from drinking. Both nurse and patient should be alerted to the fact that most tonics have an alcohol base. In small quantities these will cause nausea; in large quantities they may promote structural changes in the liver — choice of a tonic should thus be made with the utmost caution.

Sample menu (hepatitis)

Breakfast
  stewed prunes
  porridge with sugar and milk
  2 scrambled eggs or poached haddock with a little butter
  1 slice of toast, lightly buttered, liberally spread with marma-
     lade
  tea with sugar and milk
11 a.m.
  a glass of Ovaltine
Dinner
  cottage pie made with lean steak mince
  rice, peas and carrots
  fruit jelly
4 p.m.
  tea with milk and sugar and 2 plain biscuits
Supper
  grilled white fish and mash
  tomato salad
  fruit juice
9 p.m.
  a cup of warm milk and a slice of sponge cake

The above menu may appear to be excessive for the anorexic
patient but frequent meals at which small portions of the required
foods are served will encourage the individuals to take adequate
amounts.

EFFECTS OF ALCOHOL

The alcohol irregularly consumed by the social drinker is
metabolized by specific enzymes in the liver (the alcohol dehydrogenase system) and detoxified. However, chronic intake of large
quantities of alcohol by the heavy drinker results in liver injury
which markedly affects the nutritional status of the individual.
Women are more susceptible to the development of cirrhosis than
men, with a higher incidence of liver disease for a similar history of
alcohol abuse. Abnormal carbohydrate metabolism can result in
hypoglycaemia caused by impaired gluconeogenesis; reduced
protein metabolism can result in the inhibition of albumin

synthesis, and the accumulation of triglycerides in the liver cells (known as a fatty liver, discussed below) is an indication of affected fat metabolism.

Added to this, deficiencies of vitamins and minerals can occur. These may be caused by several factors including a poor diet, increased requirements, malabsorption, reduced storage or increased excretion. The vitamin B complex vitamins are particularly affected: thiamine, riboflavin, pyridoxine and folic acid deficiency are all widely seen in alcoholics. Vitamin C deficiency may also occur because of an inadequate intake.

Although alcohol theoretically contributes 29 kJ/g (7 Cal/g) when given under controlled conditions, it causes less weight gain than an isocaloric carbohydrate substitute. This is particularly true for the drinker taking large quantities of alcohol and the explanation for this phenomenon is not clear. Although the ingestion of alcohol can cause progressively more serious involvement of the liver, resulting ultimately in death, the deleterious effects of excessive alcohol intake are seen in various organs of the body.

The *neurological system* is affected both in the short term, as intoxication, and chronically. Wernicke's encephalopathy, seen as a sequel to thiamine deficiency, has been discussed in Chapter 1. Cerebral atrophy can occur and hepatic encephalopathy (discussed below) is also seen secondary to liver injury.

The *gastrointestinal tract* can be affected in several ways; cancer of the mouth and oesophagus may result from the directly corrosive effect of the alcohol, and gastritis for the same reason. Malabsorption, diarrhoea and acute pancreatitis associated with hypertriglyceridaemia are also common in alcoholics.

As discussed in Chapter 10 the major cause of *folic acid deficiency anaemia* is alcoholism.

Webster states that *fetal alcohol syndrome* resulting from alcohol abuse during pregnancy occurs in 1–2 per 1000 births. It is a condition in which the child is mentally retarded and pre- and postnatal growth retardation are seen. These infants have a high incidence of malformations; in particular, congenital heart defects. The children have a unique facial appearance with broad cheeks and thin lips. Although it has been known for some years that alcohol abuse during pregnancy is hazardous, it has only recently been recognized that alcohol intake during the first six to seven weeks after conception may have such far-reaching effects. There has been some controversy in the literature about the need for absolute abstinence from alcohol being a necessary recommendation for optimal fetal health. In general, it would seem reasonable to advise patients to refrain from taking more than the occasional glass of wine, particularly during the early months of pregnancy.

It is, however, the *liver* which is the target organ of alcoholism due to its complex structure and its diverse role in metabolism. The major short-term effect of a heavy drinking binge is a fatty liver. This is a condition where up to 50% of the tissue is affected by the infiltration of fats. This is caused by increased synthesis, decreased degradation and increased accumulation of fatty acids. It occurs after acute ingestion of large quantities of alcohol but can also be precipitated by malnutrition, by Frederickson's Type II hyperlipidaemia and uncontrolled diabetes mellitus. Although fatty liver is a benign, reversible condition it indicates metabolic dysfunction which can lead to more serious liver injury.

The chronic abuse of alcohol can result in hepatitis as discussed above, but, with continued drinking, cell death and the replacement of active cellular mass with fibrotic tissue occur. This is known as *cirrhosis*. Early functional recovery is possible in this condition if the patient stops drinking and takes adequate protein, which helps cellular regeneration. A drop in serum albumin caused by the reduced ability of the liver to make this protein is another reason for the need to increase protein in the diet. A daily intake of approximately 80–100 g protein is usually satisfactory: reference to serum protein levels will reflect the adequacy of the diet.

Worsening of the condition includes an increase in liver fibrosis with a concomitant decrease in liver function. This can result in hepatic encephalopathy (discussed below) and if this occurs the protein intake must be dramatically *lowered* to the limits of the patient's tolerance. Thus with progression of the disease the protein intake may have to be reduced: a 40 g, 20 g or ultimately a 10 g protein diet may be required. The nurse should repeatedly emphasize that permanent abstinence from alcohol is of vital importance.

Table 14 shows the alcohol and energy contents of various alcoholic drinks.

Table 14. Approximate alcohol and energy content of some alcoholic drinks.

Beverage	Kilojoules	Calories	Alcohol (g)
Beer: large glass, 250 ml			
Bitter	335	80	7.5
Lager	314	75	8
Brandy (also whisky, gin) 25 ml tot	293	70	8
Cider: large glass, 250 ml			
Dry	397	95	9.5
Sweet	585	140	9.3
Liqueurs (e.g. cherry brandy, Tia Maria, Creme de Menthe, Curacao) 20 ml	250–314	60–75	4–6
Sherry: 50 ml measure			
Dry	268	64	7.5
Sweet	300	72	7.5
Stout: large glass, 250 ml	376	90	7.5
Wine: 120 ml glass			
Dry	335	80	10.5
Sweet	376	90	12

Complications

Because the liver plays an important role in diverse metabolic activities, several other modifications of the diet may be required for the patient with hepatic insufficiency.

Ascites

Ascites is an accumulation of an abnormal amount of fluid in the abdomen and is a frequent complication. It may occur for various reasons, including a low serum albumin level, portal hypertension and increased sodium retention. Patients with ascites are given a low-sodium diet and the recommendations given in Chapter 9 for heart conditions apply. If a high-protein diet is necessary to improve serum albumin levels, a certain amount of compromise will be needed as most foods which are good sources of protein have a relatively high sodium content. As an alternative, there-fore, low-sodium high-protein proprietary products such as Casi-lan and Edosol low-sodium milk may be used to reduce the sodium content of the diet. While retaining sodium, patients usually lose potassium, so fruits, fruit juices and fresh vegetables should be emphasized to increase potassium intake. In particular, bananas, oranges, dried fruits, pineapples and tomatoes are rich sources of potassium. All-bran and wholewheat cereals, nuts, legumes and brewers' yeast supply much potassium, and they are also good sources of protein.

Hepatic encephalopathy

This complication results from an inability to handle a nitrogen load — the most common source of which is food high in protein — or a gastrointestinal haemorrhage. (It can also be caused by the administration of ammonia-containing salts.) Ammonia is formed by bacteria in the gastrointestinal tract during the digestion of protein. It is then normally transferred to the liver and converted into urea. However, increased portal blood pressure, an associated complication of liver disease, can cause dilated vessels at the junction of the portal and systemic systems. This can result in the shunting of the portal blood past the liver, thus preventing detoxification of the ammonia. The presence of ammonia in the circulation causes symptoms when it reaches the brain. The clinical assessment of this complication is determined by deterioration in intellectual ability, abnormal behaviour, a flapping tremor of the hands, a characteristic smell of the breath *(fetor hepaticus)* and an abnormal EEG, and the condition may develop into a coma in severe instances.

Dietary treatment is initially to minimize protein intake. The patient is given only fruit, vegetables, cereals and fats with minimal protein content or, if necessary, the protein-free fluid diet discussed below. With recovery from the hepatitis, protein intake may be increased to the maximum that can be tolerated without causing any symptoms or signs of relapse. Most patients at this stage tolerate at least a 40 g protein diet and many will be in nitrogen balance. A small number of patients cannot tolerate this amount and here the choice is between restricting protein, which can aggravate any ascites present, or giving protein plus drugs. Two types of drugs are used — neomycin, which kills ammonia-producing bacteria, and lactulose, a non-absorbable carbohydrate. This compound converts ammonia to ammonium in the gastrointestinal tract. Ammonium is poorly absorbed and is largely excreted in the faeces. Many drugs, including sedatives and drugs for pain, can also induce hepatic encephalopathy in patients with severe liver disease and should be avoided.

Oesophaegeal varices

This complication may result from seriously impaired hepatic function. Portal hypertension results in dilated vessels immediately under the lining of the oesophagus. Consumption of rough foods can cause tearing and bleeding from these vessels and many patients with hepatic disease will need a soft diet. Hard fibrous foods and coarse skins or pips must be avoided and in severe cases a semi-solid diet should be given (see Chapter 16).

Disturbed blood sugar levels

Both hypoglycaemia and hyperglycaemia are frequent symptoms of chronic liver disease and an abnormal glucose tolerance curve may be seen in over half the patients with cirrhosis. The term used to describe this condition is hepatogenic diabetes mellitus. It is caused by increased insulin resistance, the origin of which is unknown.

Spider naevus

This classical skin complication of liver failure is caused by the liver's impaired ability to detoxify oestrogens. The characteristic lesion is seen predominantly on the upper trunk, face and arms (the distribution of the superior vena cava). There is a central hump with dilated capillaries radiating out from it, resembling a spider. The same symptom occasionally occurs in other situations, but is usually evidence of long-standing liver disease. Although the condition does not require specific modification of the diet, its presence should alert the nurse to underlying liver disease.

DIET THERAPY IN CIRRHOSIS

Diets containing a range of protein content will be used for patients with cirrhosis, depending on the severity of the condition. A restricted-sodium diet may be required, and the consistency of the diet may have to be modified. Naturally not all possible dietary combinations can be discussed in detail in this book but given below are the principles on which the diet should be based in treating various degrees of cirrhosis.

Mild to moderately severe cirrhosis

The early stages of this condition are usually treated with a moderately high-protein diet, often accompanied by sodium restriction. A sample menu is given below. It is high in carbohydrate and fats to prevent tissue breakdown for energy purposes, which would cause an unnecessary load of protein derivates on the liver. Although the greatest proportion of sodium consumed is in the form of table salt, all foods containing this element in various forms should be considered and the stipulations mentioned in Chapter 9 should be followed. Fruit and fruit juices are emphasized for their potassium content.

Sample menu (mild to moderate cirrhosis)

Breakfast
   orange juice
   2 fried eggs
   2 slices of toast, butter and jam or marmalade
Dinner
   large helpings of meat or chicken
   large helpings of rice or potatoes, with butter
   vegetables and salad
   banana custard
Supper
   large slice fried fish with mash and tomato salad
   ice-cream
Bedtime
   milk drink with sugar

Note: It should be mentioned that the use of effective sodium-losing diuretics today often reduces the need for severe sodium restriction. Many patients are merely told *not to add* salt to their meals and to avoid excessive amounts of salted butter and bread: the consumption of four slices of baker's salted loaves and ordinary salted butter will double the amount of sodium in the basic diet. The degree of sodium restriction will thus depend on the severity of the condition, the effectiveness of diuretics and the patient's acceptance of the unsalted products.

Increasingly severe cirrhosis

In Chapter 12 a range of low-protein diets is given. Although designed for increasingly severe renal disease, these can also be applied in case of hepatic disease since the principles of protein restriction are the same. It is important to know the proportionate contribution to the diet made by the more commonly eaten foods so that one can advise the patient about variety in the diet. Severely cirrhotic patients invariably require additional potassium.

A diet plan based on fruit and fruit juice for breakfast, rice or potato and vegetables (excluding legumes) and salad followed by fruit and cream for the other two meals provides a total of approximately 10 g of protein. To meet the individual patient's requirement of, for example, 40 g or 50 g of protein the appropriate foods from the following list may be selected. Each of these portions contains *10 g of protein*:

¼ of a 250 g carton of cottage cheese
4 medium (30 g) slices of bread
1½ medium (50 g) eggs
small (50 g) piece of fish
1 chicken leg
1 thin (30 g) slice beef
1 piece (5 cm × 3 cm × 3 cm) of cheese
large (300 ml) tumbler of milk
2 cups of cooked or 60 g of raw porridge oats
2 cups of cooked macaroni

It is emphasized that the above figures are merely given as guidelines and should not be regarded as completely accurate. For more precise information use the sample menus given in Chapter 12 ignoring, of course, the comment about potassium restriction which is not relevant here.

The patient with extreme liver damage is usually confused and may even become unconscious. In cases of such severity the patient will usually require a diet of 10 g (or less) of protein but the texture of normal foods makes this unpractical. The stuporous patient may manage to swallow liquidized or semi-solid foods in which case, for instance, vegetables and salads may be replaced by thick soup, gruel or an ice-cream (made from frozen, sweetened, whipped thick cream). Should the patient be unable to consume adequate quantities by mouth, a tube feed may be used. This protein-free feed is discussed in Chapter 16.

VITAMIN K

Among the multiple functions of the liver is the production of prothrombin, which is necessary for blood clotting. Impairment of liver function is thus accompanied by a tendency to bleed, which is normally treated by intramuscular injections of vitamin K, the usual regimen being 10 mg vitamin K/day for three consecutive days. Certain foods, particularly green leafy vegetables, liver and cheese, are good sources of this vitamin. However, even emphasis of rich sources is unlikely to add more than 1 mg of vitamin K to the diet (the normal mixed diet provides 300–500 µg), which is of little significance. Moreover, anorexic patients are unlikely to enjoy large quantities of leafy green vegetables and jaundiced patients may not absorb this vitamin, so parenteral supplements are more realistic in practice.

GALL-BLADDER DISEASE

Bile acids (salts) are manufactured in the liver from cholesterol. Their prime purpose is to act as a detergent, emulsifying fats for absorption, but they are also responsible for the excretion of various substances including cholesterol. Bile collects in the canniculae in the liver which then join to form the hepatic ducts which take the bile to the gall bladder for storage. The presence of food in the gut, especially food with a high fat content, prompts the release of an enzyme, *cholecystokinin*, from the wall of the duodenum into the blood stream, which in turn initiates contraction of the gall-bladder via the common bile duct. The bile enters the duodenum where it plays a vital role in fat absorption. It is then reabsorbed from the ileum and returned to the liver where it is reconjugated and resecreted. This *enteropathic circulation* of bile acids occurs several times per day.

Gall-stones

Should the bile become supersaturated and unable to contain the cholesterol in solution, the latter will separate out, forming *gall-stones*. Although the reason for this condition is not fully understood, certain factors related to inheritance and environment appear to play a role. Gall-stones occur more extensively in obese people and menopausal women. People who live on a high-fat, high-energy diet also seem to be more prone to developing the condition. The dietary treatment of gall-stones is as follows.

1. Restrict foods which promote contraction of the gall-bladder. All fatty foods are restricted, in particular the fats derived from meat, fish, oil and margarines. These are primarily composed of long-chained fatty acids, as opposed to the dairy fats which have predominantly shorter-chain fatty acids and are often more readily tolerated.
2. Some patients cannot tolerate excessively fibrous foods such as cabbage, cucumbers, cauliflower stalks, etc., and strongly spiced dishes. Should dyspepsia be caused by these foods they should be omitted from the diet.
3. Overweight patients should adhere to a strict weight reduction regimen as weight loss may alleviate symptoms.
4. The oral use of bile acids has recently been introduced as a form of therapy for this condition. By increasing the quantity of bile acids, thus allowing for the solution of more cholesterol, the potential for gall-stone production is reduced. Interestingly, a reduction in the amount of cholesterol in the diet appears to have no effect on the formation of gall-stones.

Cholecystitis

Inflammation of the gall-bladder is usually caused by the obstruction of the cystic duct by a gall-stone. Bile trapped in the gall-bladder has an irritant effect on the wall, resulting in inflammation. Contraction of the gall-bladder causes severe pain and the dietary treatment of the condition is the same as for gall-stones (see 1–3 above), i.e. to reduce secretion of cholecystokinin by avoiding offending foods.

NURSING CONSIDERATIONS

1. Patients with a history of alcohol abuse almost invariably

need vitamin supplements, in particular vitamin B-complex (especially folic acid). However, caution must be exercised as many tonics contain alcohol and are thus totally inappropriate.

2. Cirrhotic patients require close observation for the following reasons:
   (a) Their lockers should be carefully checked for hidden liquor, often disguised.
   (b) Those with oesophageal varices should at all times be limited to soft foods. A poorly chewed hard sweet or piece of fruit can cause considerable damage to the weakened blood vessels in the throat.
   (c) Behavioural or mental changes may be symptoms of hepatic encephalopathy for which the patient requires immediate medication and a lower protein intake.

3. The anorexic patient with hepatitis is often prepared to take liquids. A jug of chilled apple juice with Caloreen to provide extra energy, ginger beer and ice-cream, or orange juice with a few tablespoons of milk powder or even well-disguised egg beaten into it, are often more acceptable than food.

4. Infectious precautions must be taken when nursing the patient with hepatitis. This includes the person serving meals as well as attention to the crockery and cutlery of the patient.

BIBLIOGRAPHY

Davidson, C.S. (1973) Dietary treatment of hepatic diseases. *J. Am. Diet. Ass.*, *62*, 515.

Hofman, A.F., Northfield, T.C. & Thistle, J.L. (1973) Can a cholesterol-lowering diet cause gall-stones? *N. Engl. J. Med.*, *288(1)*, 46.

Kirsch, R.E. & Saunders, S.J. (1978) Hepatic insufficiency. *Mod. Med. S. Afr.*, *3(6)*, 3.

Kosman, M.E. (1976) Lactulose (Cephulac) in portosystemic encephalopathy. *J. Am. Med. Ass.*, *236(21)*, 244.

Lieber, C. (1973) Liver adaptation and injury in alcoholism. *N. Engl. J. Med.*, *288*, 356.

Morgan, M.Y. (1979) Alcohol and the liver. *J. Hum. Nutr.*, *33*, 350.

Mosbach, E.H. (1972) Hepatic synthesis of bile acids. *Archs. Int. Med.*, *130*, 478.

Redinger, R.N. & Small; D.M. (1972) Bile composition, bile salt metabolism and gall-stones. *Archs. Int. Med.*, *130*, 618.

Schiff, L. (ed.) (1969) *Diseases of the Liver*. Philadelphia: J. Lippincott.

Sherlock, S. (1981) *Diseases of the Liver and Biliary System*, 6th edn. London: Blackwell Scientific.

Sturdevant, R.A.L., Pearce, M.L. & Dayton, S. (1973) Increased prevalence of cholelithiasis in men ingesting a serum-lowering diet. *N. Engl. J. Med., 288*, 24.

Tenton, J., Knight, E. & Humpherson, P. (1966) Milk-and-cheese diet in portal systemic encephalopathy. *Lancet, 1*, 164.

Visocan, B. (1983) Nutritional management of alcoholism. *J. Am. Diet. Ass., 83*, 693.

Walser, A. (1983) Nutritional support in renal failure: future directions. *Lancet, 1*, 340.

Walser, A. (1983) Nutrition in renal failure. *Ann. Rev. Nutr., 3*, 125.

Webster, W., Germain, M., Lipson, A. & Walsh, D. (1984) Alcohol and congenital heart defect: an experimental study on mice. *Cardiovasc. Res., 18*, 335.

12   The kidneys

The kidneys are highly selective filters which control the fluid, protein and electrolyte balance of the body and maintain the composition of the blood within normal limits. Impairment of function results in excessive retention or excretion of one or more of these elements.

PHYSIOLOGY

Each kidney contains about one million *nephrons*, the basic functional units responsible for the production of urine. A nephron consists of a round head (*glomerulus*), situated in the cortex of the kidney, and an extended tube (*tubule*) which leads through the medulla and discharges into the renal pelvis and thence into the ureter (Fig. 15). The glomerulus is a tuft of capillaries, ramifications of the renal artery. As blood flows through the glomerulus, some of the fluid filters out through the semipermeable walls of the arteriole into the surrounding space, inside the Bowman's capsule, which is drained by the tubule. Filtration is assisted by arterial pressure, the afferent artery having a greater diameter than the efferent one. The renal circulation is largely dependent on cardiac output but temporary reductions of volume occur with exercise, dehydration and emotional or physical trauma. Seriously diminished circulation due to severe shock or physical injury can result in acute renal failure.

Although about 120 ml of filtrate enters the tubles each minute, less than 20 ml of urine is produced per minute, because of the highly efficient and selective reabsorption at the tubule surface. Along with the fluid returned to the circulation, certain essential solutes, including sodium, potassium, phosphate and bicarbonate, are also returned as required to maintain the homeostatic acid–base balance. End products of metabolism such as urea, creatinine, inorganic salts (particularly sodium chloride) and water remain in the urine. Under normal circumstances, glucose is reabsorbed, but in diabetes mellitus, where the body is unable to maintain the blood concentration within normal limits, glucose is

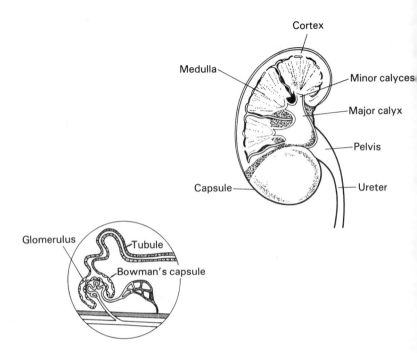

Fig. 15. *The normal kidney.*

left in the urine. Certain chemicals ingested as food additives or drugs are also cleared from the body through the kidneys

It is thus obvious that impairment of kidney function will affect the excretion of a variety of nutrients and may affect blood levels of protein, potassium, sodium and phosphate. Total body fluids may also be increased because of the kidneys' inability to eliminate surplus. Disregard of the essential principles of diet therapy in these conditions can threaten the life of the patient. The main renal disorders affected by diet and relevant to the nurse are discussed below.

ACUTE GLOMERULONEPHRITIS

The most common renal disorder is acute post-streptococcal glomerulonephritis, occurring classically shortly after a streptococcal infection such as scarlet fever, tonsillitis or an infected skin lesion. It is a fairly common disease of childhood. The symptoms are haematuria, oedema and oliguria (deficient urine output). Although in a small minority of patients the disease can lead to acute renal failure or chronic nephritis, most children recover completely. The condition has a poorer prognosis in adults: only about 50% recover completely.

Although diet plays a secondary role in this condition, most patients show signs of fluid retention and initially need salt and water restriction. Fluid intake is dependent on the current phase of the illness and the associated output of urine. It is reduced during the oliguric phase to not more than 600 ml. However, restrictions are relaxed during the later diuretic phase to compensate for the excessive output. If oedema or hypertension is present, limitation of salt intake will be an essential part of treatment.

Provision of an adequate energy intake is of particular import-ance: during the early days of the illness when the patient is anorexic and nauseous special attention should be paid to the appearance of meals and the serving of preferred foods.

Although some years ago protein restriction was considered essential to 'rest' the kidneys, this is seldom advised for children today since the study of Illingworth *et al*, who compared the prognosis of two randomly selected groups of children with nephritis. One group was given a low-protein diet whereas the other was given a standard ward diet. The children were followed up over the course of a year and no difference was seen in their recovery.

CHRONIC RENAL FAILURE (CHRONIC NEPHRITIS)

In this condition the prime disorder is inflammation of the glomeruli, impairing elimination of nitrogenous compounds from the plasma. These nitrogenous compounds are formed during the metabolism of food or, in the case of inadequate intake, from endogenous muscle stores. In cases of renal failure nitrogenous products accumulate in the blood and levels of urea and creatinine (as well as several other substances) become elevated. Checking for elevated blood urea level is thus an easy method of assessing kidney function and gives a good idea of the patient's condition. Levels above 7.5 mmol/litre are regarded as abnormal and should the level reach 30–40 mmol/litre patients will often complain of nausea, headache and malaise. These symptoms are due to the retention in the body of protein breakdown products. They are usually taken to indicate the need for dietary restriction of protein, and at this stage the protein intake will usually be reduced to 40 g/day.

A more accurate determination of kidney function is the creatinine clearance test, in which the degree of impairment of the excretory function of the kidneys can be more directly observed. A normal creatinine clearance rate is approximately 100 ml/min and implies that the kidneys are able to clear a volume of blood containing this amount of creatinine in one minute. In grossly damaged kidneys the creatinine clearance rate can drop to as little as 5 ml/min.

HAEMODIALYSIS

Today there is widespread use of haemodialysis for patients with severe deterioration in kidney function. This method of clearing abnormally large quantities of compounds from the blood has been largely responsible for prolonging life and ameliorating the condition of these patients. For those on regular haemodialysis, the diet is relatively liberal. Patients may take 50–60 g protein when in a stable condition as they are routinely assisted in excreting metabolic breakdown products which formerly accumulated unremittingly in the blood. This relative dietary freedom is a great compensation for these chronically ill patients.

In some cases the presence of *oedema* or *hypertension* will prompt the need for reduction in sodium intake and *hyperkalaemia* may necessitate a moderately restricted potassium diet. Elevated levels of serum *phosphate* are treated with the administration of aluminium hydroxide but, as these may adversely affect the bones, merely reducing phosphate intake is usually regarded as a preferable alternative. *Calcium carbonate* must be taken in large quantities by many patients to offset their poor absorption of calcium. Some of these patients have great difficulty swallowing such large quantities of unpalatable compounds, so it may be advisable to recommend that aluminium hydroxide and calcium carbonate be included in a basic biscuit dough which is then baked and served as biscuits during the day.

Another complication of dialysis is *hyperlipidaemia* due to the metabolic disturbances of uraemia and probably also the load of glucose and acetate absorbed from the dialysate thrice weekly. The appropriate regimen from Chapter 9 will be applied.

Constipation can also be troublesome and a high-fibre intake (see Chapter 8) is recommended for these patients.

Patients who are underweight are advised to take high-energy supplements and emphasize foods high in carbohydrate (glucose, sweets, cereals such as noodles, porridge and desserts) and fried foods.

An extremely serious complication of dialysis is a neurological syndrome encountered in a few patients. Encephalopathy occurs, often accompanied by bone disease, and it is suggested that this results from the accumulation of toxic levels of aluminium derived from the water used in dialysis. Currently, attention is being given to the removal of aluminium from water supplies to be used for dialysis.

PERITONEAL DIALYSIS

In haemodialysis, an artificial membrane is used to transfer solutes from the blood (where there is a high concentration) to the dialysate (where there is a low concentration). In peritoneal dialysis, the peritoneum, which has a rich capillary supply, is used as the semipermeable membrane.

One to two litres of warm dialysate fluid is run into the peritoneal cavity, left there for a short time to allow the solute exchange to take place and then drained out. This is repeated several times per day and is a relatively easy procedure which can be undertaken by the patient in his home environment; hence the name *continuous ambulatory peritoneal dialysis* (CAPD).

The major differences in dietary requirements between these patients and those having haemodialysis are:

1. patients on CAPD lose more protein in the dialysate and therefore should be given a more liberal protein intake. The usual recommendation is 1.2–1.5 g protein/kg allowance for these patients.
2. CAPD patients absorb approximately 160 g glucose/day from the dialysate. This is of considerable advantage to the underweight patient but the overweight patient will need to take cognizance of this extra source of energy.

DIETARY MANAGEMENT IN CHRONIC RENAL DISEASE

Although the use of dialysis has minimized the need for a restricted diet in many patients, for others dietary modifications are an essential part of treatment. This relatively small group includes those whose renal function is not so severely impaired as to require dialysis and those for whom dialysis can be postponed through the use of a controlled diet. In other patients whose living conditions make the use of dialysis impracticable, diet therapy is vitally important.

The symptoms and management of chronic renal disease are summarized in Table 15.

Protein

Previously, patients with chronic nephritis were given a low-protein diet largely compiled of foods making small contributions of protein to the diet. Dishes made predominantly with cereals were the major menu items. However, early in the 1960s Giordano and Giovannetti proposed a diet which provided 0.3 g protein/kg body weight. The diet provided a balanced amount of essential amino acids by use of egg protein (as this has the highest biological value) and a supplementary dosage of deficient amino acids. The rest of the diet, which was made up of foods with a minimal protein content, provided adequate kilojoules for the patient's needs. It was found that symptoms of uraemia improved, that the patient found the diet acceptable, and that nitrogen equilibrium in the body was easier to maintain. Many patients also require sodium and potassium restriction and the diet could easily be adapted to meet their needs. The modified Giovannetti diet (see below) became widely used and is still currently used for a few selected patients.

Regrettably, some practitioners regard the Giovannetti diet as being synonymous with reduced renal function and prescribe it without regard to the patient's individual filtration capacity. It must be emphasized that in most cases a higher level of protein is permissible and a more liberal diet should be introduced, as patients may in the long term develop complications such as pericarditis, bone disease and wasting on the limited Giovannetti diet. Furthermore, patients may find the diet monotonous and

Table 15. Symptoms and management of chronic renal disease.

Type	Signs and symptoms	Biochemistry	Therapy
Mild Creatinine clearance 50–100 ml/min	Asymptomatic	Normal	None
Moderate Creatinine clearance 25–50 ml/min	May have raised urea and blood pressure; mild pallor	Raised urea, serum creatinine and blood pressure may be present	Majority hypertensive – therefore antihypertensive drugs used; protein intake reduced to approx. 60 g/day
Severe Creatinine clearance 10–25 ml/min	Always symptomatic: nausea, weakness, lethargy, malaise, headache	Acidosis; raised urea, creatinine phosphate; low serum calcium	Protein restriction, drug dosage modified, phosphate restriction with or without binders
End stage Creatinine clearance 10 ml/min	Marked pallor, frequently nausea, vomiting, diarrhoea	Urea raised to over 30 mmol/l, hyperkaelaemia	Dialysis may be needed at short notice

Note: Hypertension becomes progressively more dependent on salt and fluid intake with deteriorating renal function.

difficult to maintain for a long period. Black comments that 'except in specialist centres, diets providing less protein than 0.5g/kg should not be given, and even in such centres the period and degree of protein restriction should be the minimum dictated by the local facilities for dialysis and transplantation'. However, he adds: 'But some patients must still be managed conservatively: for them low-protein diets are essential and must be properly managed'. Children particularly need adequate protein for growth and long-term severe restriction can result in serious impairment of development.

To summarize, the recommended diet should be as near to a normal intake as possible. Should symptoms of severe uraemia or complications occur, a 40 g protein diet is regarded as adequately restricted for the majority of patients, with reduction to 20 g protein (i.e. the modified Giovannetti diet)) only in a few severe cases where dialysis is not considered to be feasible. Use protein foods of high biological value.

Energy

Adequate sources of energy are essential in a low-protein diet. Black suggests 35–50 Cal/kg per day, i.e. the 65 kg patient requires over 3000 Cal (12 500 kJ). Carbohydrates are included in all meals containing protein to ensure the most favourable use of the protein because of the protein-saving effect of the carbohydrate. Children, in particular, require more carbohydrates than normal for optimum utilization of protein for growth and development.

To increase energy intake, sweetened, synthetically flavoured cool drinks, sugar, sweets, butter and other pure fats should be liberally included in the diet. Products made from special protein-free flour should also be emphasized. Patients can obtain protein-free flour, bread, pasta and biscuits on an FP 10 prescription form, but the nurse should point out to these patients that products must be *protein-free* and not merely *gluten-free*. Gluten-free products are prepared for people with coeliac disease and protein from other sources (milkpowder, soya, etc.) is added in many cases. The following three commercial products are widely used in low-protein diets to increase the energy value.

Hycal is a protein-free, flavoured glucose solution. It has the advantage of having a very low electrolyte content and can be added to foods or taken as a beverage. A 171 ml bottle provides 1776 kJ (425 Cal).

Caloreen is a glucose polymer yielding 1605 kJ (384 Cal) per 100 g. Because it is less sweet, it is more acceptable than sucrose or glucose and can thus be used in greater quantity in beverages and foods. Like Hycal it has a very low electrolyte content.

Prosparol is a 50% emulsion of fat in water. It is primarily used as a concentrated source of energy in tube feeds but is also included as an ingredient in supplementary beverages for these patients. It yields 19 kJ (4.5 Cal)/ml.

There are two other measures used today to ensure an optimum intake of essential amino acids with the minimum involvement of the kidneys. In the first place, patients may be given a very low-protein diet (15–20 g daily) to which supplementation of essential amino acids is added. These selected amino acids, including *histidine*, which appears to be essential for uraemic patients, are given in tablet form. Secondly, alpha-keto analogues of essential amino acids may be administered as a supplement to a diet containing a minimal amount of protein. These compounds combine with nitrogen derived from ammonia and urea in the body. This anabolism of nitrogen results in reduced excretion of urea through the kidney. Recycling nitrogenous breakdown products to produce protein in this way has become a feasible measure for most of the essential amino acids but the alpha-keto analogues are extremely costly to obtain, and this form of therapy will thus be impractical in most situations.

Sodium

The presence of oedema, hypertension and unexpected weight gain will alert the practitioner to decreased renal filtration capacity and the need to restrict sodium intake. The prescribed sodium intake will depend on the patient's clinical state. On the other hand, the patient unable to conserve sodium may be given additional packets of salt to sprinkle on his food as directed, or advised to eat salty foods such as ham and cheese. Sometimes salt tablets are prescribed for salt-depleted patients but as these are less effectively absorbed from the gut many practitioners prefer the administration of loose salt.

In cases where sodium retention or oliguria occurs, resulting in oedema, diuretics and a low-sodium diet are usually necessary. Where blood pressure levels are only minimally elevated, the patient may merely be advised not to sprinkle additional salt on his food. However, in more severe cases, the rules given in Chapter 9 for strict restriction of sodium may have to be applied. Salt substitutes should be used with caution as these usually contain potassium and may promote hyperkalaemia in these patients.

Fluids

With deterioration of renal function, the ability of the kidneys to concentrate urine is impaired and the patients may pass an excessive amount of hypo-osmolar (dilute) urine. At the same time, normal amounts of electrolytes cannot be eliminated and they therefore accumulate in the blood. Hypertension and oedema are direct sequelae of elevated sodium levels. In other patients, a delay in excretion of ingested fluids causes water intoxication, a condition in which plasma sodium concentration is reduced and excess ingested water is distributed throughout all body compartments. Symptoms of drowsiness, confusion and even coma can occur. Hence most patients are told to take a large quantity of fluid to promote elimination of electrolytes but it may be advantageous to reduce fluid intake in others. Patients with severe chronic renal impairment should therefore be weighed regularly to spot signs of fluid retention as early as possible. There is an optimum fluid intake for each uraemic patient, and individual management is based on renal function.

Calcium and phosphate

With progression of renal disease, the reduction in glomerular filtration rate results in retention of phosphates and *elevated* blood levels. Compensatory *lowering* of serum calcium occurs, which stimulates parathyroid hormone activity. The elevated parathyroid hormone level induces resorption of calcium from the kidneys and decalcification of bone. This osteomalacia is a component of renal osteodystrophy, which is a serious but relatively common complication of renal disease.

Primary treatment of the condition consists of administration of phosphate binders in the form of unpalatable aluminium hydroxide discussed above, plus administration of large doses of calcium. Control of plasma phosphate is followed by the administration of high doses of vitamin D. Theoretically a reduction in protein foods is advisable to reduce the phosphate level, particularly as the aluminium may affect the bones: in practice this advice is seldom necessary as these patients are invariably already fairly limited in protein intake and need all the protein they are able to utilize for tissue repair.

Table 16 shows the phosphorus content of some foods.

Table 16. Average phosphorus content of some foods.

Very high phosphorus: bran, cheese, egg yolk, walnuts

High phosphorus: milk, most wholegrain cereals, brown bread, meat (except as indicated below), fish, legumes, peanuts

Moderate phosphorus: white bread and biscuits, corn, dried apricots and peaches, mushrooms

Low phosphorus: macaroni, rice, fats and oils, vegetables, fruit, oxtail, tripe, jams and sweets

---

Potassium

In the earlier stages of renal disease, failure by the tubules to absorb potassium efficiently may very occasionally result in excessive losses of this element, and hypokalaemia. On the other hand, in severe renal failure, plasma levels may become dangerously high due to an inability to excrete normal quantities of potassium. The patient's dietary potassium intake must thus be modified according to the existing blood level and to this end a table of the comparative potassium contents of commonly eaten foods is given in Appendix C. As can be seen, many fruits and vegetables have a high potassium content, but this is markedly reduced if these foods are cut into small pieces and cooked in a large amount of water which is then discarded. This method of preparation should be used for all hyperkalaemic patients. Recommended fruit for the *hyper*kalaemic patients are stewed and drained apples and pears and canned drained fruit, particularly those which are processed sliced or cubed. For *hypo*kalaemia, orange and pineapple juice, bananas and tomatoes should be emphasized in the diet. Soups, extracts, high-protein foods (such as meat, fish and milk), wholegrain cereals and legumes also contribute much potassium to the diet.

It is clear that a wide variety of nutrients must be considered when feeding the patient with chronic renal failure; in fact, the nutritional requirements of this disease are probably more diverse than those of any other single pathological state. Furthermore, the presentation and palatability of meals must stimulate the patient to eat — theoretically perfect diets are of no use at all if refused by nauseous, anorexic, disinterested patients. The strict limitations of the diet as well as the lack of appetite which is a feature of the disease make the need for vitamin supplementation imperative in most instances, and many patients are routinely given a multivitamin preparation.

To recapitulate, it may be a useful exercise to look at the sample menu of the basic 20 g protein diet given below and consider the role of each item in terms of the patient's needs. A brief explanation of the dietary function of each food is provided. The diet can of course be used as a baseline recommendation to which additional protein is added as required. Over-conscientious protein restriction may cause protein deficiency and negative nitrogen balance in adults, and adversely affect normal growth in children.

Basic 20 g protein diet (or previously modified Giovannetti diet)

Essential daily inclusions
    180 ml milk (or 25 g cheddar cheese)
    1 egg
    Supplements of 0.5 g methionine, multivitamins and iron may be needed on this very low-protein diet but become increasingly less necessary as additional protein exchanges as listed below are included.

Sample menu

Breakfast
apple stewed with sugar   low-potassium fruit: sugar
                                 provides additional energy

Cornflour porridge with sugar and thick cream	very low in protein; energy from carbohydrate and fat
protein-free toast, butter and jam	unsalted bread and butter to be used if the patient is hyper-natraemic
sweetened tea or coffee with milk from daily ration	honey or sugar may be used to give additional energy; fluid intake may be a consideration

Dinner

fried rice and fried onions	high carbohydrate and fat content for energy; sliced onion adds flavour and is a good vehicle for fat
marrow, cabbage and runner beans	if serum sodium and potassium levels are elevated, these vegetables should be cut into small pieces and cooked in a large amount of unsalted water
butter on vegetables	use salt-free butter if necessary
canned pear slices and thick cream	in cases of hyperkalaemia, drain the pears; cream may be sweetened to provide additional energy

Mid-afternoon

tea with milk and biscuits made from special protein-free flour	the egg content of 2 or 3 biscuits can usually be regarded as insignificant when calculating daily intake

Supper

1 egg (or occasionally 30 g of cooked lamb or beef)	complete protein, contributing all essential amino acids
potato salad	home-made mayonnaise, made with one egg yolk and 300 ml of oil, contributes insignificant amounts of protein if taken in

moderate quantities; in cases of hyperkalaemia potatoes should be diced and boiled in plenty of water

salad made from lettuce, grated carrots and apple with French dressing

omit salt if necessary; oil provides extra energy

cornflour pudding

2 tablespoons of thick cream mixed with 250 ml of cold water make a useful milk replacement that adds variety

Bedtime
remaining milk plus protein-
 free biscuits if desired

It is emphasized that the above menu is merely a suggested outline including possible options which may be necessary for individual patients. The diet can be varied with the inclusion of suitable protein-free products and other fruit and vegetables chosen according to the patient's need for potassium restriction. Furthermore, a selection of dishes can be prepared using the milk substitutes described above. A savoury white sauce using butter and seasoning and thickened with cornflour can be used for vegetables, and custard (using sugar and custard powder) can be served for dessert. The puddings discussed below for acute renal failure can of course also be included for other patients where protein restriction is required.

Using this extremely limited diet as a foundation, other foods can be added to meet the patient's protein requirement and to fit in with his life-style. To this end, the following exchange lists have been compiled. However, when selecting food items from this list, two important points should be borne in mind:

1. Foods are listed according to their protein content, but cognizance of sodium and potassium content must almost invariably also be taken by patients with kidney disease. The vegetable protein exchanges each contain approximately twice as much potassium as the animal protein exchanges, *per portion.*

2. In general, preference should be given to those foods in the animal protein group, in view of the presence of all the essential amino acids.

Protein exchange lists

1. Foods containing 7 g protein.

    (a) Animal protein foods:

        1 thin slice (30 g) beef or lamb
        1 thin slice (30 g) fish
        1 small piece (30 g) chicken
        1 medium egg
        25 g cheddar cheese (high sodium content)
        200 ml milk

    (b) Vegetable protein foods:

        ½ cup (100 g, cooked weight) dried peas, dried beans or lentils
        ¾ cup (140 g, cooked weight) fresh green peas
        200 g fresh or frozen corn
        30 g almonds, peanuts or cashew nuts

2. Cereal exchanges, equivalent to 2.5 g protein:

        1 slice (30 g) white, unfortified bread
        1 cup (40 g) rice crispies or cornflakes
        4 plain biscuits, i.e. crackers or digestive type
        ½ cup (150 g, cooked weight) oat porridge
        2/3 cup (100 g, cooked weight) rice
        ½ cup (70 g, cooked weight) macaroni or spaghetti

Using the grouping above and assuming that most fruit and vegetables make little contribution to the protein content of the diet (a portion of most of these contain approximately 0.5 g protein) one can readily design an adaptable sample menu as shown in Table 17.

ACUTE RENAL FAILURE

Acute renal failure is a condition in which rapid deterioration in

Table 17. Low-protein diet: sample menu.

...........g   protein diet   Patient's name   ....

Instructions regarding intake of sodium: (e.g. omit all added salt on food OR omit salt plus bottled sauces, tinned or processed meat, fish, soups, etc.*).

Instructions regarding intake of potassium: (e.g. cook all vegetables in large quantities of water which is then discarded; avoid fresh fruit and fruit juices, etc.**)

Sample menu

Breakfast   ....   protein exchanges
                                  ....   bread exchanges
                                  ....   fruit/vegetable exchanges

Mid-morning }   ....   beverage
Mid-afternoon }   ....   bread exchanges

Dinner and }   ....   protein exchanges
Supper   }   ....   bread exchanges
                                  ....   fruit/vegetable exchanges
                                  ....   dessert suggestion

* See Chapter 9.
**See Appendix C.

glomerular filtration rate and consequent reduced excretory function occurs, resulting in major alterations in the biochemistry of the blood. There are several possible causes, of which the most common are bodily trauma, such as occurs in a car accident, and injury or shock following surgery, eclampsia or septic abortion. Acute renal failure can also be preceded by infections, by the administration of nephrotoxins such as carbon tetrachloride or by sensitivity to a specific drug.

Patients with moderately impaired kidney function will require less dietary modification than those who are more severely affected and each patient must be treated individually. In its most serious form, acute renal failure, or shut-down, is a life-threatening condition and must be treated with dialysis as soon as possible.

The condition is usually accompanied by *anuria* or severe *oliguria*, with retention of fluid and accumulation of protein and electrolytes in the blood. The top priority in dietary care of these patients is control of their fluid intake, which must be carefully controlled because of their inability to excrete any excess. The usual basic allowance for insensible loss due to sweat, respiration, etc., is approximately 600 ml. To this is added the volume of the urine excreted during a previous 24 hours to compensate for losses. Fluids given are ginger beer and cola drinks or sweetened synthetic minerals such as cream soda or raspberry, as these contain minimal quantities of potassium as well as increasing the energy intake.

Blood electrolytes are monitored regularly and the intake of several major nutrients — fluid, protein, sodium and potassium — is reduced to a minimum during the early phase of this illness. Hyperkalaemia, resulting from both impaired clearance and intracellular potassium (secondary to the hypercatabolic state, which is often a feature of the illness) is a particularly hazardous complication.

Nutritional management

This is based on similar principles to the diet in chronic renal failure and is adapted to individual renal function. Initially, many patients are unconscious or extremely nauseous and they are fed either through nasogastric tubes or intravenously. A major hazard of the latter is the risk of catheter sepsis due to reduced immune responses. Hycal, Caloreen and Prosparol discussed above, or an appropriate parenteral solution (as discussed in Chapter 16) may form the basis of the regimen. Protein-free oral feeds are then merely supplements. In these patients, dialysis is the most appropriate measure and once this is started patients may be able to tolerate up to 60–70 g protein/day.

Two common complications with a high mortality rate are *sepsis* and *gastrointestinal bleeding*. In an attempt to prevent the occurrence of gastrointestinal bleeding, it is advisable to keep food in the stomach for its buffering action. However, this is extremely difficult in practice, as the permitted diet is monotonous and unpalatable and patients are often nauseous and anorexic. The menu given below is both monotonous and seriously lacking in many essential nutrients. It is only recommended for a few days prior to dialysis. It provides minimal protein.

Sample menu (acute renal failure)

Breakfast
    porridge made from cornflour, 1 tablespoon of thick cream and water, served with sugar
    gluten-free toast, salt-free butter and honey
Lunch
    rice fried in salt-free butter
    low-protein ice-cream, made of stiffly beaten sweetened cream and melted butter or margarine
Supper
    protein-free bread fried in oil
    low-protein sago pudding using cream and water as above

Fluid intake dependent on previous day's output

Occasionally, the early oliguric phase is followed by a polyuric phase which, although indicating improvement, is not without hazard as vast quantities of fluid and essential nutrients are lost. Blood sodium, potassium, magnesium and phosphate levels drop as these electrolytes and water-soluble vitamins are lost in the urine. Intake should be adjusted to equal losses. Large quantities of fluid should be taken to avoid dehydration during this period, which may last up to a week.

THE NEPHROTIC SYNDROME

The nephrotic syndrome is a degenerative disease of the kidney characterized by increased glomerular permeability to protein, resulting in large protein losses in the urine. The condition may be precipitated by one of several diseases, which are treated independently. Diet therapy for the nephrotic syndrome is directed at replenishing protein losses and treating the oedema which is secondary to the hypoproteinaemia (low serum protein levels) caused by protein losses. These patients also frequently develop hyperlipidaemia and suffer from a high rate of coronary artery disease. This must be borne in mind when compiling the diet.

Practical dietary management

Patients who can handle a protein load satisfactorily are advised to consume up to 120 g protein/day. In view of the complicating oedema, however, the sodium present in food must also be considered although potent diuretics may be used to control the problem. As most high-protein foods contribute relatively large amounts of sodium to the diet a compromise must thus be made between the conflicting dietary needs of the patient. There is also some doubt about whether 120 g protein can be utilized by these patients and some practitioners recommend a somewhat lower intake (80–100 g/day). In most cases, the daily protein intake will be made up as follows:

> 500 ml milk, yoghurt or buttermilk (skimmed milk is advisable in cases of hyperlipidaemia)
> 2 large portions (150 g each) of meat, poultry or fish
> ⅓ carton of unsalted cottage cheese *or* two eggs (to be taken at the third meal)
> 4 slices of bread (unsalted if necessary)

Fruit, vegetables, sugars and unsalted cereals may be taken in unrestricted amounts, providing 10–15 g of protein. Also, unsalted butter (or oil if complicated by hyperlipidaemia) should be used. Enough of these foods should be eaten to meet energy requirements. Hyperlipidaemic patients should include eggs only occasionally.

RENAL CALCULI

Renal calculi are small stones, consisting of a matrix of organic material, which can cause obstruction of the kidneys or urinary tract.

Over 90% of calculi are predominantly calcium: calcium phosphate and calcium oxalate are the principal compounds involved. A small proportion of stones are composed largely of uric acid or the amino acid cystine.

Aetiology

Although the cause of the condition is still largely unknown there are several factors — including diet — which have been shown to play a role in stone formation. Environmental conditions appear to be particularly relevant in the Middle East, where the disorder occurs widely, even in children. It has been suggested that a detailed dietary history may be of value in that the onset of the condition is sometimes preceded by long-term excessive consumption of the predominant crystalline component.

Dietary management

The treatment for all types of stone formation includes the routine consumption of large quantities of fluid (3–4 litres/day) to dilute the urine and retard stone formation. Dietary modification for calculi depends on the pathogenesis of the condition and the composition of the stones. It has, however, been suggested but not proven that the megadoses of ascorbic acid being widely used by the public may promote the formation of renal calculi for two reasons. In the first place, ascorbic acid is metabolized through the formation of oxalic acid and, secondly, the resultant acid urine will contribute to the formation of uric acid — and cystine — stones in susceptible individuals.

Calcium-containing stones

Many patients with this condition have hypercalciuria (increased excretion of calcium in the urine). It may be caused either by increased absorption in the gut as a consequence of excessive intake (e.g. large quantities of milk and alkalis consumed for ulcers or dyspepsia) or possibly by disordered resorption by the kidneys. Exceptionally large doses of vitamin D may also cause high urinary levels of calcium, promoting stone formation. Whatever the cause, restriction of calcium intake will often reduce the urinary output of calcium and in such cases reduction of high-calcium foods is advisable. Milk and milk products, fish in which the small bones are eaten, and green leafy vegetables should be strictly limited in the diets of these patients. Attention must also be paid to the local drinking water. In areas with a hard water supply, 2 litres of tap water can contain 5 mmol (300 mg) of calcium. Patients with kidney stones should be advised to use a water softener or to drink distilled water. As the formation of calcium stones is aggravated by an alkaline environment, reliance on foods that are predominantly acid-forming will be less conducive to their formation. These foods are given below.

Oxalate-containing stones

Patients with oxalate-containing stones should avoid foods which have a high oxalate content. This compound is found particularly in rhubarb, beetroot and spinach, but chocolates, sweet-potatoes, cucumber, celery, chard, green beans, oranges, strawberries, endive and parsley are also relatively rich sources. Bayless and Elfert point out that these stones may occur in patients with fat malabsorption. It appears that the excess faecal fat binds calcium leaving oxalate available for absorption, thus promoting oxaluria and stones.

Uric acid stones

Excess uric excretion as a result of either an increased purine intake or the use of uricosuric drugs (administered to assist excretion of uric acid and prevent gout) may play a role in the production of these calculi. Adherence to the low-purine diet discussed in Chapter 15 may be recommended. Probably of greater importance is emphasis on foods which increase the alkalinity of the urine and retain the uric acid in solution.

Cystine stones

Cystine stones are encountered in individuals with a defective cystine transport system, resulting in the excretion of this amino acid in the urine. This is generally treated with sodium bicarbonate and a high fluid intake, with little attention to dietary manipulation. However, as acid urine aggravates the situation, patients are occasionally told to consume predominantly those foods that cause alkalinity of the urine. In rare cases, a low-methionine diet may be used.

Acid and alkaline foods

Acidic, alkaline and neutral foods may be relevant to the individual with renal calculi in counteracting an environment favourable for stone formation. Control of urine reaction by dietary modification will often at least ameliorate the condition and to this end a comparative list of foods is given below.

Acid-reacting	*Neutral*	*Alkali-reacting*
cheddar and sweet milk cheese	margarine, oil boiled sweets,	parmesan cheese
eggs	liquorice,	milk
all meat and fish	peppermints	all fruit except olives
peanuts and walnuts	white sugar	almonds, brazil nuts, chestnuts
asparagus	tea and coffee	all vegetables except as indicated
mushrooms	lemon and orange squash	toffee, treacle
		Bovril
		Horlicks

NURSING CONSIDERATIONS

1. Patients on salt-restricted diets should not be given salt substitutes, which are made with a potassium-containing compound, without the doctor's permission.
2. Dehydration and over-hydration are major problems resulting from renal disease; hence, intake and output must be carefully monitored in these patients.
3. Uraemic patients are often extremely nauseous and reject the high-fat diet which is routinely given as part of restricted protein regimen. As an optimal kilojoule intake is needed for protein-sparing, alert the dietitian immediately so that other acceptable foods can be tried.
4. The volume of Hycal or other glucose polymers must be

included in the fluid allowance.

5. All ward personnel must be aware of the stringent dietary restrictions required by these patients. A 'SPECIAL DIET' notice at the foot of the bed will prevent the routine serving of tea with milk (thus adding to both protein and fluid intake), fruit (contributing potassium) or milky nightcaps to the patient.

BIBLIOGRAPHY

Acchiardo, S., Moore, L. & Latour, P. (1983) Malnutrition as the main factor in morbidity and mortality of hemodialysis patients. *Kidney Int., 24* (Suppl. 16)

Bayless, T. & Elfert, G. (1984) Modifications of fat. In: *Nutritional Management: The Johns Hopkins Handbook*. London: W.B. Saunders.

Berlyne, G., Epstein, N. & Booth, E. (1973) Reduction of incidence of renal osteodystrophy associated with low protein diet in early renal failure. *Nutrition, 27*, 34.

Black, D.A.K. & Jones, N.P. (1979) *Renal Disease*, 4th edn. London: Blackwell Scientific.

Blainey, J.D. (1972) The biochemistry of renal failure. *Nutrition, 26*, 142.

Booth, E.M. (1973) Dietary treatment in renal disease. *Nutrition, 27*, 375.

Burton, B. (1974) Current concepts of nutrition and diet in diseases of the kidney. *J. Am. Diet. Ass., 65*, 623.

Drume, W., Laggner, A., Widhalm, K., Kleinberger, G. & Lenz, K. (1983) Lipid metabolism in acute renal failure. *Kidney Int., 24* (Suppl. 16), 139.

Giordano, C. (1963) Use of exogenous and endogenous urea for protein synthesis in normal uremic subjects. *J. Lab. Clin. Med., 62*, 231.

Giordano, C., Phillips, M., De Pascale, D., De Santo, N., Fürst, P., Brown, C., Houghton, B. & Richards, P. (1972) Utilisation of keto-acid analogues of valine and phenylalanine in health and uraemia. *Lancet,1*, 178.

Giovannetti, S. & Maggiore, Q. (1964) A low-nitrogen diet with proteins of high biological value for severe chronic uraemia. *Lancet, 1*, 1000.

Gretz, N., Korb, E. & Strauch, M. (1983) Low protein diet supplemented by keto-acids in chronic renal failure: A prospective controlled study. *Kidney Int., 24* (Suppl. 16), 263.

Illingworth, R., Philpot, M. & Rendle-Short, J. (1954) Controlled investigation of the effect of diet on acute nephritis. *Archs. Dis. Childh., 29*, 551.

Ing, T.S. & Kark, R.M. (1977) Renal disease. In: Schneider, H., Anderson, C. & Cowsin, D. (eds.) *Nutritional Support of Medical Practice*. London: Harper and Row.

Lancet (1976) Dialysis osteodystrophy. *Lancet, 1*, 451.

Leaf, A. & Cotran, R. (1976) *Renal Pathophysiology*. New York: Oxford University Press.

Pacey, N. (1975) Living with a renal diet. *Nutrition, 29*, 3.

Schoolwerth, A. & Engle, J.E. (1975) Calcium and phosphorus in diet therapy of uraemia. *J. Am. Diet. Ass., 66*, 460.

Vetter, L. & Shapiro, R. (1975) An approach to dietary management of patients with renal disease. *J. Am. Diet. Ass., 66*, 158.

Walser, M., (1983) Nutritional support in renal failure: future directions. *Lancet, i*, 340.

Walser, M. (1983) Nutrition in renal failure. *Ann. Rev. Nutr., 3*, 125.

13 The diet in surgery and burns

The nutritional demands of minor surgical trauma in well nourished patients are easily met by body reserves for a period of a few days. However, there are a variety of debilitating metabolic consequences of serious injuries such as major surgical procedures and burns which require specialized nutritional support. Surgical complications, infection and sepsis also make severe demands on the body's nutritional resources.

THE BODY'S RESPONSE TO INJURY

Immediately following the injury there is a brief period of catabolism, followed by a longer recovery period of accelerated metabolism, increased heat production and local anabolic processes at the site of injury.

In the 1940s, Cuthbertson introduced the terms 'ebb' and 'flow' for these two phases of body reaction. Moore has defined four phases of convalescence following injury. The *first* phase is injury accompanied by suppressed insulin production, glycosuria, depressed heat production and retention of sodium and water. Catabolism, the chemical breakdown of complex substances in the body to form simpler ones with a release of energy, occurs in patients with sepsis. There is extensive breakdown of body protein and considerable losses of nitrogen in the urine. This may last for several days, after which the *second* phase or turning point occurs: metabolism shifts to gradually increasing anabolism accompanied by a diuresis and increasing losses of sodium in the urine. Nutrient reserves are mobilized for use at the site of injury, and elsewhere if necessary, and there is a sudden drop in urinary nitrogen losses. The patient's appetite usually returns and the diet rapidly progresses through a stage of light, easily digestible foods to a full diet. The foods emphasized are those high in protein and those contributing large amounts of vitamin C, both necessary for tissue repair. Energy intake is very important in the promotion of protein synthesis. The *third* phase is the period during which muscular strength returns as a result of continued anabolism and resynthesis of muscle. The *final* period is that in which fat is deposited and the patient returns to his normal weight and vitality.

THE SURGICAL PATIENT

The dietary problems of the surgical patient are three-fold:

1. The building-up of preoperative reserves presents a dietetic challenge, particularly in those patients who are admitted to hospital debilitated and malnourished and who, with little appetite, are required to replenish body stores.
2. Following surgery, the patient's needs for a variety of nutrients, but particularly protein and energy, are greatly increased by the need for tissue repair. There may be practical problems in meeting these postoperative needs in patients who are either unable or unwilling for any prolonged period to take adequate food by mouth.
3. The sequelae of surgery may create the need for specific dietary management, e.g. low-carbohydrate diets are used in the treatment of the post-gastrectomy 'dumping syndrome' and the low-residue diet is used for patients who have had bowel surgery.

Preoperative nutrition

There is an increased risk of intercurrent infections and surgical complications in patients who are either underweight or considerably overweight preoperatively and it is thus necessary to take appropriate steps as early as possible. Regarding the obese patient, the moderate weight reduction diet discussed in Chapter 5 will usually be adequate, but should an even lower energy intake be required, the fruit portions can be omitted as the daily consumption of salads will supply adequate amounts of vitamins and minerals. For the underweight patient, the recommendations made in Chapter 6 will be appropriate but optimal body stores of protein and ascorbic acid are also a prerequisite of preoperative diet therapy.

With regard to the protein requirements of these patients,

Bistrian *et al* recently conducted a survey which investigated the nutritional status of surgical patients in hospital. They found that half the patients had clinical manifestations of protein-calorie malnutrition which clearly indicated that the nutritional support of these patients had been seriously neglected. It was particularly disturbing that in three out of ten patients studied, serum albumin levels dropped below normal *after* their admission to hospital, i.e. during their dependence on medical and nursing expertise. Hill *et al*, who undertook a similar study in England, confirmed that malnutrition was extremely common with the manifestation of two out of three indices of malnutrition present in 55% of patients who had undergone major surgery and were in hospital for more than a week postoperatively. The investigators point out that the fact that this serious situation had gone unrecognized and had thus not been treated was the most disconcerting aspect of the survey. Progressive weight loss, increased incidence of infection, prolonged weakness and malaise, slow wound healing and muscle wasting can all result from deficient nutrient intake.

It is thus emphasized that the nurse should play an extremely positive role in the dietary management of these patients, in an attempt to compensate for previous inadequacies as well as to provide reserves for immediate postoperative needs. These include protein (for plasma and tissue replenishment), adequate energy (to increase glycogen stores and spare protein) and optimal amounts of necessary minerals and vitamins. Ascorbic acid in particular plays an important role in wound healing, and to ensure saturation of tissue stores preoperatively the patient is usually given ascorbic acid supplements, especially where previous intake may have been inadequate.

Where adequacy of food consumption prior to hospitalization is in doubt, particular attention should be given to the intake of hospital meals. Patients should be encouraged to take mid-meal snacks of milk drinks, fruit or fruit juice, and food preferences should be given consideration whenever possible.

In the immediate preoperative period, food is withheld for at least eight hours prior to surgery to allow all foods to leave the stomach. Vomiting, aspiration of food during anaesthesia and postoperative complications such as dilatation and gastric retention may result from non-compliance with this precautionary measure. Patients undergoing surgery to the digestive tract are given a low-residue diet (see Appendix A) or a residue-free diet (see Chapter 16) for several days preoperatively. In the presence of severe obstruction, cancer of the digestive tract or fistulae, elemental diets or parenteral feeding may be necessary (see Chapter 16).

In a study by Zagoren *et al*, the progress of patients on a dextrose infusion was compared with a group on an amino acid parenteral feed. Although the study was undertaken for only a few days there was a significantly lower incidence of postoperative complications in the latter group.

As soon as normal peristalsis returns and bowel sounds can be heard, feeding is commenced with clear, residue-free fluids to replace losses and stimulate gastric secretion. The patient progresses to a full fluid diet as bowel motility and gastrointestinal function improve: milk forms the basis of this diet, and ice-cream, milk soups and strained gruel are usually included. Progress to a normal diet will depend on the severity of the surgery, the state and age of the patient and the absence of complications. However, the inclusion of progressively larger quantities of more concentrated food is necessary to ensure dietary adequacy. If this is impractical and the patient is unable to consume a relatively normal diet by the end of the first postoperative week, supplementary nutrients in the form of nasogastric feeds, an elemental diet or parenteral feeding is usually commenced (see Chapter 16).

Postoperative nutrition

Adequate *protein* intake is of the utmost importance. It is necessary for satisfactory wound healing and to replenish the losses resulting from surgery. This loss of protein is directly related to the degree of injury. Hence although minor or moderate surgical procedures present less of a challenge to the body, and the majority of patients suffer from no long-term ill-effects, the catabolic response to major complicated surgery is a serious sequel requiring active nutritional support. Exceptional breakdown of tissue protein occurs, which in situations of extreme physiological stress can approach 1 kg of muscle tissue per day. A protein-deficient diet will also result in low serum protein levels which can lead to oedema.

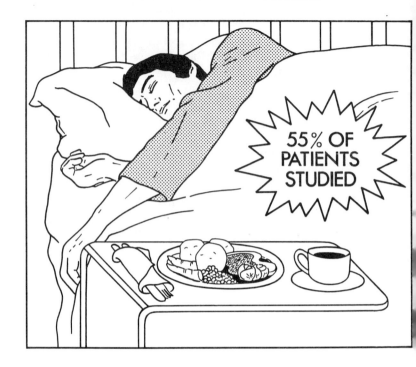

Fig. 16. *Malnutrition after major surgery.*

Energy requirement is also increased. Although energy expenditure may increase to only 110–120% of normal in uncomplicated surgery, the requirement can increase to 150% of normal in the event of sepsis, inflammation, etc. Furthermore, intake in the immediate postoperative period is minimal and the deficit has to be made up as soon as practical. Carbohydrate, in the form of glycogen, is the first-call energy source, after which the body depends on fat and endogenous (muscle) protein. Interestingly, elevation of the environmental temperature to about 30 °C arrests the catabolism of both protein and energy reserves and the patient's requirement is considerably reduced.

A *potassium* supplement may be given postoperatively to compensate for increased losses during the phase immediately after the operation. *Phosphorus* is also lost during this phase but the early consumption of milk will usually rapidly replace any deficit. With regard to *vitamins*, supplementary *vitamin C*, recommended preoperatively as a precautionary measure, is obviously required postoperatively, too. Furthermore, as *vitamin B complex* requirement is proportional to carbohydrate intake it may initially be given as a supplement, as food sources of this vitamin may be very limited. A recent survey of the nutritional status of hospital patients found reduced blood levels of two or more vitamins in 60% of patients, the most common deficiency being folate. Supplementation of this vitamin is often advisable.

Postoperative dietary management

The problems of postoperative feeding may be compounded by difficulties such as lack as appetite, losses resulting from haemorrhage and vomiting and a temporary reduction of digestive enzymes causing malabsorption and diarrhoea. The need to exclude specific foods from the diet due to limitations imposed by the particular operation may also restrict the patient's intake.

The immediate postoperative needs are *fluid replacement* and *replenishment of energy reserves*. These are met quite adequately after minor surgical procedures with a rapid progression through a transitional diet to a full diet within as little as a day. However, the patient undergoing major surgery or any surgery to the gastrointestinal tract presents a greater feeding challenge. Initially, the patient is given only sips of water, but this is rapidly increased in volume and variety to include other clear fluids, e.g. sweetened tea, jelly, clear fruit juice and clear broth or meat extracts dissolved in boiling water (the latter items being useful sources of sodium and potassium). If the patient is unable to take any, or an adequate amount of, fluid orally or if progression to a nutritionally adequate diet will take more than a day or two, parenteral supplementation (as discussed in Chapter 16) is imperative.

Immediately normal bowel sounds are heard the diet should progress through the following transitional diets at a rate dependent on the site and severity of surgery. The details of each stage are to some extent also dependent on hospital policy.

'Clear fluids' are followed by a 'free' or 'full' fluid diet. Here eggs and milk (in the absence of lactose intolerance) form the basis of the diet. Egg-flips, custard, milk, jelly, ice-cream and cream soups are liberally included. Orange juice is an excellent source of the vitamin C and potassium needed in increased quantities for tissue repair. Soup made with a pea flour basis adds both protein and variety to the regimen. The diet is liberalized to the light or low-residue diet with the introduction of more, but relatively easily digestible, fibre. Suitable foods are included in Appendix A.

Until the patient's capacity and recovery warrants the introduction of three normal meals from the standard hospital diet provided, food should be served in the form of six smaller nutritious snacks rather than three large meals. Routine assessment to determine whether the nutritional regimen is promoting optimal weight gain and recovery is essential in these patients.

SPECIFIC SURGICAL PROCEDURES

Following certain surgical procedures, specific dietary modification is required either as a result of the site of surgery or because of untoward complications.

Mouth and throat surgery

Fluids play a prominent role postoperatively and either a fluid or a semi-solid diet (see Chapter 16) will usually be suitable in the early period. Ice-cream is emphasized in the diet; patients find the consistency and temperature soothing and ice-cream also contributes a number of essential nutrients. Patients are often sensitive to sour fruits and juices which must initially be avoided. Although previously the tonsillectomy patient was usually given light bland food for the first few days postoperatively, today there is a trend to give patients coarse food as soon as possible. The consumption of toast, chicken, minced meat and cooked vegetables appears to remove sloughing and helps with scab formation and healing. However, older people, who often experience more pain following this operation, usually commence on a soft bland diet (including such foods as scrambled egg, soup and mash) and may take a week before their diet approaches normal.

Temporary dysgeusia (abnormal taste sensation) is often a postoperative consequence of surgery to this area and patients' whims should be understood and used to encourage a greater food intake.

Gastrectomy

A large proportion of patients undergoing gastrectomy experience food-associated problems postoperatively and many fail to regain their previous weight. Reduction of the output of digestive enzymes and acid and removal of part or all of the food reservoir causes both anorexia and a variety of postprandial symptoms. Flatulence, a feeling of fullness and discomfort after eating are all common postoperative symptoms. In the majority of patients there is a gradual recession of the symptoms and within about two months of the operation they are able to take moderate amounts of normal foods without ill-effects. However, in some patients these symptoms continue over a prolonged period and can be debilitating, usually because of a serious complication known as the 'dumping' syndrome, for which diet is the main form of treatment.

Dumping syndrome

Dumping syndrome can be classified as early or late: both conditions have specific symptoms related to the mechanism of reaction.

Early dumping occurs within a very short time of ingesting food as a result of the response of the jejunum to provocative undigested foods. In particular, those dietary items with hyper-osmolar pressure — such as high-carbohydrate and heavily salted foods — can cause retention of fluid and distension of the jejunum. The patient feels weak and nauseous 15–30 minutes after ingestion and has epigastric discomfort. Insulin output is increased and the patient may have symptoms of hypoglycaemia.

Late dumping syndrome occurs 1½–2 hours after the ingestion of the same foods. It is caused by a rapid drop in blood sugar following overstimulation of insulin output after a high-carbohydrate meal. The patient looks pale and feels weak. This complication is treated with the consumption of readily available carbohydrate, and patients who are prone to this reaction are advised to carry glucose sweets with them.

In view of the fact that the syndrome is observed to some extent in a fairly large number of patients undergoing gastric resection, it seems reasonable that all the patients should be well informed

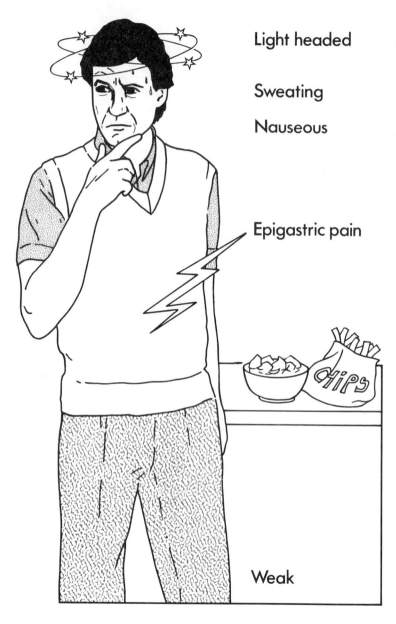

Fig. 17. *Early dumping syndrome.*

about the possibility of this complication occurring. They should be aware of which foods may precipitate dumping, know of the observable symptoms and understand how they can actively participate in the prevention or, at least, amelioration of the condition. However, the nurse should be extremely tactful when discussing this possible complication with the patient. Not only may the patient readily infer non-existent ill-effects from the word 'dumping', but he or she may become apprehensive about eating, attributing any minor feeling of discomfort to this complication.

The recommended diet consists initially of small dry meals, minimally salted, and the replacement of sugar with artificial sweeteners. Liquids are taken at least 45 mins before or after food consumption. If symptoms occur after the introduction of questionable foods the regimen detailed below should be applied for some months.

Sample menu (dumping syndrome)

06.30	*On awakening* weak tea without sugar
07.30	*Breakfast* 2 scrambled eggs, tablespoon mince, half slice of well buttered toast
09.00	synthetically sweetened milk drink (100 ml), cream added if possible
10.30	2 small biscuits, butter and grated cheese
11.30	unsweetened weak tea
12.30	*Lunch* small portion roast chicken, few brussels sprouts, slice of marrow
13.30	artificially sweetened baked custard
15.00	weak tea, water or artificially sweetened soft drink
16.30	2 small biscuits and grated cheese
18.00	liquid — water, unsweetened tea or artificially sweetened soft drink
19.00	*Supper* baked fish with melted butter and parsley small portion of tomato salad grated carrot and apple salad
20.00	junket, artificially sweetened
21.00	beverage as at 18.00

Intestinal surgery

Patients with chronic inflammatory disease or carcinoma of the intestine are often underweight and debilitated on admission to hospital. In a study by Hill *et al* (1981) the patients who developed major septic complications after surgery were relatively protein deficient preoperatively, compared to controls. Limited dietary intake coupled with malabsorption can directly affect the patient's prognosis. The nurse will be confronted with two conflicting dietary problems. She has to encourage the patient to eat the optimal amount to increase preoperative nutritional reserves, but for three or four days before surgery the patient's intake must be limited to those foods producing minimal bulk in the digestive tract, to facilitate surgery. Furthermore, surgery to specific sites in the intestine may be followed by diarrhoea resulting from malabsorption and enzyme deficiency. In particular, lactose intolerance may occur. Should this be suspected as the cause of diarrhoea, milk withdrawal may be tried. However, this will create a greater nutritional deficit and may precipitate further weight loss.

Bowel surgery

It is of the greatest importance that the bowel is adequately cleansed preoperatively. The presence of unnecessary faecal matter hinders surgery and increases the risk of complications. Three to four days preoperatively, a residue-free diet is given (see Chapter 16). Miles and Stevens recommend the following residue-free fluid diet for the last two preoperative days: it makes a quantity of 1500 ml, for consumption at three daily meals, and provides 8363 kJ.

> *Ingredients:* 300 ml cream, 30 egg whites, 150 g sugar, 120 g Caloreen, juice of 6 lemons. *Blend and serve chilled.*

Clear soup, black tea and coffee and diluted fruit cordials may be taken in addition to the above.

Postoperative dietary management

It is usual to introduce fibrous foods slowly into the postoperative diets of these patients to prevent unnecessary bulk and pressure at the resection site. Following the standard routine of administering clear and then free fluids, the patient may be given a residue-free diet for several days, or hyperalimentation or elemental diets may be used as fibre-free alternatives. However, in view of the fact that these patients have a relatively long perioperative period of impaired nutrition, the nurse should encourage a normal intake at the earliest opportunity.

Rectal surgery

For the patient undergoing a haemorrhoidectomy, a residue-free diet for up to a week postoperatively is of particular importance to prevent a bowel action during the early phase of healing.

Cholecystectomy

Following the loss of the bile reservoir, patients sometimes experience long-term discomfort following ingestion of large amounts of fat. They should therefore be given a low-fat diet, fats included being those of dairy origin which are more digestible. Other patients readily tolerate fat within a few weeks.

Liver surgery

Following resection of part of this organ, the remaining liver tissue regenerates rapidly and consequently postoperative nutrition is of enormous importance. Initially, these patients are usually fed parenterally, but as soon as they are able to take food orally they should be given an easily digestible high-protein diet. This is usually accompanied by intravenous albumen to promote tissue regeneration, which occurs extremely rapidly in the liver.

DIETARY REQUIREMENTS FOR BURNS

Major burns result in a greater extent of catabolism and energy utilization than any disease process. A feature of this hypermetabolism is the redistribution of nutrients, particularly protein, in the body. Catabolism of tissue in various unaffected parts (such as the gut, muscle and skin collagen) takes place to effect anabolism in the injured tissue. Increased gluconeogenesis (i.e. the conversion of non-carbohydrate energy reserves to glucose) results in increased uptake of glucose by the cells. The patient's needs are therefore exceptionally high with regard to requirements of protein and energy. The patient's needs are considerably increased with regard to requirements of *energy* (plus additional *vitamin B complex* for optimal energy utilization); *protein* (for tissue repair): vitamin C (required in wound healing) and *potassium* (to replace excessive urinary losses in the early post-injury stage).

Energy

The body's response to this type of injury is characterized by an elevated basal metabolic rate. Weight loss is a common feature of the condition and the patient's energy demands may increase to 150–300% of normal requirements, depending on the extent of the burn area and the patient's pre-burn nutritional state. Curreri *et al* have suggested a formula which may be useful to the nurse for rapidly calculating the needs of these patients. They suggest that the ideal energy intake expressed as Calories is estimated at 25 times the patient's weight in kilograms plus 40 times the percentage total body surface burnt: thus a 70 kg patient with 40% burns would require

$$(25 \times 70) + (40 \times 40) = 3350 \text{ Cal } (14\ 000 \text{ kJ})$$

Some authorities suggest even higher requirements.

Protein

There are extensive losses of nitrogen due to generalized catabolism, urinary nitrogen excretion and losses through the exudate. Lee suggests that with severe burns over 120 g of body protein may be lost per day, resulting in enormous demands in terms of replacement. Pennisi suggests the following formula for calculating the protein requirement of these patients.

Adult's daily protein requirement (g)
= body weight in kg + (3 × percentage burns)
Child's daily protein requirement (g)
= (3 × body weight in kg) + percentage burns

Thus for a 70 kg adult patient with 40% burns the daily protein requirement is

$$70 + (3 \times 40) = 190 \text{ g}$$

The rate of wound healing is accelerated with adequate protein intake, and the generalized catabolism is arrested. Like the surgical patient, the burnt patient benefits from increased environmental temperatures. Studies have shown that there is less nitrogen excreted in the urine and less protein catabolism in patients treated in a warm dry environment.

Vitamins

Ascorbic acid in particular is required in increased amounts for optimal wound healing and routine supplementation is usually advisable. Vitamin B complex requirements are increased, including raised thiamine and niacin needs due to the high carbohydrate and kilojoule intake of these patients, higher folic acid needs for tissue synthesis and repair, and raised riboflavin requirements for the efficient utilization of the protein consumed. Vitamin A supplementation is often recommended due to its role in maintaining the integrity of epithelium cells and membranes and as it appears to have a protective effect against stress ulceration in these patients.

Minerals

Owing to extensive urinary potassium losses, supplementation is often necessary. Haemoglobin levels in these patients are also often depressed, in which case additional iron is required. Zinc and magnesium requirements are increased, because of significant urinary losses and also losses from the sites of injury.

Fluids

These patients lose a large amount of fluid through dehydration, which must be replaced either orally or parenterally. If practical, regular three-hourly milk-based feeds offer an excellent vehicle for fluid and a variety of essential nutrients.

Practical dietary management

The patient should be given six small nutritious and attractively served meals a day. They should be easily digestible, with a low fibre content, because fibrous foods have a relatively low nutritive value and to restrict the need for defecation. If there is an exposed surface around the mouth, sour and salted foods should be avoided to prevent local pain. Burn patients are frequently anorexic and preferred foods should form the basis of the diet, modified where necessary to increase food value. A frequent complication encountered in these patients is paralytic ileus (i.e. paralysis of the muscles of the digestive tract). When this occurs, patients need to be maintained on a clear fluid diet, often for a prolonged period. Supplementary parenteral feeding is implemented to ensure adequate nutrient intake. One of the major problems in feeding these patients is the lack of precise knowledge regarding the extent to which the patient's theoretical nutritional needs are met in practice. Patients may be anorexic and have difficulty manipulating cutlery or chewing, and frequent observation, encouragement and assistance are an essential part of treatment. Pennisi has devised a nutritional management record which details the patient's weight, protein and energy requirement, and daily intake. She suggests that an arbitrary maximum weight loss of 10% should be imposed: should the patient cross the limit, possible improvements in the current method of feeding should be considered.

Sample menu (burns patients)

Daily intake: approximately 180 g protein; 16 300 kJ (3900 Cal)
On wakening
　　glass of milk from ration
Breakfast
　　oat porridge mixed with 10 g butter, served with sugar and milk
　　2 eggs scrambled in 10 g butter
　　thin slice well buttered bread
　　glass of milk from ration
10 a.m.
　　glass of high-energy milk from ration
11.30 a.m.
　　glass of high-energy milk from ration

Dinner
  100 g fried calf's liver
  100 g chips
  small serving carrots and peas
  100 g sago pudding
  glass of milk from ration
4.0 p.m.
  glass of high-energy milk from ration
Supper
  75 g mashed canned sardines in oil
  1 slice well buttered bread
  small helping avocado salad
  stewed apple with sugar
  egg custard

Daily ration
  1 litre full-cream milk + 1 litre high-energy milk made from 750 ml milk, 150 g milk powder, 2 eggs, sugar (or Caloreen), synthetic colouring and flavouring

NURSING CONSIDERATIONS

1. As discussed in this chapter many patients admitted to hospital for surgery are protein deficient, resulting from pre-existing disease, malabsorption, etc. Recognition of these patients, who are at greater risk of developing complications, is of paramount importance.

   (a) Weight loss since the onset of the illness is a good indicator of nutritional status: a loss of more than 15% suggests significant protein malnutrition (Morgan).

   (b) Observe the patient's body stores of protein and fat. Wasting, if present, is particularly noticeable in the triceps, biceps, shoulders, buttocks and thighs.

   (c) Anorexia and dysgeusia (perversion of taste sensation) in hospital should alert the staff to the possibility of the need for immediate supplementation, either enterally or parenterally.

2. Fruit juice, in particular orange juice or juices fortified with vitamin C, will help to meet increased demands of ascorbic acid in the postoperative diet. However, the frequent serving

of manageable quantities to patients is preferable to the single large glassful, as losses of vitamin C occur rapidly on exposure to air and light.

3. During the early postoperative period, the patient has a high nutrient need and a low capacity. Cooked vegetables are of minimal importance, particularly as most patients are given vitamin supplements; rather encourage the patient to take the high-protein foods first and then to eat the balance of the meal, if their appetite allows.

4. Intake and bowel losses of these patients should be recorded to ensure that the planned nutritional support is being both received and absorbed. Malabsorption due to reduced enzyme output resulting from severe physiological stress may result in diarrhoea. Routine accurate weighing may not be feasible, owing to the immobility of the patient, differences in weights of dressings and the presence of oedema.

BIBLIOGRAPHY

Bistrian, B., Blackburn, G., Hallowell, E. & Heddle, R. (1976) Protein status of general surgical patients. *J. Am. Med. Ass., 230(6)*, 858.

Blackburn, G., Flatt, J., Clower, G. & O'Donnell, T. (1973) Peripheral intravenous feeding with isotonic amino acid solutions. *Am. J. Surg., 125*, 447.

Butterworth, C.E. (1974) Malnutrition in the hospital. *J. Am. Med. Ass., 230(6)*, 879.

Carswell, S. (1975) Changes in aerobic power in patients undergoing elective surgery. *Proc. Phys. Soc., 251*, 42.

Clark, R. (1971) Calorie requirements after operation. *Proc. Nutr. Soc., 30*, 150.

Collins, J. & Alley, P. (1981) Indications for nutritional therapy after major surgery. In: Hill, G. (ed.) *Nutrition and the Surgical Patient.* London: Churchill Livingstone.

Curreri, P., Richmond, D., Marvin, J. & Baxter, C. (1974) Dietary requirements of patients with major burns. *J. Am. Diet. Ass., 65*, 415.

Cuthbertson, D.P. (1971) Nutrition after injury. *Proc. Nutr. Soc., 30*, 150.

Davies, J. & Liljedahl, S-O. (1971) The effect of environmental temperature on the metabolism and nutrition of burned patients. *Proc. Nutr. Soc., 30*, 165.

Fortier, R. (1977) Nutrition and the burn patient. *Can. Nurs. Hosp. Rev., 73* (Aug.), 30.

Halburg, J. (1961) The patient with surgery of the colon. *Am. J. Nurs., 61(3)*, 64.

Hill, G., Blacket, R., Pickford, I., Birkinshaw, L., Young, G., Warren, J., Schorah, C. & Morgan, D. (1977) Malnutrition in surgical patients. *Lancet, 1*, 689.

Hill, G., Pickford, I. & Birkinshaw, L. (1981) Malnutrition — risk factor in surgical sepsis. *Proc. on Adelaide Surgical Conference.* London: Churchill Livingstone.

Immelman, E. (1976) Routine, early post-operative fluid therapy. *S. Afr. Med. J., 50*, 1663.

Klug, T., Ellensohn, J. & Zollinger, R. (1961) Gastric resection. *Am. J. Nurs.,* *61(12),* 73.

Lancet (1975) Postoperative feeding and metabolism. *Lancet, 2,* 263.

Lee, H.A. (1974) Intravenous nutrition. *Br. Med. J., 11,* 719.

Lieber, H. (1961) The jejunal hyperosmolic syndrome (dumping) and its prophylaxis. *J. Am. Med. Ass., 176,* 208.

Miles, A. & Stevens, P. d'E. (1977) A suggested method of preparation of the large bowel for investigation and surgery. *S. Afr. Med. J., 52,* 639.

Molander, D. & Brasfield, R. (1961) Liver surgery. *Am. J. Nurs., 61(7),* 73.

Moore, F.D. (1959) *Metabolic Care of the Surgical Patient,* pp. 25–48. London: W.B. Saunders.

Pennisi, V. (1976) Monitoring the nutritional care of burned patients. *J. Am. Diet. Ass., 69,* 531.

Schwartz, P.L. (1970) Ascorbic acid in wound healing — a review. *J. Am. Diet. Ass., 56,* 497.

Sevitt, S. & Stoner, H.B. (eds.) (1970) *The Pathology of Trauma.* London: Royal College of Pathologists.

Willmore, D.W. (1974) Nutrition and metabolism following thermal injury. *Clin. Plast. Surg., 1(4),* 60.

Zagoren, A., Waters, D., Sonn, R. & Silverman, D. (1982) Protein-sparing nutrition in post-operative management. *Nutr. Support Services, 2,* 61.

14 Cancer and the diet

In recent years it has become increasingly obvious that environmental conditions, and dietary factors in particular, play a major role in the causation of cancer. There is considerable circumstantial evidence relating to these dietary components and current opinion on this subject will be briefly summarized here. Furthermore, diet plays a role in the treatment of specific cancers and the appropriate modifications will be discussed in the second part of this chapter.

DIET IN THE PATHOGENESIS OF CANCER

There are numerous examples of epidemiological studies which indicate that diet is closely related to the incidence of cancer in various populations. It is now clear that at least 50% of all cancers have an important nutritional component in their aetiology (Van Rensburg). A lack or imbalance of nutrients creates an environment conducive to the development of certain tumours. Epidemiological studies show that cancer of the stomach is encountered predominantly in developing countries and cancer of the colon in industrial societies. On a worldwide basis, however, cancer of the stomach is declining in incidence, while there is an increase in the incidence of cancer of the pancreas: a dietary correlation is being sought as a possible explanation. Currently, the high incidence of cancer of the colon in populations consuming refined, low-residue diets is invoking considerable interest: there is a significantly lower incidence in communities where a high-fibre diet is eaten. The higher transit rate of faecal material through the digestive tract resulting from a high fibre intake reduces the time for absorption of potentially harmful substances into the body. Other theories about the correlation of fibre and colon cancer are that the bacterial content of the bowel may be modified by the high fibre content, or that the latter may dilute the bowel contents and reduce the irritation to the colon wall. However, the subject remains controversial in that other researchers relate the incidence to associated differences in fat intake as this cancer occurs predominantly in populations eating diets high in polyunsaturated fats. Still others have suggested that a high-fat, high animal protein diet is generally characteristic of countries in which bowel cancer is encountered most frequently.

The high incidence of breast cancer in Caucasian women is being studied in relation to dietary components. Japanese and Negro women living in their countries of birth and eating traditional foods have a considerably lower incidence of this condition. Hill has found that a change from a Western to a vegetarian-type diet is accompanied by a reduction in the nocturnal release of prolactin, a hormone which is elevated in communities where there is a high incidence of breast cancer. He suggests that cholesterol may also play a role in this disease. Disturbances of carbohydrate metabolism, with associated obesity, have been shown to be present in a high proportion of women with uterine or breast cancer. Furthermore, cancer of the prostate occurs predominantly in communities where there is a high saturated fat and cholesterol intake and pancreatic cancer has also been related to a high fat consumption. Interestingly, in migrants from one area to another, there is a change in probability of cancer development to that present in their new country of adoption, another factor which emphasizes the role of environmental influences. For instance, there is a higher mortality rate of cancer of the pancreas among Japanese immigrants to the USA than among Japanese living in Japan. Phillips has pointed out that the incidence of cancer in Seventh Day Adventists, who are ovolactovegetarians by faith, is lower than in comparable populations with different religious beliefs.

It appears that food components may influence the development of cancer in two ways: firstly by the ingestion of specific carcinogenic factors which, through constant irritation, are causative of the condition, and secondly by the consumption of foods which can predispose the individual to develop cancer by increasing cell vulnerability in the host. Alcohol in particular has been related to the incidence of cancer and Wynder suggests that the assault of carcinogens is facilitated by increased susceptibility created by excessive alcohol ingestion. Thus the risk of cancer of the oesophagus in smokers is considerably increased if excessive alcohol is also consumed.

There is considerable evidence to suggest that certain types of carcinoma occur more frequently in overweight people. In a review article, Van Rensburg points out that breast, colon, prostate, endometrial, ovarian, pancreatic and possibly skin cancer occur with higher incidence in overweight individuals. Ross and Bras found that there was a higher incidence of tumours in heavier rats when compared with a similar but lighter group. They also compared protein intake and found that in rats with the same energy intake, the rats on a higher protein diet had a greater risk of malignancy than the other group. The lowest incidence and greatest life expectancy was seen in those rats with low intakes of protein, carbohydrate and energy. However, there is unfortunately no information available which indicates whether weight loss in obese individuals has a beneficial effect in this respect. Other workers suggest that malnutrition is an important predisposing factor and although it is not known whether this is due to the suppression of immunological pathways or the altering of detox-ification pathways in the body, it seems apparent that vulnerability is increased.

The above comments are of course largely of academic interest. However, they re-emphasize the importance of a prudent diet, i.e. the long-term intelligent selection of good food taken in moderate quantities and the avoidance of overweight.

FOOD ADDITIVES AND CONTAMINANTS

The following are a few of the additives and contaminants encountered in foods which are carcinogenic in effect.

AFLATOXINS. Aflatoxins are produced by a fungus (*Aspergillus flavus*) which develops in peanuts, certain cereals, peas and beans. They are carcinogens which affect the liver. Because aflatoxins occur in a variety of foods which are stored at high moisture levels and particularly in products eaten in large quantities by underpri-vileged people, the FAO/WHO have laid down standards of maximum acceptable levels of aflatoxins in foods. Strict control of the drying and storing conditions of susceptible products helps control this toxin, which is encountered predominantly in tropical countries.

NITROSAMINES. These can be produced in foods to which nitrite is added as a preservative (such as bacon and smoked fish) or can be formed in the stomach from such nitrites and amines taken in the diet. Nitrosamines have been shown to induce tumours in various parts of the body, but particularly the stomach, and have been implicated in the high incidence of cancer of the stomach in Japan, where dried fish is a common item of the diet: it is thought that the nitrate naturally present in the fish is converted to nitrosamines by bacteria. The role of vitamin C as a protective factor is currently being studied, as it appears that a high vitamin C intake is associated with a reduced risk of stomach cancer.

SACCHARIN AND CYCLAMATES. Extensive studies have been undertaken on these two widely used and, until recently, readily available substances. It appears that saccharin is carcinogenic if given as 7.5% of the total diet through two generations of experimental animals. The implications, at this stage, appear to be insignificant for the average user of this artificial sweetener, which is still routinely prescribed.

Cyclamate, however, has been banned as an additive because an active metabolite, *cyclohexamine*, is formed in variable amounts in the people who ingest it, and it has been shown to produce bladder cancer in rats if administered in large quantities.

POLYCYCLIC HYDROCARBONS. These substances, found in smoked foods, barbecued beef, cooking oils and coffee, have been incriminated as carcinogenic substances affecting the digestive tract. The practical relevance of these studies is still being investigated.

Various dyes added to foods have also been found to be carcinogenic, as well as saffrole, a flavouring agent which affects animals. Future studies by toxicologists may well implicate other food additives, but a realistic approach to this subject is essential. Unless there is some possibility that the quantity found to be carcinogenic may be consumed by at least one individual, there is little need for concern and emotionalism.

Summary

The widespread incidence and high mortality of cancer often

prompts the question 'If I change my diet is there reduced risk of developing cancer?'. Several nutrients have been studied in this connection and it would appear that the risk of developing particular types of carcinoma can be lowered, both in experimental animals and in epidemiological studies in man. However, caution must be exercised in the extrapolation of these results to the individual: for example, in any community there is a specific incidence of several different cancers occurring in that group (partly due to environmental factors) but the risk to the individual is not necessarily the total of all the various rates. Nevertheless, when looking at the role of diet in the causation of cancer one should at least be aware that certain dietary practices appear to be advantageous in this regard; hence the following points:

1. Reduction of alcohol in heavy drinkers markedly reduces the risk of cancer of the liver. As discussed earlier, females are more prone to liver damage at a lower level of intake than males. Cancer of the oesophagus also occurs more widely in individuals with a history of drug abuse.
2. A high vitamin C intake appears to have a protective effect in gastric cancer and colorectal cancer because of its antioxidant properties. The conversion of nitrites to nitrosamines in the digestive tract is blocked in the presence of this compound.
3. Recently there has been considerable interest in the role of vitamin A and carotene. Deficiency of vitamin A is related to increased incidence of gastric, lung, salivary gland and nasopharyngeal cancer, whereas high levels appear to inhibit epilethial cancer. Improved risks for smoking-related cancers have been observed in individuals taking diets high in carotene (Wenck et al).
4. Energy imbalance correlates with increased incidence of cancer; particularly overweight but also malnutrition are risk factors in this regard.
5. A high intake of raw vegetables may reduce risk of gastric cancer. In a study by Graham et al, the controls who did not develop cancer ate substantially more raw vegetables than those who developed gastric tumours. This may be due to fibre or micro-elements present.

In conclusion, although it would be premature to directly implicate specific nutrients as causes of cancer, the advice to follow a diet containing optimal amounts of fibre, carotene and vitamin C, predominantly in the form of raw salads, maintain weight within normal healthy limits and take only limited amounts of alcohol would be prudent to follow. Awareness of the hazards of ingesting large quantities of the additives and contaminants discussed above and avoidance of smoking must surely add to our nutritional defence and the maintenance of optimal health.

DIET AND THE CANCER PATIENT

The patient with progressive cancer suffers from *weight loss, anorexia* and *cachexia*. These symptoms may be aggravated by the nausea associated with radiotherapy or chemotherapy, or debilitation resulting from related surgical procedures. The patient becomes wasted in the presence of uncontrolled growth of the tumour, which develops preferentially at the expense of the patient's needs. Currently the nursing approach to this has been to encourage the patient to eat, emphasizing preferred foods attractively served. Protein plays a major role in the diet in an attempt to arrest weight loss.

Recently, however, certain workers are questioning whether this is theorctically the most advantageous procedure, as the rate of growth of the tumour may be accelerated by optimum nutrition. It is suggested that perhaps limitation of specific nutrients essential for tumour growth may be advisable and that in the future it may be feasible to modify the diet to effect a nutrient imbalance which will be to the patient's advantage in the tumour–host competition for nutrients described by Munro. Other workers suggest that in patients with rapidly growing tumours increased intakes of food are accompanied by acceleration of tumour development whereas, with slowly growing tumours, forced feeding is to the patient's advantage. Watkin and Steinfield confirmed this suggestion with the use of hyperalimentation, showing that large increases in kilojoule administration were followed by increased disease activity in patients with rapidly growing neoplasms. In patients where the disease was quiescent, such increases resulted in increased retention of nutrients by the host.

However, this research is largely of academic interest to the nurse: in practice the patient should be as well nourished as possible to ensure maximum resistance to the effects of the malignant disease as well as the debilitating effects of treatment (i.e. chemotherapy and radiotherapy). An interesting use of nutritional control in the therapy of cancer is the administration of methotrexate, a folic acid antagonist in the treatment of leukaemia. Folic acid plays an essential part in the synthesis of nucleic acids in cell nuclei. The latter are necessary for the multiplication of cells, a situation which occurs very rapidly in the development of cancer. Methotrexate blocks the availability of folic acid in this process but unfortunately only temporarily, as with prolonged use the body overcomes this effect.

Therapy

Repletion of muscle nitrogen stores which are expended by the demands of the tumour results in improved response to therapy. The nurse's role is all-important in encouraging the patient to eat sufficient to maintain and if possible to gain weight. The patient who is debilitated and frequently depressed and cachexic presents an enormous challenge to the nurse who has to encourage him to realize that progressive weight loss is *not* an inevitable part of the illness and that by active participation in this aspect of therapy the patient can play a positive role in his own treatment.

A detailed dietary history is taken and the patient is encouraged to have frequent, small, concentrated meals within the limitations created by his disease and the type of therapy undertaken. Many cancer patients have low serum albumin levels and a high protein intake is necessary to correct this. Others may develop ascites which aggravates their anorexia as they feel distended. For them a light fluid diet is often more acceptable.

Patients with advanced cancer may have impaired taste perception (dysgeusia) and the nurse will have to take cognizance of temporary individual idiosyncrasies. Some patients go through an unfortunate stage when they cannot tolerate sweetened foods, whereas others find that even mildly spiced or salted foods are unpalatable. These attitudes may well change over a short period and the nurse who finds her patience and compassion strained must realize that these are unavoidable aspects of the disease.

Food should be attractively presented to ensure acceptance by the patient, with emphasis on preferred foods. The use of alcoholic beverages to stimulate appetite (sherry, beer, etc.) is often helpful to those patients who have this form of appetizer at home.

A large proportion of patients will be totally unable to consume more than a grossly inadequate intake, and for them supplementary nasogastric feeding or hyperalimentation (discussed in Chapter 16) is the most appropriate alternative. This has been found to be particularly valuable in ensuring satisfactory postoperative progress in patients requiring surgery and in increasing response to chemotherapy.

Practical dietary management

The following sample menu includes food items which may be helpful in selecting suitable foods for debilitated patients.

Breakfast
   fruit yoghurt
   orange juice whisked with a raw egg and served chilled
   oatmeal porridge cooked with milk instead of water, served
      with sugar and a little butter
Mid-morning snack
   concentrated beverages (see liquid diets in Chapter 16)
   cheese and biscuits
   ice lollies made with chocolate milk
   junkets
Dinner
   egg dishes such as cheese or ham omelette
   Welsh rarebit, soufflés or chicken pie
   chips if acceptable
   milk-based desserts such as cream caramel, custard jelly or
      banana custard and cream
Mid-afternoon snack as mid-morning
Supper
   pea soup with croutons
   chicken liver paté with well buttered toast
   herring served with biscuits
Bed-time snack as mid morning

CANCER OF THE DIGESTIVE TRACT

In addition to the general debilitating and organic effects of this condition, cancer can be accompanied by various localized complications requiring dietary adaptation.

Cancer of the upper digestive tract

If the malignancy is in the area of the mouth, pharynx or oesophagus, a semi-solid diet will be required. In particular, those patients with cancer of the oesophagus in whom a Celestin or similar tube has been inserted require dietary advice, as the tube can easily become clogged with food particles. Even foods that are smooth and devoid of particles can cause obstruction. In most cases foods will be puréed or blended, but patients are often depressed and discouraged by the presentation of sloppy unidentifiable blended mixtures. Food items served should be well selected and include only those that are normally fairly liquid, have a high nutritive value and retain a true flavour when blended. For instance, it is unrealistic to serve liquidized cabbage or carrots which contribute minimal nutrients and have little interest value!

A valuable adjunct to the diet of these patients is the use of gelatin; 3 teaspoons gelatin, dissolved in 600 ml of boiling liquid, can be added to savoury mixtures to improve presentation. Mixtures of cooked fish or chicken blended with mayonnaise, cottage cheese or cream and well seasoned can be mixed with the gelatin mixture and chilled. These moulds are attractive when set and solid when eaten, but on contact with the warmth of the mouth they naturally become more liquid. This gelatin base or dissolved jelly can be used for nutritious desserts by mixing with cold milk, custard or yoghurt, using only a small amount of boiling water to dissolve the gelatin and making up the balance with other more nutritious liquids. Cool dissolved gelatin should be added to the cool milk mixture to prevent curdling.

Another useful culinary manoeuvre for these patients is to make a custard mixture of an egg in 200 ml of milk and to use this as a basis for either savoury or sweetened dishes. Fish or meat blended with a little stock and well seasoned, or grated cheese and breadcrumbs, can be added to this and baked in a warm oven. Alternatively, it can be sweetened and served as a baked custard, or converted to a 'Queen's pudding' with a few tablespoons of cake crumbs and smooth jam. The following sample menu includes a selection of food items recommended for these patients.

Sample menu (cancer of the upper digestive tract)

Breakfast
puréed sweetened stewed apple
strained oatmeal porridge with sugar and a generous amount of creamy milk
2 lightly scrambled eggs
Mid-morning snack
high-energy supplementary drink (for recipe see Chapter 6) *or* yoghurt *or*
buttermilk *or* ice-cream
Lunch
fruit juice
jellied chicken mould or liquidized cottage pie
baked custard
liquidized banana and milk
Mid-afternoon snack as mid-morning
Supper
pea soup blended with a little minced meat
fish custard
chocolate mould blended with cream
Evening snack as mid-morning

Cancer of the stomach

Many patients with cancer of the stomach undergo surgery as soon as practical. Postoperatively, the dumping syndrome may be a complication and a modified diet — as discussed in Chapter 13 — will be given as the major form of therapy. The reduced output of intrinsic factor can result in megaloblastic anaemia unless vitamin B_{12} is administered by injection. In those patients where surgery is not feasible, there will be reduced capacity caused by the lesion. Patients should be advised to have frequent, small, easily digestible meals. Meat intolerance is a common feature, and milk, eggs and protein supplements are often the cornerstones of the diet.

Cancer of the intestine

Resection of a large proportion of the small intestine can result in the 'short bowel syndrome'. Diarrhoea and malabsorption of sugars, protein and fat, caused by the loss of absorptive surface, results in weight loss. Medium-chain triglycerides (MCT), which bypass the digestive tract, are sometimes used with success in an attempt to increase weight. However, only a small amount of these compounds is acceptable to and tolerated by many patients, and MCT will thus be of limited value.

Ileostomies and colostomies

When a piece of bowel is resected, the end of the remaining section of digestive tract may be secured to an opening in the wall of the abdomen. A bag is firmly attached to the body and the intestinal contents are eliminated into this container. The stoma may be made either from the lumen of the ileum (ileostomy) or at the right or left side of the colon (colostomy) (Fig. 18). The greater the length of the remaining intestine, the greater the storage and concentration capacity and the more formed and predictable are the eliminated contents. Thus the patient with an ileostomy is the most handicapped; regularity of discharge is almost impossible to achieve and the intestinal contents are watery and irritating to the skin owing to the concentration of enzymes present. The patient with a right-sided colostomy has similar problems but they are less severe because of the longer portion of remaining intestine. The left-sided colostomy is far more manageable; elimination normally occurs on a reflex basis at regular, predictable intervals, and the discharge is more solid and less irritating to the skin.

In the early postoperative period, the patient will be given a low-residue diet but will soon progress to as near a normal range of food as possible. Initially the patient is usually apprehensive about diet but he should be encouraged to ascertain by trial and error which foods adversely affect him.

In 1970, a study was undertaken by the Ileostomy Association of Great Britain in which members were asked to record their experiences with various food items. Several useful comments were made by participants. It was found that an offensive odour was caused by fish in about one-third of participants. Both fats and milk — particularly unboiled milk — were incriminated by many colostomy patients as being responsible for 'spillings'. Many participants reported that the consumption of cheese and boiled milk resulted in constipation. Foods with a high fibre content such

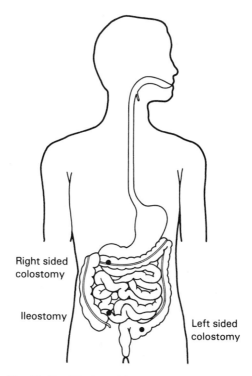

Fig. 18. *Possible sites of ileostomies and colostomies.*

Right sided colostomy

Ileostomy

Left sided colostomy

as pineapple, cucumber, cabbage, etc., were implicated as gas producers, onion being listed as the most troublesome food: the participants in this survey reported that it caused both flatulence and a strong odour.

Many colostomy patients point out that with simple dietary changes they can regulate the consistency of their discharge. In particular, a block of chocolate often alleviates constipation and the consumption of alcohol causes a watery flow in many patients. Aerated drinks and nuts can also adversely affect the discharge.

It is emphasized that the above comments are intended merely as guidelines and that individual experimentation, encouragement and reassurance are all important rehabilitative measures for these unfortunate patients.

BIBLIOGRAPHY

Berg, J. (1976) Nutrition and cancer. *Semin. Oncol., 3,* 17.

Breckman, B.E. (1979) Role of the nurse specialist in stoma care. *J. Hum. Nutr., 33,* 383.

Calman, K.C. (1978) Nutritional support in cancer patients. In: Johnston, T. & Lee, H.A. (eds.) *Developments in Clinical Nutrition.* Tunbridge Wells: MCS Consultants.

Copeland, E., MacFayden, B., Lanzotts, V. & Dudrick, S.J. (1975) Intravenous alimentation as an adjunct to cancer therapy. *Am. J. Surg., 129,* 167.

Cummings, J. (1978) Dietary factors in the aetiology of gastrointestinal cancer. *J. Hum. Nutr., 32,* 455.

DeWys, W.D. (1978) Changes in taste sensation and feeding behaviour in cancer patients: a review. *J. Hum. Nutr., 32,* 447.

Dickerson, J. (1979) Nutrition and breast cancer. *J. Hum. Nutr., 33,* 17.

Fong, Y. & Walsh, O'F. (1971) Carcinogenic nitrosamines in Cantonese salt-dried fish. *Lancet, 2,* 1032.

Gori, G.B. (1977) Diet and cancer. *J. Am. Diet. Ass., 71,* 375.

Graham, S., Schotz, W. & Martino, P. (1972) Alimentary factors in the epidemiology of gastric cancer. *Cancer, 20,* 2234.

Haenszel, W., Kurinara, M., Segi, M. & Lee, R. (1972) Stomach cancer among Japanese in Hawaii. *J. Nat. Cancer Inst., 49,* 969.

Harman, D. (1971) Free radical theory of aging. Effect of the amount and degree of unsaturation of dietary fat on mortality rate. *J. Geront., 26,* 451.

Hegedus, S. & Pelham, M. (1975) Dietetics in a cancer hospital. *J. Am. Diet. Ass., 67,* 235.

Hill, P. (1976) Diet and prolactin release. *Lancet, 2,* 806.

Lanzotti, V., Copland, E., George, S., Dudrick, S. & Samuels, M. (1975) Cancer chemotherapy response and intravenous hyperalimentation. *Cancer Chemother. Rep., 59,* 437.

Johnston, I. (1979) Parenteral nutrition in the cancer patient. *J. Hum. Nutr., 33,* 189.

Macdonald, J. & Schein, P. (1976) Malnutrition states in patients with cancer. *Clin. Gastroent., 5(3),* 809.

Morrison, S.D. (1975) Origins of nutritional imbalance in cancer. *Cancer Res., 35,* 3339.

Munro, H. (1977) Tumour–host competition for nutrients in the cancer patient. *J. Am. Diet Ass., 71,* 380.

Phillips, R.L. (1975) Role of life-style and dietary habits in risk of cancer among 7th Day Adventists. *Cancer Res., 35,* 3513.

Ross, M. & Bras, G. (1975) Tumour incidence and nutrition in rat. *J. Nutr., 87,* 245.

Shubik, P. (1975) Potential carcinogenicity of food additives and contaminants. *Cancer Res., 35,* 3475.

Soukop, M. & Calman, K.C. (1979) Nutritional support in patients with malignant disease. *J. Hum. Nutr., 33,* 179.

Theologides, A. (1972) Pathogenesis of cachexia in cancer. *Cancer, 29,* 484.

Thomson, T., Runchie, J. & Khan, A. (1970) The effect of diet on ileostomy function. *Gut, 11,* 482.

Van Rensburg, S. (1982) Nutritional factors in human carcinogenesis. *S. Afr. Cancer Bull., 26,* 153.

Watkin, D. & Steinfield, J.L. (1965) Nutrient and energy metabolism in patients with and without cancer during hyperalimentation with fat administered

intravenously. *Am. J. Clin. Nutr.*, *16*, 185.
Wenck, D., Baren, M. & Dewan, S. (1983) *Nutrition: The Challenge of Being Well Nourished*, 2nd edn., pp. 438–447. Virginia: Reston.
Wynder, E. (1977) The dietary environment and cancer. *J. Am. Diet. Ass.*, *71*, 385.

15 Uncommon metabolic disorders

Disorders caused by defective metabolic pathways resulting from an absence of specific enzymes or hormones are known as *diseases of metabolism*. In this chapter the major conditions in which dietary modifications form an essential part of treatment are briefly summarized. The most commonly seen metabolic disease, diabetes mellitus, is covered in Chapter 7. A comprehensive discussion of the dietary management of these rare disorders is to be found in *Diets for Sick Children* by D.E.M. Francis. A list of products used as the basis of dietary treatment is given at the end of this chapter.

PHENYLKETONURIA (PKU)

Phenylketonuria is an inherited disease occurring in approximately 1 in 12 000 births. In this condition, the enzyme phenylalanine hydroxylase is lacking, thus preventing the normal conversion of phenylalanine to tyrosine. Characteristically, phenylpyruvic acid is excreted in the urine, and can usually be detected by the appropriate urine dipstick (Phenistix). However, the condition is identified more accurately with the help of a blood test. The major feature of the illness is mental retardation, due to the effect of high levels of circulating phenylalanine on the developing brain.

Aetiology

The patient is born with this enzyme defect and mental deterioration can begin within the first few months. In countries where routine screening is not undertaken the condition frequently remains undiagnosed until it becomes obvious that 'normal milestones' are not being attained (Fig. 19). During this crucial period irreversible brain damage may occur and it has been suggested that 1% of institutionalized mental defectives suffer from PKU. It is for this reason that in many countries, including Britain, infants are routinely examined for the condition. This is usually undertaken when the baby is six to ten days old, as false negative results have been obtained in neonates.

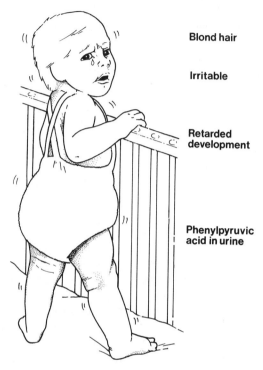

Blond hair

Irritable

Retarded development

Phenylpyruvic acid in urine

Fig. 19. *Effects of phenylketonuria.*

The metabolism of the amino acid tyrosine is dependent on phenylalanine, and as tyrosine is essential for the formation of skin pigments, PKU patients are usually fair and blue-eyed, even in dark-skinned families. With treatment, skin colouring returns to normal. Some workers suggest that PKU occurs predominantly in people of Norwegian or Irish descent.

Affected children are irritable, hypersensitive and developmentally slow, and treatment must commence as early as possible in an attempt to minimize these unfortunate sequelae. If the appropriate diet is initiated within the first few months, a favourable prognosis can be anticipated, but if the condition is neglected for more than about the first 18 months of life, full mental capacity is seldom achieved.

Therapy

Phenylalanine is an essential amino acid which is required by the body for growth. It is thus an essential component of all diets, even for those who are unable to metabolize it normally. The optimum diet for such children must contain a calculated quantity of phenylalanine, sufficient for growth and development but too little to precipitate toxic effects. The diet must be regularly reassessed to confirm that the changing needs of growth and development are met, not only by the phenylalanine content of the diet but also with regard to the other essential nutrients. Requirements are determined from tables of normal recommended allowances. Approximately 5% of protein in natural sources is phenylalanine. The basis of the diet is a milk substitute and the most commonly used products are listed at the end of this chapter. The 'milk' should be given in divided amounts at meal times. The rest of the diet consists of a variety of foods selected from a table of food exchanges, each equivalent to 50 mg of phenylalanine. High-protein foods are given in carefully measured quantities which are adjusted regularly to the needs of the growing child. In infancy the entire amount of phenylalanine is normally given in the special milk substitute. In older children, some fruits and vegetables are included in unrestricted amounts (in spite of the small amount of protein present) as are sugar, boiled sweets, honey, oil and a few other concentrated energy sources. This usually ensures an adequate consumption of these foods. Vitamin and mineral supplements are routinely included to prevent deficiency.

The purpose of therapy is to maintain serum phenylalanine levels within normal limits: 200–500 μmol/litre of blood (3–8 mg/dl) is generally acceptable in early childhood. The young infant is given a higher intake of phenylalanine than the older child: the daily requirement has been estimated to drop from approximately 50 mg/kg body weight at birth to 15 mg/kg subsequently. Calculating the amount needed requires the skill of several experts, and in Britain the paediatrician, dietitian and biochemist work together, with the support of a psychologist or psychiatrist when necessary. Routine monitoring of blood levels of phenylalanine is executed by the laboratory staff with blood that the mother obtains from a heelprick and drops on to the absorbent section of a special form which is sent through the post.

Parents are also supported and informed about various aspects of the regimen by the National Society for Phenylketonuria and Allied Disorders, 26 Towngate Grove, Mirfield, West Yorkshire. This organization also gives parents the opportunity to discuss mutual problems with other affected families. This contact is most valuable as the most problematic aspects of the diet concern parent education: the mother must understand the need for the regimen and be prepared to administer a measured-out diet relentlessly, year after year.

In the short term, the main benefit is a more manageable, less unhappy child. However, a recent study has shown that even with early treatment PKU children had more impaired emotional and social behaviour than children with most other handicapping conditions. Boys were particularly affected, with a high rate of neurotic, antisocial and psychiatric disorders prevailing. The researchers comment that this may be a direct effect of raised phenylalanine levels on brain cell metabolism, brain growth and development, and they suggest that a low-phenylalanine diet should be given during pregnancy, or even prior to conception in predisposed individuals.

It has not yet been clearly established just when the diet should be relaxed, but as the brain has almost reached its growth potential by the age of five years, the regimen is sometimes discontinued between the ages of five and ten. However, there is good evidence to suggest that a life-long regimen is advisable in some patients and that offending foods should at least be restricted indefinitely. Regular follow-up of children who have returned to a normal diet and routine monitoring of their blood phenylalanine levels is important.

GALACTOSAEMIA

Galactosaemia is an inherited condition caused by the absence of the enzyme galactose-1-phosphate uridyl transferase, which is necessary to convert galactose to glucose in the body. Milk contains large amounts of the disaccharide lactose, which is hydrolysed to the monosaccharides glucose and galactose. Normally, the latter is converted to glucose, but in the presence of this defect the galactose accumulates in the blood. The condition becomes apparent early in life owing to the ingestion of milk, and the main features are liver damage, enlargement of the spleen and ascites. There is also a high incidence of cataracts which are cured by a galactose-free diet. The brain will become affected if the condition is not treated quickly, and there is a high rate of early mortality.

Although overt galactosaemia occurs only in approximately 1 in 25 000–50 000 births, the significance of asymptomatic carriers in older patients or their families is currently receiving attention.

Although some workers have suggested that the diet may be discontinued in older children, recent work has indicated that a low-galactose diet may be necessary for life. The need for screening of the family and adherence by carriers to a low-galactose diet during pregnancy is suggested.

Therapy

Treatment consists of the use of a non-dairy milk substitute and the exclusion of all foods containing milk or milk products. Specially manufactured 'milks' (listed at the end of the chapter), containing only a trace of lactose, are usually used in this condition. Although a soya milk replacement is sometimes recommended, many workers question its usefulness, because of the galactosides produced during hydrolysis in the gut. In the UK, commercially produced low-lactose 'milks' are generally used. Calcium replacements and supplementary vitamins are necessary, particularly for older children who drink minimal quantities of the milk substitute.

Mothers should be cautioned to be especially wary of processed foods and confectionery which may contain small amounts of milk powder or whey. Foods containing soya, peas, beans and lentils are also doubtful inclusions in the diet, and as lactose is often used as a filler in pills, the composition of such items should be investigated before administration to the galactosaemic child.

OTHER DISORDERS OF AMINO ACID METABOLISM

Although phenylketonuria is perhaps the best known and most widely recognized amino acid disease, the absence of other amino acid splitting enzymes causes similar disorders of metabolism. Examples of these are tyrosinaemia, homocystinuria and Maple Syrup Urine disease. This last disorder is due to an inability to metabolize the essential branched-chain amino acids valine, leucine and isoleucine, and derives its name from the characteristic odour of the urine of these patients. In all these diseases, diet therapy is the sole form of treatment and must be commenced as early as possible. Initially, a diet free of the offending amino acid is given. When plasma levels return to normal, the diet is supplemented with the individual amino acid(s) as required for growth and development. The basis of the diet for Maple Syrup Urine disease is a special milk from which the three branched-chain amino acids have been removed.

SPONTANEOUS HYPOGLYCAEMIA

It is not known whether this metabolic abnormality results from excessive insulin production or decreased breakdown of insulin, but it is prompted by the consumption of a precipitating substance by the sufferer. Symptoms are similar to the hypoglycaemia encountered in diabetics: weakness, lightheadedness, excessive hunger and agitation occur. The varied causes of this disorder are discussed below.

Ketotic hypoglycaemia

This is a relatively common syndrome occurring in children aged between two and eight. It is caused by an inability to maintain normal blood sugar levels during fasting because of impaired release of amino acids (in particular alanine) from muscle tissue for gluconeogenesis. These children have low serum insulin levels and the treatment consists of frequent high-carbohydrate, high-protein, low-fat meals and prevention of prolonged fasting, especially during febrile childhood illnesses. As ketonuria always precedes the hypoglycaemic attack, urinary ketones should be monitored at night and in the early morning during times of stress.

Functional hyperinsulism

Functional hyperinsulinism is also known as reactive hypogly-caemia or carbohydrate-induced hypoglycaemia. Patients with this disorder over-react to a carbohydrate load, i.e. their insulin output is excessive, causing an abnormal drop in blood sugar after meals.

Ingestion of large amounts of alcohol with a predominantly carbohydrate diet may be one of the causative factors. The diet must be modified to minimize the amount of carbohydrate, which triggers the reaction. Foods which are predominantly protein and fat, and low-carbohydrate vegetables, form the basis of the diet, which is usually given as six small meals rather than three large ones per day.

Leucine-sensitive hypoglycaemia

This condition occurs particularly in children under the age of five. Although drug administration may form a major part of therapy, some workers have successfully used exclusively dietary treatment. The basis of the diet is a special leucine-free milk formula and a low-protein diet in which the leucine-containing foods are restricted to the minimum required for health and development. The daily intake is distributed over three meals, each followed by a feeding of sugar 20–30 minutes after the meal to elevate the depressed blood sugar level. The composition of the diet was originally described by Roth and Segal in 1964, who suggested that the leucine content should not exceed 80 mg/kg body weight.

Fructose intolerance

This rare inherited disease causes severe hypoglycaemia when fructose is consumed. The acute attack is treated by intravenous glucose. Long-term treatment is omission of all foods containing fructose (or sucrose, since each molecule of sucrose consists of one molecule of fructose and one molecule of glucose).

JOINT DISEASES

Though not uncommon, these disorders are most appropriately included in this chapter. They are perhaps more fraught with dietary misunderstanding and quackery than any other disease state. This probably results from the fact that spontaneous remission is a feature of this group of conditions. Such remissions will often be quite erroneously related to an item of food which has been either eaten or avoided in the preceding period. Furthermore, the constant pain and discomfort of these conditions prompts the patients, and often health workers, to attempt any possible environmental manipulation to alleviate the symptoms. Added to this, the aetiology of the disease is not well understood and the emotional opinions of faddists and quacks are readily accepted by sufferers.

To date, there is no substantiated evidence to support the opinion that specific food items play a direct role in the aetiology or treatment of any of the arthritides other than gout (discussed below). The author recently undertook a study which included a literature review and a survey of patients with osteo-arthritis and rheumatoid arthritis attending the out-patient department of a large teaching hospital. Patients were questioned with regard to their dietary history, their food preferences and their beliefs about the role of food in their disease. Over 100 articulate patients were interviewed in this rather fruitless study in which no dietary item could be incriminated.

However, weight reduction is an essential part of treatment of overweight arthritic patients, particularly where the weight-bearing joints are affected. Patients should follow the recommendations made in Chapter 5, with the warning that because of their limited capacity for physical exercise weight loss will be extremely slow without strict adherence to the regimen.

Gout

Gout is a disorder of purine metabolism leading to the accumulation of sodium urate crystals (tophi) in the joints. It is a hereditary disease characterized by acute attacks of painful inflammation of the joints, particularly in the big toe. It is seen predominantly in men, but occasionally in postmenopausal women.

Aetiology

Gout was originally correlated with the consumption of large amounts of rich foods and alcoholic beverages. More recently, it has been suggested that it may be an individual response to a specific food allergen. Neither of these opinions is generally accepted today, but the pathogenesis of the condition is still not completely understood. Although it does occur predominantly in regular alcohol drinkers, it is also associated with obesity and hypertension.

Metabolism

The cell nuclei of plant and animal tissue are broken down in the digestive tract to nucleic acid. This is converted to purines, which are then oxidized to uric acid, the basis of the sodium urate crystals encountered in gout. Nuclear proteins are found particularly in foods which have a dense cellular structure, and this provides the theoretical premise for the dietary modification for gout. However, uric acid can be manufactured from a wide range of other compounds in the body, and in the gouty patients, where high levels of uricaemia occur, the role of purine-rich foods is less important. Furthermore, there are extremely effective drugs to increase the excretion of uric acid, and nowadays diet plays a secondary role in the treatment of this condition. However, certain gouty individuals are sensitive to a purine load. In such cases, a low-purine diet is recommended.

In most cases, merely the restriction of high-purine foods will suffice; these are organ meats, such as liver, kidneys and brains, meat extracts and gravies. Fish roe and small fish such as anchovies and sardines also have a dense cellular structure and should be avoided. Meat, fish, legumes and oatmeal have a relatively high purine content and those patients who have found purine restriction to be effective in reducing the frequency of their acute attacks should limit the intake of these foods too. Items which have a low purine content are fruit, vegetables, cereals, fats and sugar. Dairy products and eggs have a very low purine content and should be used as the main source of protein in the diet, if hypercholesterolaemia is not an associated problem.

PRADER–WILL SYNDROME

This is a relatively rare endocrine disorder causing impaired motor development and mental retardation from a young age. The child rapidly becomes obese due to an insatiable appetite; the body fat is characteristically deposited on the trunk and the buttocks. Hypogenitalism occurs in boys.

Children with this disorder are difficult to control as they steal food or make up reasons to manipulate their mothers into giving them far more food than necessary. The mother is also likely to be sympathetic to her retarded child.

The obesity is thought to be caused by increased appetite, low metabolic rate and restricted exercise and it is essential for a weight reduction regimen to be instituted as early as possible. A dietary history will disclose the child's previous intake and associated weight gain. A diet is then compiled restricting food consumption to the minimum for the age, consistent with including adequate amounts of all necessary nutrients. A large amount of low-kilojoule, high-fibre food is included. Inclusion between meals of 'diet' cool drinks, soup containing a large amount of high-fibre vegetables, and a variety of salads such as carrots, celery sticks, radishes and tomatoes, all helps to satisfy the child's voracious appetite. It is sometimes necessary to lock away or hide food and to arrange eating times away from the parents to prevent the patient seeing forbidden food being consumed.

FAVISM

This metabolic disorder occurs predominantly among people living in Mediterranean countries. It is precipitated by the consumption of fava beans, *Vicia fava*, raw or cooked, or the inhalation of the pollen. Clinical manifestations — haemolysis, jaundice and haemoglobinuria — result from a deficiency of an essential enzyme (glucose-6-phosphate dehydrogenase). Affected individuals become pale and weak soon after contact. Male children are particularly vulnerable and remain susceptible for life. A number of unrelated drugs (e.g. antimalarials and antiseptics) may also precipitate these attacks.

GLYCOGEN STORAGE DISEASES

These are rare conditions in which the normal conversion of glycogen to glucose cannot occur normally due to a deficiency of one or more essential enzymes. The symptoms, prognosis and treatment vary according to which enzyme is involved. These disorders are rare and only the two most commonly seen are discussed below.

Glucose-6-phosphatase deficiency (von Gierke's disease)

This is the most severe form of glycogen storage disease, with a high mortality rate. The effect of the disease is that glucose is the only carbohydrate that can be metabolized normally, as glycogen cannot be readily converted to glucose. This means that starch, glucose and maltose (which consists exclusively of glucose) must be taken regularly day and night as sources of immediate energy, to prevent hypoglycaemia and its sequelae and permit normal growth and development. Even short periods of fasting cause hypoglycaemia and patients are fed at intervals of approximately three hours during the day with a high-starch snack containing glucose. Initially this may be continued throughout the night. More recently a continuous nasogastric feed at night has been recommended, which appears to improve growth and development. By adolescence, most patients can omit the snacks required by younger children in the night. As patients cannot break down other sugars, these must be omitted from the diet. Hence, fruit, cane sugar and milk (because of its lactose content) must be avoided.

A major difficulty of this condition is the high serum lactic acid levels caused by the incomplete breakdown of carbohydrate, a situation which is treated by routine administration of sodium bicarbonate.

Secondary hyperlipidaemia is a feature of the condition and is effectively treated with a high-carbohydrate, low-fat diet in which polyunsaturated fats are emphasized and medium-chain triglycerides may be included.

Phosphorylase enzyme deficiency

A deficiency of one of the enzymes in the phosphorylase system causes mild symptoms, usually seen in early childhood. The milestones of development may be retarded, because of inadequate muscle strength, but may return to normality later. Hypoglycaemia may follow prolonged fasting and these children are usually given a high-protein, high-carbohydrate meal on retiring to counteract this situation. Hyperlipidaemia is also a secondary complication and is treated by partial replacement of the carbohydrate in the diet with polyunsaturated fat.

EPILEPSY

Epilepsy is a neurological disease characterized by seizures with convulsions and loss of consciousness. There are several types of clinical manifestation of the condition but the disorder is mainly classified as *grand mal* (major attacks) or *petit mal* (milder attacks).

The disorder is not in itself a metabolic disorder, but is included in this chapter because diet therapy for the condition promotes distortion of a normal metabolic process (i.e. fat absorption) and the ketosis produced causes improvement of the condition. The mechanism of this effect is unknown.

Over 60 years ago, the ketogenic diet was widely used to reduce the severity and frequency of epileptic seizures. Although the long-term use of such diets, with an abnormally high fat content and a low carbohydrate content, was difficult to manage and unpalatable, they were relatively successful, particularly in children with minor motor seizures. With the subsequent widespread use of suitable drugs, diet therapy lost popularity, but there has recently been a resurgence of interest in these diets for young patients with whom drug administration has been ineffective. The availability of medium-chain triglycerides (MCT) has considerably eased the practical problems of management as MCT is considerably more ketogenic than dietary fats, thus smaller quantities are required, allowing the inclusion of proportionately larger quantities of protein and carbohydrate. As MCT is tasteless, it is also tolerated better by many children.

The diet suggested by Huttonlocher *et al* is generally applied. The basis of the diet is MCT, which provides 60% of the child's kilojoule requirement. The remaining 40% is used primarily for meeting the protein needs and the balance is given as small quantities of preferred foods. The diet for a four- or five-year-old child would thus be made up as follows:

Daily energy requirement: 6270 kJ
MCT should provide 60% of 6270 = 3762 kJ
MCT yields 35 kJ/g, thus daily requirement is

   $3762 \div 35 = 107$ g MCT

Remaining energy requirement = $6270 - 3762 = 2508$ kJ
The daily protein requirement is 40 g, which provides 669 kJ
The energy balance to be made up with other foods is therefore
$2508 - 669 = \underline{1839 \text{ kJ}}$

Note: It has been observed that these children often require a greater energy intake than their theoretical requirement, in which case the energy content of the diet will have to be increased.

The suggested method of administration of MCT is to whisk it into skimmed milk with the addition of synthetic sweetener, colouring and flavouring. Served cold, this makes a palatable milkshake. 550 ml of skimmed milk, containing 20 g of protein, is divided over three meal-times. MCT can also be included in gelatin desserts or ice-cream. The balance of food can be varied with the use of 200 kJ portion exchange lists, and adapted to fit in with the family's eating habits.

There are disadvantages to the use of MCT diets. In the first place, the oil is extremely expensive. Secondly, the child may experience osmotic diarrhoea, especially if the oil is introduced rapidly into the diet. In such cases, the standard 3:1 or 4:1 ketogenic diet, based on the ratio of ketogenic to non-ketogenic factors, may be more appropriate. 'Ketogenic factors' make up 90% of the fat and 50% of the protein in the diet; the 'antiketogenic factors' are derived from the carbohydrate plus the other 50% of the protein and 10% of the fat. This diet is calculated as follows:

Daily energy requirement: 6270 kJ
The daily protein requirement of 40 g provides 669 kJ
Energy to be supplied from carbohydrate and fat:
$6270 - 669 = 5601$ kJ

We allow the child 14 g of carbohydrate, which provides 234 kJ
Energy to be supplied from fat: $5601 - 234 = 5367$ kJ
5367 kJ requires a daily fat intake of $5367 \div 38 = 141$ g

The total intake of ketogenic factors (fatty acids)
$= (50\%$ of $40) + (90\%$ of $141) = 147$ g
The total intake of non-ketogenic factors (available glucose)
$= (50\%$ of $40) + (10\%$ of $141) + (100\%$ of $14) = 48$ g
Ketogenic : non-ketogenic intake $= 147 : 48 = 3 : 1$

It is clear from the following sample menu that the diet is restricted, monotonous and likely to be nauseatingly rich for a young child.

Sample menu (ketogenic diet)

Breakfast
    1 large fried egg in 10 g butter
    60 g unsweetened apple sauce mixed with 60 g thick cream
Dinner
    60 g fatty meat (pork or mutton)
    50 g each of two of the following vegetables: cabbage, cauliflower, tomatoes, spinach, lettuce, marrow
    10 g butter on vegetables
    jelly made from lemon juice, artificially sweetened, and set with gelatin with 60 g thick cream
Supper
    clear broth or bouillon cube mixed with boiling water
    50 g cheddar cheese
    50 g of low-carbohydrate vegetables or salads given above
    jelly as at dinner with 60 g thick cream

COMMERCIAL DIETARY PRODUCTS

The following products are commonly used in the dietary management of metabolic diseases.

Phenylketonuria
    Aminogran (Allen and Hanburys)
    Lofenalac (Mead Johnson)
    Albumaid XP (Scientific Hospital Supplies)
    Minafen (Cow and Gate)
    PK Aid 1 (Scientific Hospital Supplies): this is an amino acid mixture specially prepared for phenylketonurics over two years of age
Galactosaemia
    Nutramigen (Mead Johnson)
    Galactomin (Cow and Gate)
Leucine-induced hypoglycaemia
    S-14 (Wyeth Laboratories) (available only in the USA)
    LSHG mixture (Scientific Hospital Supplies)
Homocystinuria
    Albumaid Methionine Low (Scientific Hospital Supplies)

Tyrosinaemia
  Albumaid XPXT (Scientific Hospital Supplies)
Maple Syrup Urine Disease
  MSUD Aid (Scientific Hospital Supplies)

Rite-Diet protein-free bread and flour are available from

Welfare Foods (Stockport) Ltd
63/65 Higher Hillgate
Stockport
Cheshire SK1 3HE

BIBLIOGRAPHY

Coutts, J. & Fowler, B. (1967) Low methionine diets for homocystinuria with reference to two cases. *Nutrition*, *21*, 35.

Di George, A., Auerbach, V. & Mabry, C. (1960) Elevated serum insulin associated with leucine-induced hypoglycaemia. *Am. J. Dis. Childh.*, *100*, 543.

Fishler, K., Donnell, G., Bergren, W. & Kock, R. (1972) Intellectual and personality development in children with galactosemia. *Pediatrics, Springfield*, *50*, 412.

Folk, C. (1984) Dietary management of type I glycogen storage disease. *J. Am. Diet.*, *84*, 293.

Francis, D.E.M. (1974) *Diets for Sick Children*, 3rd edn. Oxford: Blackwell.

Francis, D.E.M. (1979) Inborn errors of metabolism: the need for sugar. *J. Hum. Nutr.*, *33*, 146.

Huttenlocher, P., Wilbourn, A. & Signore, J. (1971) Medium-chain triglycerides as a therapy for intractable childhood epilepsy. *Neurology*, *21*, 1097.

Komrower, G.M. & Lee, D.H. (1970) Long-term follow-up of galactosemia. *Archs. Dis. Childh.*, *45*, 367.

Lancet (1976) Gout for gourmets. *Lancet*, *2*, 777.

Mutton, P., Gupta, J., Yu, J., Crollini, C. & Harley, J. (1977) Impaired galactose tolerance in older patients with galactosemia. *Austr. Paediatr. J.*, *13(1)*, 7.

Pipes, P.L. & Holm, V.A. (1973) Weight control of children with Praeder–Willi Syndrome. *J. Am. Diet. Ass.*, *62*, 520.

Raine, D.N. (ed.) (1975) *The Treatment of Inherited Metabolic Disease*. Lancaster: MTP Press.

Smith, I. & Wolff, O. (1974) Natural history of phenylketonuria and influence of early treatment. *Lancet*, *2*, 540.

Starfield, B. & Holtzman, N.A. (1975) A comparison of effectiveness of screening for phenylketonuria in the United States, United Kingdom and Ireland. *N. Eng. J. Med*, *293*, 118.

Stevenson, J., Hawcroft, J., Lobascher, M., Smith, I., Wolff, O. & Graham, P. (1979) Phenylketonuria: behaviour deviance in children with early treated phenylketonuria. *Archs. Dis. Childh.*, *54*, 14.

16 Transitional diets

When patients are unable to consume natural food in its normal form there are several alternative ways of feeding them. Nutrients should always be administered in the most effective way for the individual, allowing optimal utilization and minimal hazard of complications. The preferred method is always by mouth; hence if patients are unable to consume and digest even totally inadequate amounts of food they should be encouraged to do so, with tube feeding as supplementary, not the exclusive, form of nutrient intake.

Diets may be adapted in the following ways.

REDUCTION OF FIBRE. This is necessary in the treatment of certain diseases of the digestive tract. Appropriate use of this diet is discussed in Chapter 8 and suitable foods are listed in Appendix A. This diet is also used pre- and postoperatively as part of the dietary management for patients undergoing surgery, as well as for those patients who are anorexic and disinterested in eating a normal diet. This low-residue diet merely consists of those foods which are not particularly fibrous, and the fibre which is present is often broken down by mincing or chopping to make it more easily digestible.

The fibre content of the diet needs to be even more restricted for patients with obstructive disease of the bowel or prior to surgery to the digestive tract. The prescribed diet will consist predominantly of tender meat, broiled or baked fish, eggs, refined cereal, fruit juices, and butter or margarine. These are foods with minimal fibre producing a very limited residue of faecal matter. This diet is intended for short-term use only and is deficient in several nutrients.

MODIFICATION OF CONSISTENCY. Whereas the above *light* diets are not necessarily soft (for example, cheese or a steamed veal chop may be included), the following diets are intended for patients with reduced capacity to chew and/or swallow. If only moderately affected (e.g. following the removal of teeth or a tonsillectomy) the patient will still manage to eat foods like mincemeat, eggs, cottage cheese, porridge, soft fruits and cooked vegetables, mashed if necessary. Soups, ice-cream, fruit juices, etc., are also obviously important inclusions in this diet.

The semi-solid or blended diet is intended for patients who are more incapacitated. For example, the patient with advanced oesophageal varices may develop a haemorrhage on a soft diet, and the patient with obstructive carcinoma of the oesophagus may choke unless the food is fine in texture and fluid in consistency. Foods which are normally like this are generally more acceptable to patients; hence soups, custards, strained porridge, milk beverages and jellies (which will liquefy at body temperature) should form a major part of the diet. Liquidized cottage pie or cauliflower cheese, for example, are less tempting but highly nutritious inclusions. This diet is also suitable for patients with mouth injuries and splinted or wired jaws but, in many cases, food will have to be made more liquid if it is to be sucked through a straw. For these latter patients six small concentrated meals are preferable to three larger ones, as patients tire quickly from sucking. Feeds should be prepared with the optimum consistency; if too thick they will be difficult to suck into the mouth, if too liquid the kilojoule value per millilitre will be disproportionately low. A prerequisite for this type of feeding is palatability of the beverages used and patient motivation is essential. Practical details of preparation and menu suggestions of suitable foods are discussed in Chapter 14.

'Free fluids' are mainly given as part of the postoperative feeding regimen but are also of some value for patients with severe mouth injury; for example, following mouth surgery or severe burns (see Chapter 13). Sour-tasting beverages such as fruit juices and soups flavoured with tomato purée should be omitted for these patients, as they cause pain or discomfort.

'Clear fluids' refers to beverages that are residue free and used specifically pre- and postoperatively. A few days before bowel surgery this diet will be prescribed as part of the cleansing procedure. Postoperatively, before the recommencement of peristalsis, the clear fluid regimen will supply liquids, some sugar and no residue (as discussed in Chapter 13).

ENTERAL FEEDS

This refers to the feeding of patients with a functional digestive tract as compared to parenteral feeding, which is clearly used when bypassing of the digestive tract is necessary.

Administration

Enteral feeding is administered as follows.

Orally

Drinks may be selected from the free fluid regimen, the preparation of choice being the one which meets the patient's nutritional needs and is palatable enough to be taken throughout the day. Formula feeds (p. 349) are often used to supplement the diet of a seriously debilitated patient whose appetite and capacity at meal-times do not allow an adequate intake of nutrients. Examples of such patients are the severely burned patient, the patient with cancer and the elderly or anorexic patient.

Tube feeding

THE NASOGASTRIC ROUTE. This is employed if the patient is unable to take sufficient food by mouth. This group includes comatose or disorientated patients or those who, as a result of radical surgery, have obstruction to the mouth or throat or diffuse mouth sores and are unable to take even adequate liquids. In fact, any patient who cannot or refuses to take an adequate oral diet is tube fed in this way — providing the digestive tract is functional. Nasogastric feeding is of particular value in paediatric practice when oral feeds may be rejected and the intravenous route presents difficulties, such as dislodgement and sepsis.

GASTROSTOMY FEEDS. These are usually preferred for patients where long-term enteral feeding is anticipated. By placing a tube directly into the stomach there is reduced incidence of regurgitation and aspiration of vomit. Jejunostomy tubes are also generally more acceptable and manageable for patients discharged on tube feeds. The composition of nasogastric and gastrostomy feeds is the same.

JEJUNOSTOMY FEEDS. The tubes for administering these feeds bypass the stomach and duodenum, hence the feed composition must be such that it is readily absorbable, and for this purpose elemental diets (discussed below) are sometimes preferred. Jejunostomy feeds are used, for example, in patients where caustic soda or other highly irritating compounds have been ingested and where the upper region of the digestive tract has been damaged.

Calculation of preparation

The approximate quantity administered to patients is 2000–3000 ml/day depending on the composition of the feed and the environmental temperature. Tube feeding is commenced with about 1 kJ/ml but with gradual increase in concentration, until after 3–4 days the patient is receiving 3–4 kJ/ml (i.e. 1 Cal/ml). There are three main forms of liquid feed that may be administered: commercial preparations, hospital prepared feeds and blended whole food.

Commercial preparations

Elemental diets

In these highly specialized diets the nutrients are provided in a readily absorbable form, i.e. the proteins are as amino acids, the fat is in the form of triglycerides or medium-chain triglycerides, and carbohydrates are included as glucose or other easily assimilable sugars. Vitamins and minerals are included in quantities to meet the recommended allowances. Elemental diets are used either for direct administration to the jejunum or in patients with a short bowel syndrome resulting in poor digestion. Elemental diets are also used in the preoperative period of digestive tract resection. Examples of elemental diets available in the UK are Vivonex and Flexical; in the latter 30% of its kilojoules are as fat; Vivonex, however, has a very low fat content. These are hyperosmolar and may cause diarrhoea; hence they should be given at a slow steady rate and initially dilute.

Formula diets

These are preparations made either from food components and added vitamins and minerals or balanced combinations of specific nutrients. They may be flavoured and/or lactose free. They may be complete combinations used as sold or administered with water, or they may require supplementation prior to use. Caloreen and Hycal, both glucose polymers, and Prosparol, a fat emulsion, may be added for extra energy to feeds supplying inadequate energy for specific needs.

Milk is often used as a vehicle for the feed instead of water. Milk provides additional protein and energy but should be used cautiously. Commercially produced compounds often have a high protein content and the supplementary protein from milk creates a high protein-to-energy ratio which is inadvisable, particularly for paediatric use. Furthermore, although milk is an extremely nutritious food, it is an outstanding culture medium for bacteria and readily causes diarrhoea unless the most stringent aseptic measures are applied in the preparation and administration of feeds. Another hazard of using milk in liquid feeds is the problem of lactose intolerance; either primary lactose intolerance or the mild lactose intolerance sometimes seen in debilitated patients, which will promote diarrhoea if large amounts of milk are given.

The use of alcohol in feeds as a concentrated source of energy is not recommended. Known, or as yet undiagnosed, liver damage will be aggravated by the toxic effects of alcohol, and the sedative effect of alcohol is inadvisable in comatose patients.

It is emphasized that, although a few of the recommended commercial products are comprehensive, others are intended specifically for improved protein intake and require supplementation with carbohydrate, fat, vitamins and minerals for adequate nutrient intake. Several of these preparations are also unpalatable if taken by mouth and should oral administration be anticipated they should be well flavoured and served chilled.

Hospital-prepared liquid feeds

Liquid feeds can also be made up in the hospital or ward kitchen to the individual needs of the patient. The most commonly used basis for these feeds is milk to which eggs are added for supplementary protein and iron. Both these foods, however, are easily contaminated and strict hygienic measures are essential in the preparation and administering of these feeds. It is also advisable to bring the two ingredients to boiling point, strain, cool rapidly and refrigerate until used. The use of 3 eggs in a 2-litre feed will not thicken the milk to an unmanageable consistency. Ingredients which are commonly included in these feeds for patients with normal requirements are given in Table 18. Protein and energy values are included to facilitate the calculation of the required feed. A concentrate supplying the recommended daily amounts of vitamins and minerals is added to the feed prior to use. An advantage of this type of made-up feed is that it is cheaper than the commercially prepared feeds; major disadvantages are that they are imprecise, time-consuming to prepare and must be made fresh each day as they are readily contaminated.

Table 18. Protein and energy contents of ingredients used in feeds.

Ingredient	Protein	Energy
Milk (full)	34 g/litre	2750 kJ/litre
Milk (skimmed)	35 g/litre	1463 kJ/litre
Eggs	6.8 g/egg	385 kJ/egg
Milk powder (full cream)	27.0 g/100 g	2200 kJ/100 g
Milk powder (skimmed)	34.5 g/100 g	1260 kJ/100 g
Casilan (Glaxo)/protein hydrolysate	87.0 g/100 g	1526 kJ/100 g
Glucose	Nil	1640 kJ/100 g

Blended whole food

Although it is considered old-fashioned and impractical by some, many workers still consider the blended whole food feed to be most suitable for meeting the normal nutrient requirement of their patients. Although more time-consuming than the scientifically balanced, sterile and considerably more expensive formulated feeds, there are certain advantages in feeding merely by blending the components of a standard, varied diet and administering it in a nasogastric tube. This type of feed has a low lactose content and seldom causes diarrhoea. It may also contain micro-elements, as yet unidentified, which are helpful to the unconscious patient and absent in milk-based feeds.

A special food pump which can administer a continuous drip supply of food at a constant rate is a useful piece of ward equipment under such circumstances. Alternatively, a wider bore tube may be used.

Recipes for modified liquid feeds

High-protein, high-energy drink

Some patients merely need additional protein and energy presented in a liquid form. The recipe for a most palatable supplementary drink is given in Chapter 6. It supplies over 80 g protein and 6500 kJ (1550 Cal) per litre and can be varied with the use of different synthetic colourings and flavourings — cocoa, coffee, etc. Should patients find this drink too rich, the milk can be replaced with orange juice but then, naturally, the protein and kilojoule content will be considerably lower, i.e. 55 g protein and 4500 kJ (1070 Cal) per litre.

Protein-free feed

For renal or hepatic failure, the following feed is sometimes used:

    1.2 litre water
    50–100 g fat
    50–100 g sugar
    40 g starch

The *fat* used in this feed may be oil or salt-free butter. If fluid retention is not a problem, salted butter may be considered.

The *sugar* may be sucrose or glucose. However, glucose polymers such as Hycal and Caloreen are often preferable as they considerably reduce the possibility of hyperosmolar diarrhoea.

Starch is added for extra energy from a non-irritant source and to improve the consistency of the feed. Cornflour is usually used, but custard powder, which is merely coloured and flavoured cornflour, may be preferable if the feed is to be taken partly by mouth.

The method of preparation is to heat most of the water, the fat and sugar and to stir the starch, mixed to a paste with the balance of water, into the boiling liquid.

Initially, the smaller quantities of fat and sugar are used. These are increased over a three to four day period to 100 g of each. The feed will then supply 6120 kJ (1460 Cal).

Note: The nutrients supplied by this feed are totally inadequate and it should thus only be used for a short time.

Administration of nasogastric feeds

(Tube feeding is also discussed in Chapter 4.)

Tube feeds are administered preferably by constant drip or occasionally a bolus every 2–3 hours. With this latter technique patients are given 200–250 ml each time, followed by a small amount of water to rinse through the tube. Unless the patient is critically debilitated the midnight feed is usually omitted. Between feeds the preparation is retained in a covered container in the refrigerator, being brought to body temperature on administration. Although this method is most convenient for home use, the constant drip administration is, however, the preferable method of administration in hospitals. It removes the uncertainty about precise and regular administration of feeds, reduces nursing time and minimizes complications. Furthermore, compromised patients are less likely to develop diarrhoea with this method. The feed is administered through the smallest bore tube that will allow the free flow of feed, thus ensuring maximum patient comfort.

Complications

DIARRHOEA. The most serious problem of tube feeding is diarrhoea which can occur for a number of reasons. Hyperosomolarity is a frequent precipitating factor, i.e. the administration of a too concentrated feed too quickly, and occurs particularly with bolus feeding. However, dilute tube feeds are usually introduced at the start and gradually increased to full strength over a few days. If sugar concentration is too high, hyperosmolar diarrhoea can also occur. However, in a recent study undertaken by Keohane *et al.* the value of 'starter' (more dilute) feeds was questioned. Their findings showed that not only was the nutrient uptake inadequate on the dilute feed, but also that diarrhoea was significantly related to treatment with antibiotics and not the administration of an undiluted hypertonic feed.

Bacterial diarrhoea can be caused by inadequate hygiene in the preparation and administration of the feed. The use of contaminated utensils and inadequate protection from airborne bacteria can be a serious threat to compromised patients who are particularly vulnerable to bacterial invasion. Lactose intolerance or simultaneous administration of antibiotics can also cause diarrhoea. Codeine phosphate is usually effective in treating this.

OESOPHAGITIS. This may occur because of the pressure of the tube and acid reflux. It occurs more readily with a larger bore tube, and seldom with a fine-bore tube.

NAUSEA, VOMITING AND INHALATION PNEUMONIA. These can occur with tube feeding. These complications occur more readily when the patient is horizontal while being fed.

PARENTERAL FEEDING (HYPERALIMENTATION)

Although it is not the role of the nurse to prescribe these nutritive preparations nor the function of this book to discuss the minutiae of administration, it is relevant in this context to discuss the outlines of this vital procedure.

Parenteral feeding is complete intravenous nutrition, supplying an adequate amount of essential nutrients in the form of an amino acid mixture, fat emulsions and glucose, with added electrolytes and vitamins. Parenteral feeding is used when other routes of nutrition are unsuitable and is strictly a last resort measure of nutritional support. It is used when the oral or enteral route is unavailable or inadequate. For instance, the comatose patient who is vomiting is in serious danger of aspiration if nasogastric feeding is used here: the intravenous route is clearly indicated. Patients with absolute pyloric or intestinal obstruction, or chronic disabling digestive tract disorders (such as massive bowel resection) are also usually fed in this way. Parenteral feeding is also used for patients with severe anorexia nervosa or depressive illness, or for patients suffering from hypercatabolic states such as serious burns. In such cases, parenteral feeding may be used to supplement oral intake.

Preparations used for parenteral feeding

Amino acid mixtures

These are widely used as a basis for parenteral feeding and are available as protein hydrolysates. Protein hydrolysates are composed not only of amino acids but also other useful compounds (such as phosphates) which are of value in the metabolism of these patients. Preparations are usually combined with *glucose* before use to provide additional energy.

Carbohydrate

An adequate amount of sugar is necessary, both as an energy source and for its protein-sparing effect (discussed in Chapter 1). The preferred sugar is glucose, in solutions ranging from 5% to 50%, though the more dilute solutions are of little use as energy sources. To ensure optimum kilojoule intake, 25% solutions are normally administered. A disadvantage of the 50% concentration is that it may easily elevate the blood sugar levels and the patient may need insulin injections to retain these levels within normal limits. Some patients appear to handle glucose less efficiently following trauma — it is thought that this results from either a lack of insulin output or increased insulin resistance in the body. Severe hyperglycaemia and ultimately coma may result and the condition, known as *hyperosmolar hyperglycaemic non-ketotic coma*, has an extremely high mortality rate. For this reason, caution must be exercised in administering concentrated solutions of glucose, and blood sugar levels must be monitored regularly.

Glucose and fructose

Fructose was, until recently, widely used as the carbohydrate of choice in intravenous feeding. The main advantages were thought to be that it was not insulin-dependent for utilization and that it could be given in higher concentrations than glucose. However, recent work has shown that not only is a large percentage of fructose converted to glucose (which requires insulin for utilization) but it also increases the blood lactate level. There is thus a danger of lactic acidosis in patients being fed with intravenous fructose, children being particularly vulnerable. For this reason, glucose is generally regarded as the most satisfactory form of intravenous carbohydrate and fructose is rarely used today.

Alcohol

Alcohol is not recommended. Although it is a concentrated source of energy, it can only be used in relatively small amounts because of its intoxicating effect. There are also other disadvantages: elderly, debilitated patients appear to have a reduced tolerance and it is contra-indicated in patients with liver damage and pancreatic disorders. It is seldom used today.

Fat

Fat is an essential aspect of parenteral feeding. The effects of a deficiency of essential fatty acids have been reported in patients given long-term fat-free parenteral feeds. They continued to improve and gain weight during the period of administration but developed clinical evidence of essential fatty acid deficiency within six or eight weeks. The condition occurs more rapidly in infants and young people.

Fat is also the most concentrated source of energy (37 kJ/g). Although previously in disfavour because of toxic effects caused by fatty emulsions (which are no longer available), fat is now regarded as an essential part of parenteral feeding. However, fats should be used with care and no drugs should be added to the fat emulsion for simultaneous administration.

Vitamin and mineral concentrates

These are routinely included in this regimen. In particular, potassium is required where extensive tissue repair is a major aspect of therapy.

Administration of parenteral feeding

As with enteral feeding, intravenous feeding is initiated with a dilute solution, i.e. approximately 1 litre of 10% glucose over the first 24 hour period. Glucose tolerance is monitored over the next few days as the volume and concentration of the infusion is increased until 2–3 litres of fluid per day is given. If dehydration, vomiting or diarrhoea are present, additional fluid is required.

A debilitated patients' needs for tissue regeneration may be met with the following combination of parenteral feeds: 1 litre of 10% fat emulsion (e.g. Intralipid) providing 4600 kJ (1100 Cal), plus 2 litres of half-strength 8.5% amino acid solution (e.g. Travasol). This concentration of 4.2% amino acid solution, providing a total of 1420 kJ (340 Cal), is mixed with a 25% glucose solution which provides 8400 kJ (2000 Cal). Total daily intake: 14 450 kJ (3440 Cal).

Electrolytes are routinely added for long-term parenteral feeding, with weekly trace element supplementation.

Patients with severe burns or extensive surgery are usually given the 20% fat emulsion to increase their energy intake, which is inadequate on the above feed. Amino acid solutions of high concentration are also often administered to these patients.

The infusion is administered through a peripheral vein if weak concentrations of sugar are given but if more than 10% glucose solutions are used, or if long-term parenteral feeding is anticipated, a large central vein (usually the superior vena cava) is used and an in-dwelling catheter is maintained in position. Introduction of pathogenic bacteria at the infusion site is an extremely serious risk and meticulous care and sterile procedure is all-important to reduce the risk of infection.

Gastrointestinal losses are accompanied by losses of sodium, potassium and chloride. Thus serum levels are routinely monitored if the patient has diarrhoea or is vomiting profusely, and supplementary electrolytes are given. The patient should also be regularly weighed if possible and the urine tested for sugar.

Complications

Sepsis is the most important problem resulting from parenteral feeding and in a severely compromised patient with increased vulnerability this can be an extremely hazardous complication. It can be caused by contamination of the feed or the catheter and aseptic procedures are essential to minimize its incidence. Immediate withdrawal of the catheter is necessary and often results in resolution of the situation without the use of antibiotics.

Incorrect positioning of the catheter can have life-threatening sequelae. Whilst the dislodgement of the peripheral tube into the tissues is obvious from the swelling at the site, and is easily remedied, the use of the vena cava for the administration of the feed is more hazardous. Puncture of the wall resulting in *pneumothorax* and *embolism* are serious complications.

Hyperosmolar non-ketotic hyperglycaemic coma can occur because of impaired glucose tolerance when an overload of glucose is given to a patient who is unable to handle it efficiently. It occurs secondary to hyperglycaemia and it is thus essential that caution is exercised in administering concentrated solutions of glucose. Blood and urine sugar levels must be monitored routinely.

Nutrient deficiency, while seldom encountered, occurs usually either if the selected preparation supplies an inadequate amount of a specific nutrient or where needs of a particular nutrient are inordinately high, i.e. during periods of growth. The three deficiencies most likely to occur are:

1. linoleic acid deficiency resulting in typical dermatitis;
2. zinc deficiency which may cause alopecia (loss of hair), reduced taste sensitivity and a scaly dermatitis;
3. hypophosphataemia causing abnormal sensation, weakness and fits.

Acidosis may result from an inability to maintain homeostasis following administration of amino acid solutions. However, today some mixtures are formulated with acetates to prevent this.

It is of great importance to administer intravenous fluids at the optimal rate. If they are given too slowly progress will be adversely affected and the patient will lose weight. Too rapid an administration may result in *dyspnoea* (laboured breathing) or *orthopnoea* (difficulty in breathing in the horizontal position). Routine charting of intake and output will minimize this problem. The tubing must also be regularly checked for kinking to ensure a continuous flow.

NURSING CONSIDERATIONS

1. Regular observation and monitoring of patients on enteral and parenteral feeds is essential. Preferred administration is

by steady continuous flow. However, if the speed is too slow the patient will not receive an optimal nutrient intake; if too fast, diarrhoea (in patients on tube feeds) and hyperglycaemia (in the parenterally fed patient) are likely complications.

2. Supplementary sip feeding, if practical and permissible, can markedly increase nutrient intake. Patients are told to routinely drink some of the beverage retained next to their bed, every 15 minutes. Such drinks should be carefully selected to contribute optimal nutritional value to the patient. Milk-based formulae are more acceptable for oral consumption than elemental diets, which patients reject due to the unpalatable taste of the amino acids.

3. Patients discharged on tube feeds need detailed instruction about the application of this technique at home. Maintenance of optimal standards of hygiene and holding the feed in the refrigerator when not in use are major considerations of management.

4. Dislodgement of the drip in the tissues is a common complication in comatose patients being infused peripherally. Close observation and immediate response will minimize the discomfort and nutrient loss.

5. Rebound hypoglycaemia is occasionally seen in patients when parenteral feeding with a concentrated glucose solution is suddenly terminated. Patients should be observed for any untoward effects.

6. 'Wishful-thinking feeding' must be avoided. It occurs all too frequently when a patient is given totally inadequate nutritional support in the hope that tomorrow the improved situation will allow for increased intake. This delay may continue for weeks while the patient becomes progressively more debilitated.

BIBLIOGRAPHY

Barron, J., Prendergast, J. & Jocz, M. (1956) Food pump: new approach to feeding. *J. Am. Med. Ass.*, *161*, 621.

Biebuyck, J. (1976) Substrate availability and utilization in normal man: effects of starvation and trauma. *S. Afr. Med., J.*, *52*, 1638.

Black, D.A.K. (1973) Intravenous infusion therapy. *Br. J. Hosp. Med.*, *9*, 765.

Crooks, P.E. (1975) Intravenous feeding and the dietitian. *Nutrition*, *29*, 357.

Imbembo, A. (1984) Parenteral nutrition. In: *Nutritional Management. The Johns Hopkins Handbook*. London: W.B. Saunders.

Jones, D.C. (1975) *Food for Thought — a Report of the Nutritional Nursing Care of Unconscious Patients*. Rcn Series: Study of Nursing Care. Whitefriars Press.

Jones, D.C. & Dickerson, J. (1976) Decision-making in the nutritional care of unconscious patients. *J. Adv. Nurs., 1*, 359.

Keohane, P., Attrill, H., Love, M., Frost, P. & Silk, D. (1984) Relation between osmolarity of diet and gastrointestinal side effects in enteral nutrition. *Br. Med. J., 288*, 678.

Lee, H.A. (1974) Intravenous nutrition. *Br. J. Hosp. Med., 11*, 719.

McMichael, H.B. (1978) Physiology of carbohydrate, electrolyte and water absorption. In: Johnston, I.D.A. & Lee, H.A. (eds.) *Developments in Clinical Nutrition*. Tunbridge Wells: MCS Consultants.

McWilliam, D., Robinson, M. & Sherwood Jones, E. (1977) Planning nutrition in acute illness. In: Mallick, N.P. (ed.) *Glucose Polymers in Health and Disease*. Lancaster: MTP Press.

Platt, B., Eddy, T. & Pellett, P. (1963) *Food in Hospitals*. London: Oxford University Press.

Porter, S.W. (1978) Feeding critically ill patients. *Nurs. Times, 74*, 355.

Richardson, T. & Sgoutas, M. (1975) Essential fatty acid deficiency in four adult patients during total parenteral nutrition. *Am. J. Clin. Nutr., 28*, 258.

Russell, R.I. (1975) Progress report: elemental diets. *Gut, 16*, 68.

Williams, K. & Walike, B. (1975) Effect of temperature of tube-feeding on gastric mobility in monkeys. *Nurs. Res., 24(1)*, 4.

Woolfson, A.M., Saour, J., Ricketts, C., Pollard, B., Hardy, S. & Allison, S. (1976) Prolonged naso-gastric tube feeding in critically ill and surgical patients. *Postgrad. Med. J., 52*, 678.

Yeung, C. (1981) Enteral nutrition — practical aspects. In: Hill, G. (ed.) *Nutrition and the Surgical Patient*. London: Churchill Livingstone.

17 Food Sensitivity

Food sensitivity, or allergy as it is commonly called, is the clinical manifestation of hypersensitivity to certain ingested substances to which most other people are normally immune. May (1984) classifies food sensitivity as shown in Table 19.

Table 19. Adverse reactions to food.

Biochemical
    (a) Enzyme deficiency
    (b) Toxic substances (occurring naturally or as additives in foods)
Immunological
Psychological

BIOCHEMICAL RESPONSES. In the first place, these are caused by known enzyme deficiencies. Lactose intolerance and gluten enteropathy are discussed in Chapter 8, and reference to several other metabolic defects such as favism and phenylketonuria are to be found in Chapter 15. Secondly, toxic substances which induce a reaction due to the release of mediators, particularly histamine, are encountered in strawberries, egg white, tomatoes, seafood and other common foods. Bronchospasm or asthma, gastrointestinal reactions, urticaria and pruritus(itching) are all symptoms seen in hypersensitive individuals.

IMMUNOLOGICAL RESPONSES. These can affect any aspect of bodily function but most generally affect the digestive tract (diarrhoea, vomiting, abdominal cramps), the skin (urticaria, eczema, etc.) and the respiratory tract (asthma and rhinitis). Other clinical manifestations of food allergy, such as oedema, tachycardia and neurological reactions, may occasionally be encountered.

PSYCHOLOGICAL RESPONSE. The nurse should avoid the common misconception that food sensitivity is *generally* a psychological or neurotic reaction rather than a physiological response. A recent editorial in the *Lancet* makes the point that dietary manipulation was a major therapeutic manoeuvre for many centuries but was relegated to the background with the technological progress of the pharmaceutical industry and the production of effective drugs. It is suggested that this trend may have gone too far and that more attention should be paid to the short-term effects of diet in susceptible individuals, rather than immediate reliance on drug therapy.

As early as 1924, Spain and Cooke proposed that *inheritance* was an important predisposing factor. They demonstrated that children whose parents were both allergic had a 69.4% risk of becoming allergic, and children with one hypersensitive parent a 58% risk. There is a strong correlation between the presence of food allergy in members of a family and the manifestation of asthma, hayfever or eczema in other family members due to provocative substances in the environment.

Infants and young children are at much greater risk than adults of exhibiting allergic reactions to food. It has been suggested that this may be due to the increased permeability of the gut to protein compounds which then land in the bloodstream undigested, or to the comparatively large quantity of allergen ingested in relation to body weight. Food allergy is the most common cause of hypersensitivity in young children and is considered to be responsible for 25% of asthma encountered in this age group. As the child gets older, inhalants become more important in this respect.

Dannaeus *et al* suggest that the most commonly encountered allergens of young children are *cow's milk, eggs, tomatoes, citrus fruit, bananas, chocolate* and *fish*. Corn, cola drinks, legumes (peas, beans and soya) and peanuts have also been incriminated. These foods frequently cause reactive responses in adults, too, although consumption of *alcohol, strawberries* and *shellfish* also often precipitates a reaction in older people. Raw foods are more likely to cause a reaction than cooked ones as allergens are sometimes denatured by heating. However, May comments that although any food can cause food sensitivity occasionally, 90% of food sensitivity is caused by four foods; namely, milk, eggs, nuts and wheat.

MILK ALLERGY

Intolerance to milk occurs more widely than with any other food. It has been suggested that it is encountered in half the world's population, either as a result of an enzyme defect (lactose intolerance) or as a hypersensitive reaction to milk protein, causing eczema, asthma, digestive tract disorders and rhinitis (Fig. 20). Breast-feeding for the first six weeks of life promotes immunity and it has been suggested by Walker and Hong that the antibodies secreted in the breast milk may coat the intestine, providing passive immunity until local active immunity is established. However, during the period of breast-feeding nursing mothers in hypersensitive families should avoid those foods (*chocolates, pork, strawberries*, etc.) that commonly cause allergic reactions, as it has been shown that provocative substances can be secreted in the breast milk and affect the baby.

A recent study by Atherton *et al* showed considerable benefits resulting from withdrawal of *eggs* and *cow's milk* from the diet of a group of young children with eczema. Children who are allergic to cow's milk usually tolerate goat's milk or soya milk without symptoms and many practitioners routinely recommend such replacement as initial therapy in children presenting with allergic symptoms, particularly eczema. However, up to 25% of infants may become allergic to *soya milk* as well. Those with severe allergy to milk may need to avoid *beef* and those with egg sensitivity may react as well to *chicken* or *vaccines grown on egg*, owing to the similar protein type in these related foods.

It has been suggested that food fads encountered in children may in many cases be a protective mechanism against food sensitivity. Many allergies are life-long and although there may be a period of remission, manifestation of another hypersensitive symptom may occur later in life. The infant with milk allergy may later develop symptoms related to other environmental factors. The diagnosis of milk allergy is thus of life-long relevance.

FOOD ADDITIVES

There is an increasing awareness that chemical additives such as flavour enhancers and dyes used in the food industry can be harmful. Grater has pointed out that the average person consumes

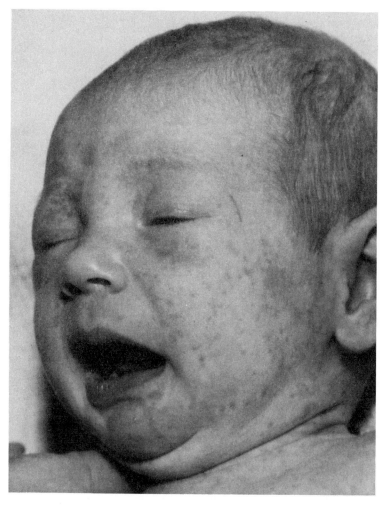

Fig. 20. *A baby with milk allergy. After only four days without milk the reaction had virtually disappeared.*

30 lbs of 'junk chemicals' per year. Antioxidants, concentrated flavouring compounds, dyes and even spices have been implicated in causing gastrointestinal, respiratory and cutaneous reactions.

Sodium benzoate, used as a preservative, and *tartrazine*, a yellow colouring agent used in sweets, margarine, toothpaste and drugs, can both cause asthma. This hypersensitivity has also been shown to cause skin reactions and is more frequently encountered in people who are sensitive to aspirin.

Allergy to *monosodium glutamate*, commonly used as a flavour enhancer in salty foods, is sometimes encountered. Within 15–20 minutes of ingestion, the individual develops a numbness at the back of the neck, radiating down the arms and back. Sweating, palpitations, headache and general weakness are features of the attack, which usually lasts for about 45 minutes but may persist for up to two hours. It occurs more frequently in women than in men and was first described by Kwok who called it the 'Chinese Restaurant Syndrome'. The term is still used to describe this allergy.

Cutaneous reactions are sometimes encountered following the ingestion of food additives. Hypersensitivity to *quinine* in tonic water can result in a skin eruption and, as mentioned above, tartrazine can also cause a cutaneous reaction. Contact dermatitis can be caused by the use of *dyes* in the food industry, although it appears to occur only in skin which is already damaged or eczematized. In 1958–1960 an epidemic of 'Dutch Margarine Disease' occurred in Germany and Holland when the emulsifier used in the margarine industry in these countries caused an outbreak of an urticaria-like rash. *Cinnamon oil*, used in food, chewing gum and toothpaste, has been incriminated as an eczema-producing allergen and *black pepper* has been found to cause pruritis ani (intense itching around the anus).

Coffee and *tea* have been repeatedly implicated as potential allergens. The caffeine found in these beverages and in *cola drinks* can produce a hypersensitivity response, resulting in headache, tension, arrhythmias and digestive tract symptoms. Neurological symptoms have also been encountered in people drinking excessive quantities of coffee and in more sensitive people taking smaller quantities. Replacement of coffee with a decaffeinated variety usually — but not always — causes improvements, but patients are often advised initially to avoid all types of tea and coffee to determine the effect, also the cola drinks and medicines containing caffeine, e.g. many analgesic tablets.

HYPERKINESIS

Hyperkinesis or *hyperactivity* is a behavioural disorder characterized by increased motor activity, excitability, aggression and irritability. Although it is frequently encountered in children with a high IQ, the associated decreased attention span and learning disability result in poor achievement. The number of children suffering from the condition has markedly increased in recent years and although environmental factors are generally considered to play a major aetiological role, there is considerable controversy as to the cause of the disorder.

In 1973 Feingold raised the question of artificial food additives as a primary cause, commenting that 'with the thousands of food chemicals in the environment, it seems remarkable that their influence on behaviour has not been suspected sooner'. He also suggested that these children may not be able to tolerate foods containing naturally occurring salicylate. He pointed out that certain drugs can affect human behaviour and that food chemicals of similar low molecular weight may produce the same effect. Feingold maintains that a favourable response to the elimination of artificial food additives and naturally occurring salicylates may be obtained in about 50% of hyperkinetic children. He proposes a diet containing only naturally occurring foods, excluding those containing salicylates. Labels of processed foods must be carefully scrutinized for content of artificial additives, and commercially produced confectionery and sweets must be avoided. Foods containing salicylates are listed in his article in the *American Journal of Nursing* (Feingold 1975) and include most fruits. Pears, bananas, grapefruit and quinces are among the few fruits permitted. Foods to be avoided include almonds, cucumbers, pickles, tomatoes, tea and oil of wintergreen.

The implications of these dietary changes are nutritionally, socially and therapeutically of the greatest importance as they demand major life-style changes.

However, Feingold's theories have met with a storm of opposition. Many workers have criticized his theory, for various reasons. In the first place, they suggest that the treatment is entirely empirical: the mechanism is not understood nor is it scientifically substantiated. They claim that the body cannot determine between 'natural' and 'artificial' chemicals. Secondly, these children often come from homes where there are family problems. Major changes in the diet affect the whole family and the inter-relationships of its members. As observations of improvement are subjective, teachers or parents assessing dietary success may be biased in their assessment. Conservative medical opinion is hesitant to advise patients on such a change in life-style in the absence of controlled trials which demonstrate that hyperkinesis is clearly related to ingestion of food additives.

In a recent review article (Lipton & Mayo) the authors 'refute the claims that artificial food colourings and salicylates frequently produce hyperactivity and/or learning disabilities'. However, they found that the additive-free diet has no harmful effects and the non-specific placebo effects of this dietary treatment are frequently very beneficial to families.

MIGRAINE HEADACHES

Migraine is a condition of neurological origin. About 10% of the British population suffer from the condition and a positive family history of migraine is reported by the majority of sufferers.

The episodic headaches can last several hours and are often associated with visual and/or gastrointestinal disturbances. A variety of triggering mechanisms can cause an attack: stress, oral contraceptives, exposure to bright flickering light, onset of menstruation and excessive tiredness. Furthermore, it is becoming increasingly apparent that food intake is an important causatory factor; indeed Dalessio refers specifically to 'dietary migraine'. Prolonged fasting or adherence to a stringent weight reduction regimen resulting in hypoglycaemia can induce a migraine headache which can be considerably alleviated with the return to a greater intake of food preferably distributed as six small meals.

Tyramine, a compound in various foods, has been incriminated in the causation of migraine headaches. As discussed in Chapter 18, monoamine oxidase normally inhibits the vaso-active effect of tyramine, but in sensitive individuals where the breakdown of tyramine is incomplete, a migraine headache can occur because of loss of tone in the cranial arteries. High-tyramine foods include chocolate, mature cheese, pickled herrings, red wine (in particular chianti), yeast extracts (e.g. Marmite) and sour cream; these are major precipitating foods in susceptible individuals.

Excessive sodium intake either as salt (in crisps, bacon, etc.) or as monosodium glutamate may also trigger a migraine headache as discussed earlier in this chapter. A symptom of the Chinese

Restaurant Syndrome is a headache which may well be part of the migraine picture. Other reports incriminate alcohol, citrus fruits and megadoses of vitamin A, reinforcing the conclusion that patients should be alerted to note the meals preceding their migraine in an attempt to ascertain whether or not there is a dietary correlation in the aetiology of their specific condition.

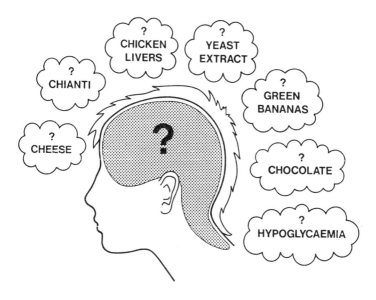

Fig. 21. *Possible causes of migraine headache.*

PSORIASIS

Psoriasis is a chronic inflammatory disease characterized by red patches on the skin covered with dried white scales. Over the years, many workers have correlated the condition with specific nutrients. Initially, protein was implicated and patients were advised to adhere to a low-protein diet. Subsequently it was thought that sulphur caused the reaction and patients were told to avoid the sulphur-containing amino acids. More recently, psoriasis has been linked to the amino acid tryptophan, and marked improvements have been experienced on a low-tryptophan diet.

DIAGNOSIS

Food allergies are extremely difficult to diagnose. In the first place, the quantity of allergen necessary to cause a reaction varies from person to person. Furthermore, psychosomatic factors may influence the reaction and hypersensitivity may occur only when the individual is particularly tired, tense or upset. To add to the complexity of the subject, not only may a wide range of environmental factors other than food be the cause of a reaction, but a specific allergen can precipitate a variety of symptoms in different people.

Various methods are employed to determine the causes of an allergy.

DIETARY HISTORY. This is most important. Often, merely sitting down with a patient and questioning him about the details of his food intake may give the interviewer — or the patient — insight into the precise role of specific foods in the condition.

RADIO ALLERGO SORBENT TEST (RAST). This important clinical test is regarded as a great advance. It is widely used to measure specific serum antibodies to a variety of individual food allergens. Sensitivity to the injected substance is demonstrated by diverse symptoms, including anaphylaxis (increased response), urticaria, asthma, eczema, diarrhoea, allergic rhinitis, etc. Although the diagnosis is time-consuming and problematic to establish, such symptoms are regarded as an accurate indication of allergy.

SKIN TEST. This is also commonly used. A drop of the suspected allergen is placed on the forearm and the skin then pricked superficially. A positive reaction is an inflammatory weal within ten minutes, fading within half an hour. Unfortunately, results are not always reliable.

The Ad Hoc Committee on Provocative Food Testing of the American College of Allergists has commented 'positive responses to subcutaneous provocative tests are not reliable and thus cannot be valid. Negative responses to the test are reliable but do not predict responses to food challenge and, therefore, are not valid indications of food allergy'.

FEEDING TESTS. These were suggested by Miller for migraine but are also applicable for other types of sensitivity. They consist of deliberately feeding the suspected food under controlled conditions. However, the technique can be used only when symptoms of allergy are not too profound. The patient is asked to compile three lists of food. The first list details all foods which the patient considers result in hypersensitive reactions if ingested; the second lists foods that are particularly enjoyed or make the patient feel better; and the third list is of those foods most frequently eaten. Foods are tested in order of those noted, commencing with the first group. The first four foods listed are avoided for four days, then they are tested simultaneously on the 5th day, the patient being told to eat these four foods at all three meals of the day. This procedure is continued, with patients paying particular attention both to remission of symptoms during the four-day withdrawal of selected foods and aggravation of symptoms on the 5th or 6th day. If the test is positive the patient is advised to reintroduce the group containing the provocative foods, but only one each day, after a four-day abstention period. In this way the offending food can be pinpointed and the patient advised to avoid this food (at least temporarily), as well as all other made-up foods containing it. Some patients may find that small quantities eaten irregularly cause no reaction, and challenge in this way may be advisable later.

ELIMINATION DIETS. These were first proposed by Rowe in 1944 and although the classical Rowe diet is still used, various other elimination diets are also currently recommended. The regimen consists of the administration of a collection of diets, in which common allergens are included under controlled conditions. Commencing with diet I — the diet least likely to precipitate reaction — the patient will progress (one to three weeks later) to diet II, and so on. When a hypersensitive reaction occurs another diet is tried. This diagnostic test is a cumbersome, time-consuming procedure, but it is effective and still used.

ELEMENTAL DIETS. These are occasionally used as a last resort in severely affected individuals for determining whether reactions result from food allergy. Patients are fed either by mouth or through a nasogastric tube (as these formulas are often most unpalatable) and observed for improvement over a few days. Suspected foods are added singly and the reaction is noted.

MANAGEMENT

Elimination of the offending food components is the basis of treatment of food allergy. The patient must avoid the consumption of the food, even in processed foods. Lists of combination foods likely to cause a reaction in allergic subjects are given by Speer. If symptoms are not completely alleviated by the withdrawal of the suspected allergen, Speer suggests that a minimal diet made up of only five selected basic food items is given for two weeks. Thereafter other foods are included individually every second day and the patient observed for a hypersensitive response. Densitization is sometimes used to reduce the reaction. Commencing with minute quantities of allergens, increasingly larger amounts are administered, with progressive reduction in allergic response. This too is a long-term procedure, but it is justified in some cases.

BIBLIOGRAPHY

Amos, H. & Drake, J. (1976) Problems posed by food additives. *J. Hum. Nutr., 30*, 165.

Atherton, D., Soothill, J., Sewell, M., Wells, R. & Chilvers, C. (1978) A double-blind controlled crossover trial of an antigen avoidance diet in atopic eczema. *Lancet, 1*, 401.

Breakey, J. (1978) Dietary management of hyperkinesis behavioural problems. *J. Hum. Nutr., 32*, 303.

Dannaeus, A., Johansson, S. & Foucard, T. (1978) Clinical and immunological aspects of food allergy in childhood, II. *Acta Paediat. Scand., 67*, 497.

Feingold, B. (1975) Hyperkinesis and learning disabilities linked to artificial food flavours and colours. *Am. J. Nurs., 15*, 797.

Fisher, A. (1975) Contact dermatitis due to food additives. *Cutis, 16*, 961.

Fisher, A. (1976) Reactions to antioxidants in cosmetics and foods. *Cutis, 17*, 21.

Grater, W. (1976) Hypersensitive skin reactions to F.D. and C. Dyes. *Cutis, 17*, 1165.

Institute of Food Technologists' Expert Panel (1976) Diet and hyperactivity: any connection? *Fd. Trade Rev.*, (Oct.), 591.

Kandela, P. & Blau, J. (1980) Second opinion: A patient suffering from migraine. *Mod. Med., 5*, 61.

Kwok, R. (1968) Chinese-Restaurant syndrome. *N. Engl. J. Med., 278*, 796.

Lancet (1979) Food allergy. *Lancet, 1*, 249.

Levantine, A. & Almeyda, J. (1974) Cutaneous reactions to food and drug additives. *Br. J. Derm., 91*, 359.

Lipton, M. & Mayo, J. (1983) Diet and hyperkinesis — an update. *J. Am. Diet. Ass., 83*, 132.

MacLaren, W. (1974) Food allergy in adults. In: Frazier, C.A. (ed.) *Annual Review of Allergy*. New York: Med. Exam.

May, C. (1984) Food sensitivity: facts and fancies. *Nutr. Rev., 42*, 72.

Miller, J. (1974) Management in migraine headaches. In: Frazier, C.A. (ed.) *Current Therapy of Allergy*. New York: Med, Exam.

Speer, F. (1974) Food and gastrointestinal allergy in children. In: Frazier, C.A. (ed.) *Current Therapy of Allergy*. New York: Med. Exam.

Spiera, H. & Lefkovitis, A.M. (1967) Remission of psoriasis with low dietary tryptophan. *Lancet, 2*, 137.

Walker, W. & Hing, R. (1973) Immunology of the gastrointestinal tract, Part I. *J. Paediat., 83*, 517.

18 Diet and drug interaction

The reciprocal effects of food and drugs are currently evoking much interest and research. It has only recently become apparent that the absorption of some drugs is influenced by the nutritional status of the patient as well as the specific food items eaten concomitantly. The ingestion of certain drugs, many of them widely used, can impair nutritional status and promote toxicity in malnourished patients. The erratic response to a particular drug encountered in some patients may be due to the interaction between the drug and dietary components. The patient is entirely dependent on the nurse for food intake and drug dosage and it is thus essential that the nurse understands the correlation between the two.

EFFECTS OF DRUG ACTION ON NUTRITION

Apart from the diarrhoea or vomiting that certain drugs can precipitate in some individuals, there are other direct ways in which the nutritional status can be directly affected by drug administration. A single transport or enzyme system may be blocked, or the integrity of the villi may be affected, resulting in reduced absorption of certain nutrients. Furthermore, the optimum amount of drug to be administered bears an important relationship to the general state of nutrition. Malnourished patients may have a reduced enzyme activity in the tissues, making them less competent to metabolize certain drugs. Thus the standard dose could be toxic, and for this reason malnourished patients should be given a lower dosage of many drugs than those who are well nourished.

Taste acuity can be impaired (dysgeusia) resulting in a reduced intake of food due to poor appetite. This, in turn, can markedly affect nutritional status.

Impaired absorption, transport and utilization of *Vitamin B_{12}* and *folic acid* are seen with a growing number of drugs. Oral contraceptives, antibiotics, chemotherapeutic drugs for cancer, antimalarials, drugs used for psoriasis and immunosuppressive drugs have all been implicated in this way. Alcohol also impairs the absorption of these vitamins. Although the resulting deficiencies may not be pronounced in most patients, megaloblastic anaemia has been encountered in patients with minimal stores taking a high dosage of these offending drugs over a long period. The duration of medication and the simultaneous administration of several drugs may both affect the absorption and metabolism of nutrients. Poorly nourished patients with tuberculosis, treated with INH, may develop pellagra if on a marginal intake of niacin, owing to impairment of the endogenous conversion of tryptophan to niacin.

Diuretics may be potassium-losing as well as promoting fluid loss and patients frequently need to modify their diet to effect replacement. High-potassium foods are listed in Appendix C. The situation can be further aggravated by the simultaneous administration of *digitalis* to these patients as they readily develop cardiac arrhythmias if they become hypokalaemic because of inadequate replacement of diuretic-induced potassium losses.

The routine ingestion of mineral oils as laxatives is strongly discouraged, as the absorption of the fat-soluble vitamins ingested at the same time is adversely affected and deficiency of vitamins A and D can be caused by excessive losses in the stool.

Side-effects of the administration of certain drugs are *anorexia* and *vomiting*, which may result in weight loss. A wide range of drugs cause destruction of the villi and microorganisms of the gut and result in *malabsorption, diarrhoea, steatorrhoea* and *lactase deficiency*. In the case of hypocholesterolaemic drugs such as cholestyramine, the mode of action is based on malabsorption causing increased breakdown of cholesterol to bile acids and removal of these compounds in the faeces. However, cholestyramine also inhibits iron transport, and the possibility that long-term use of this drug may promote the development of iron deficiency anaemia is now being considered.

Antibiotics may affect nutritional status in two ways. In the first place they bind with calcium or cholesterol, as mentioned below. Secondly, they may cause destruction of the intestinal flora resulting in malabsorption and reducing the synthesis of vitamin B complex. For this reason vitamin B complex is usually administered with antibiotics. Many practitioners routinely advise the supplementation of yoghurt in an attempt to replace deficient flora but the advantages of this are controversial. *Neomycin* is an antibiotic but also affects fat digestion and reduces the serum cholesterol level. However, it also causes malabsorption of other nutrients; *sugars* such as lactose (causing diarrhoea), *vitamins* (carotene and vitamin B_{12}) and *iron*.

Long-term use of *colchicine* may be accompanied by losses of various nutrients in the faeces. This is thought to result from disturbed epithelial cell function and depressed enzyme production. Apart from fats, lactose, bile acids and sterols, which are lost because of reduction in enzyme action, carotene and vitamin B_{12} are also less effectively absorbed.

There are several adverse effects of *anticonvulsant drugs* on nutritional status. Vitamin D absorption is severely impaired: rickets has been encountered with long-term use of these drugs in children. The higher the dose and the lower the vitamin D intake, the greater the risk of deficiency. Lack of sunlight and a black skin both reduce the synthesis of vitamin D, increasing the risk of deficiency and ultimately osteomalacia. Vitamin B_6, vitamin K and folic acid deficiencies may be encountered in patients taking anticonvulsants. This appears to be a result of both increased requirement and antagonism to these drugs. These patients are often given routine supplementation of vitamin B_{12} and folic acid. However, excess folic acid will adversely affect the metabolism of the anticonvulsant and cause an increase in seizures.

Oral contraceptives

Several studies have emphasized the need for additional vitamin B_6 (pyridoxine) for women taking contraceptive drugs. It appears that the requirement for this nutrient increases dramatically and that the depression that sometimes accompanies the routine use of oral contraceptive agents can be reversed with the administration of vitamin B_6. The use of oestrogens also results in a drop of normal serum vitamin C and B_{12} levels, as well as folic acid. With regard to minerals, oral contraceptives generally have a favourable effect. Calcium deposits in the bones are increased and iron needs are reduced (especially when the menstrual flow is diminished).

Table 20 summarizes the major effects of some common drugs on nutritional status.

Table 20. The major effects of some common drugs on nutritional status.

Drug	Side-effect	Usual dosage recommendation
Laxatives		
Mineral oils	Excretory losses of carotene, vitamins A and D	Long-term use inadvisable
Phenolphthalein	Increased losses of calcium and vitamin D; hypokalaemia, dehydration	High-K foods usually recommended
Diuretics		
Thiazide, Frusemide	Increased excretion of Na, K, Mg and water, resulting in electrolyte imbalance, dry mouth, and hypokalaemic symptoms of lethargy, tiredness	Take single morning dose to reduce night urination; High-K foods usually indicated; low-salt diet if appropriate for hypertension and cardiac failure; intake with food delays absorption of Frusemide.
Spironolactone	As with above diuretics *except* no hypokalaemia, K-sparing therefore contra-indicated in renal failure	More efficiently absorbed and less gastric irritation if taken with food
Antibiotics		
Antibiotics in general	Destroy gut flora causing malabsorption of sugars (hence diarrhoea) and reduced production of several B vitamins	Vitamin B supplementation often recommended with prolonged use; antidiarrhoea measures may be necessary
Tetracycline	Chelates Ca and Fe in foods	Not to be taken with milk or other major Ca and Fe sources
Neomycin	Binds bile salts; less effective absorption of fat, also Fe	

(cont. overleaf)

Table 20. *(Cont.)*

Drug	Side-effect	Usual dosage recommendation
Oral contraceptives		
Oestrogens	Salt and fluid retention (hence oedema); nausea; increased need for vitamins B_6, C, B_{12} and folic acid	Take with food to minimize nausea; monitor weight; vitamin B_6 supplementation may be necessary
Anti-inflammatory		
Indomethacin	Indigestion; even acute ulceration	Must be buffered with food to reduce gastric irritation
Aspirin (also analgesic, antipyretic)	Can cause gastric pain or bleeding; increased requirements for vitamin C	Although delayed absorption if taken with a meal, this must always be taken with milk or water to reduce gastric irritation; vitamin C supplementation may be indicated
Penicillamine (also used as heavy metal antagonist)	Chelates Cu, Fe and Zn; dysgeusia; loss of appetite	Take on an empty stomach and not at the same time as mineral supplements
Anticonvulsants		
Phenobarbitone, phenytoin	Decreased deposition of calcium, hence rickets, osteomalacia; dysgeusia; decreased serum folic acid and vitamin B_6 levels	Take with food to reduce gastric irritation; optimal vitamin D intake necessary; supplementation with folic acid and vitamin B_6 may be necessary
Other		
Methotrexate (cancer chemotherapy)	Folic acid antagonist; disturbed mucosal function, hence malabsorption of fat and vitamin B_{12}; dysgeusia; sore mouth; hyperuricaemia; peptic ulceration	Increased fluid intake may be recommended to aid excretion of uric acid; frequent small meals may be advantageous *but* milky meals may reduce absorption

(cont. on facing page)

Table 20. *(Cont.)*

Drug	Side-effect	Usual dosage recommendation
Hydralazine (antihypertensive)	Loss of appetite, vitamin B_6 antagonist	Take with meals to enhance absorption; vitamin B_6 supplementation may be indicated; also recommendations for hypertension
Isoniazid (antitubercular)	Dyspepsia; vitamin B_6 antagonist	Take on an empty stomach; vitamin B_6 supplementation may be recommended
Cholestyramine (cholesterol binder; bile-acid sequestrant)	Malabsorption of fat-soluble vitamins, also Fe; causes constipation	Take with fruit juice, crushed pineapple or canned peaches to mask unpalatability; high-fibre diet
Aluminium hydroxide (antacid; phosphate binder)	Reduced phosphate and vitamin A absorption destruction of thiamine	For ulcer therapy, administration between meals; for phosphate-binding therapy, take with meals
Colchicine	Disturbed mucosal function, hence reduced lactase activity (diarrhoea), reduced absorption of fats, carotene and vitamin B_{12}	Take with meals to reduce gastric irritation

EFFECTS OF NUTRITION AND FOOD ON THE METABOLISM OF DRUGS

Foods can affect absorption of drugs from the digestive tract and their utilization by the body in several ways.

SLOWED ABSORPTION. The presence of food in the stomach can slow down absorption. Examples of this are when methylphenidate (Ritalin) or aspirin is taken; however, in the latter case, the gastric irritation which can result from ingestion of aspirin on an empty stomach makes it imperative to buffer it with milk or, at least, water. Some antibiotics are adversely affected by gastric acid and are thus administered at times when minimal secretion of acid occurs, i.e. between meals. The absence of food allows for accelerated passage through the stomach, thus limiting the impact. Alkalis administered to ulcer patients to neutralize the outpouring of acid and protect the mucosa lining are taken particularly as a buffer when there is no food in the stomach to dilute the effect of the acid.

PROMOTED ABSORPTION. On the other hand, food may promote absorption, e.g. of spironolactone. Prolonged contact with food allows pills to break down into a more assimilable form. It also spaces out the entry of the dose into the small intestine, allowing delayed uptake. Certain potentially ulcerogenic drugs are given with meals so that the food can buffer their effects in the stomach. Indomethacin (Indocid) is given in the middle of a meal — the 'indomethacin sandwich' — because of its otherwise irritating effect on the gastric mucosa.

AMOUNT OF DRUG ABSORBED. This may be affected by a specific food component, e.g. the interference by foods that are high in iron or calcium in tetracycline absorption. Tetracycline is a chelating agent and attaches itself to the large Ca^{2+} ion. Simultaneous ingestion of milk and cheese products, for example, which have a high calcium content, causes chelation of the calcium by tetracycline, thus inhibiting the absorption of both the calcium and the tetracycline. A similar binding also occurs with certain organic acids as discussed in Chapter 1. Hence, supplementation with oral iron will be adversely affected by the simultaneous ingestion of a high phosphate, phytate or oxalate diet. In practice, probably the most important implication is that patients should not eat large quantities of wholewheat bread while taking supplementary oral iron.

Furthermore, a high-fat meal and, to a lesser extent, a meal high in protein, delays gastric emptying, thus slowing down the passage of drugs to the small intestine. A diet high in fibre may both increase the motility of the digestive tract and also adsorb drugs, preventing absorption. However, fat-soluble drugs, such as griseofulvin, are better absorbed when taken with fat. Broccoli which has a high vitamin K impairs the efficacy of warfarin sodium and excessive quantities should be avoided when this drug is prescribed.

SIDE EFFECTS. Nausea and vomiting (resulting in gastric losses of the precipitating drug) can sometimes be prevented if taken with food.

ANTAGONISTIC EFFECTS. Specific drugs may have an antagonistic effect on certain nutrients, e.g. isoniazid administration can result in vitamin B_6 deficiency, and supplementation of vitamin B_6 is often recommended. This antagonism can, however, also be used to the benefit of the patient, as in the case of methotrexate (discussed in Chapter 14) where folic acid antagonism is used as therapy in leukaemia.

DIET–DRUG TOXICITY. This is another hazard of drug administration and can occur, for example, between food containing tyramine and certain antidepressant drugs. Parnate, Nardil, Parstelin and Marsilid are monoamine oxidase inhibitors (MAOI). They combine irreversibly with monoamine oxidase (MAO) in the liver. MAO is necessary to break down tyramine, which therefore accumulates in the circulation displacing large quantities of noradrenaline. This affects the blood flow and causes hypertension, severe headaches and nose bleeds. Cheese, in particular, is a rich source of tyramine, the name being derived from *tyros*, the Greek word for cheese. People taking these drugs must be clearly informed not to take foods that are rich in free amines which promote the production of tyramine in the gut. Cheese, chicken livers, Chianti wines, chocolate, Bovril, Marmite and other similar yeast extracts must be avoided. Tyramine has also recently been implicated in the causation of migraine headaches, a subject which is discussed in Chapter 17.

ALCOHOL. Alcohol adversely affects the utilization of a variety of drugs. When consumed with antihistamines, antidepressants or tranquillizers it can cause excessive drowsiness. When taken with antidiabetic drugs or insulin, alcohol can potentiate the hypoglycaemic effect. Also, it should never be taken by people taking monoamine oxidase inhibitors.

NUTRIENTS AS DRUGS

Nutritionists are particularly concerned today about the current practice of the ingestion of megadoses of vitamins. These huge doses are taken — usually self-prescribed — as treatment for an ailment, either real or perceived, or for the promotion of health. Massive doses of vitamin A are currently being swallowed to prevent sunburn, vitamin B for psychiatric illnesses and emotional states, and vitamin E to promote longevity. The use of megadoses of vitamin C to prevent and cure colds is highly controversial. In general these claims are unsubstantiated, costly to implement and, most important, potentially toxic. As discussed in Chapter 1 excessive intakes of fat-soluble vitamins result in hypervitaminosis with accumulation of these compounds in the liver and fatty tissues of the body. Although it was previously thought that if taken in excess, water-soluble vitamins would merely be excreted in the urine, more recently the risks of such administration are becoming evident. Rebound scurvy has been encountered in infants of mothers taking megadoses of vitamin C in pregnancy, or in others when they stop such massive intakes. Kidney stone formation is possibly another hazard of excessive vitamin C intake. Vitamin B_6 toxicity has also been described (see Chapter 1).

In conclusion, there is no evidence to support the reasoning that if small amounts of vitamins are good for you, large amounts must be better! The accepted RDA have been studied in depth before being made available and used by health professionals. They are also regularly updated. Patients should thus be cautioned against the potentially harmful practice of self-prescription of megadoses of vitamins, the more so because they get a false sense of security about their state of health and may delay seeking orthodox medical advice.

PHARMACOLOGICAL EFFECT OF FOOD

This chapter would be incomplete without some reference to the unique physiological effect of certain foods. An example of this is fava beans and favism, which has been discussed in Chapter 15. Other substances have been found to have pronounced *hypoglycaemic* effects and occasional references to teas made from herbs or the leaves of certain trees will be found in the popular press.

However, the enormous quantities of these compounds that need to be consumed for such effects, the lack of accuracy of dose and the lack of year-long supply make these substances totally impractical for pharmacological use.

A food which is of some practical relevance in this respect is liquorice, because of its hypertensive effects. The consumption of large quantities of this sweet (i.e. 100 g/day) has been shown to induce hypertension due to excessive fluid and salt retention. This condition is reversed by withdrawal of liquorice from the diet.

In the chicken industry tetracycline is often administered to birds before slaughter to prevent contamination of the carcases by pathogenic bacteria. Individuals with an extreme sensitivity to tetracycline may therefore suffer from gastrointestinal side-effects when eating chicken.

In conclusion, the need for astute observation by the nurse — to be able to recognize not only untoward symptoms related to the illness of patients but also reactions to the therapy given — is stressed.

BIBLIOGRAPHY

Adams, P.W., Folkard, J., Wynn, V., Seed, M. & Strong, R. (1973) Effect of pyridoxine hydrochloride (vitamin B_6) upon depression associated with oral contraception. *Lancet, 1*, 897.

Christiakis, G. & Miridjanian, A. (1968) Diets, drugs and their inter-relationships. *J. Am. Diet. Ass., 52*, 21.

Conney, A. & Burns, J. (1972) Metabolic interactions among environmental chemicals and drugs. *Science, 178*, 576.

Dickerson, J. & Labadarios, D. (1972) Inter-relationship between nutrition and drugs. *Nutrition, 26*, 297.

Faloon, W. (1970) Drug production of intestinal malabsorption. *N.Y. St. J. Med., 70(2)*, 2189.

Gray, G. (1973) Drugs, malnutrition and carbohydrate absorption. *Am. J. Clin. Nutr., 26*, 121.

Hamilton Smith, C. (1984) Dietary concerns associated with the use of medications. *J. Am. Diet. Ass., 84*, 901.

Hartshorn, E. (1977) Food and drug interactions. *J. Am. Diet. Ass., 70*, 15.

Ioannides, C. (1979) Effect of diet on the metabolism and toxicology of drugs. *J. Hum. Nutr., 33*, 357.

Kempin, M. (1983) Warfarin resistance caused by broccoli. *N. Eng. J. Med., 308*, 1229.

Koster, M. & David, G. (1968) Reversible severe hypertension due to licorice ingestion. *N. Engl. J. Med., 278*, 1381.

Krondl, A. (1970) Present understanding of the interaction of drugs and food during absorption. *Can. Med. Ass. J., 103*, 360.

Kunin, C. & Finland, M. (1961) Clinical pharmacology of the tetracycline antibiotics. *Clin. Pharmac. Ther.*, *2*, 51.

Massey Stewart, M. (1976) MAOI's and food — fact and fiction. *Adv. Drug Reaction Bull., (June)*, 58.

Race, T., Paes, I. & Faloon, W. (1970) Intestinal malabsorption induced by oral colchicine. *Am. J. Med. Sci., 259*, 32.

Roe, D. (1983) Drug and nutrient interactions. In: Schneider, H., Anderson, C. & Coursin, D.B. *Nutritional Support of Medical Practice*, 2nd edn. London: Harper and Row.

Roe, D. (1984) Nutrient and drug interactions. *Nutr. Rev., 42*, 141.

Theuer, R. (1972) Effect of oral contraceptive agents on vitamin and mineral needs: a review. *J. Reprod. Med., 8*, 13.

Theuer, R. & Vitale, J. (1977) Drug and nutrient interactions. In: Schneider, H., Anderson, C. & Coursin, D.B. (eds.) *Nutritional Support of Medical Practice*. London: Harper and Row.

Waxman, S., Corcino, J. & Herbert, V. (1970) Drugs, toxins and dietary amino-acids affecting vitamin B_{12} or folic acid absorption or utilisation. *Am. J. Med., 48*, 599.

General bibliography

Beck, M.E. (1980) *Nutrition and Dietetics for Nurses*, 6th edn. London: Churchill Livingstone.

Conn, H.F. (1971) *Current Therapy 1971*. London: W.B. Saunders.

Davidson, S. & Passmore, R. (1979) *Human Nutrition and Dietetics*, 7th edn. London: Churchill Livingstone.

Dickerson, J.W.T. & Lee, H.A. (1978) *Nutrition in the Clinical Management of Disease*. London: Edward Arnold.

Francis, D.E.M. (1974) *Diets for Sick Children*, 3rd edn. London: Blackwell Scientific.

Goodhart, R. & Shils, M. (1980) *Modern Nutrition in Health and Disease*, 6th edn. Philadelphia: Lea & Febiger.

McCance, R.A. & Widdowson, E.M. (1960) *The Composition of Foods*. London: HMSO.

McLaren, D.S. & Burman, D. (1976) *Textbook of Paediatric Nutrition*. London: Churchill Livingstone.

Proudfit, F.T. & Robinson, C.H. (1961) *Normal and Therapeutic Nutrition*, 12th edn. New York: Macmillan.

Schneider, H.A., Anderson, C.E. & Coursin, D.B. (1983) *Nutritional Support of Medical Practice*, 2nd edn. London: Harper & Row.

Turner, D. (1970) *Handbook of Diet Therapy*, 5th edn. London: University of Chicago Press.

Williams, S.R. (1977) *Nutrition and Diet Therapy*, 3rd edn. St. Louis: C.V. Mosby.

Appendix A: The low-fibre diet

The low-fibre diet is also called a bland, light or low-residue diet.

Cereals

Include refined cereals, e.g. flour, rice, cornflour, macaroni, sago and tapioca; also white bread, plain cakes, biscuits and rusks.
Avoid wholewheat products, bran and other coarse cereals such as sweetcorn.

Dairy products

Include milk, butter, cream, eggs and mild cheeses.
Avoid cooked and strong cheeses (e.g. Roquefort).

Meat

Include all tender meat and poultry.
Avoid tough overcooked meat and highly seasoned dishes (e.g. curried and pickled meats), sausages and fried meats.

Fish

Include all fresh or plain tinned fish (e.g. pilchards and salmon).
Avoid obvious bones (such as backbone of pilchards), also smoked fish such as kippers and dishes made with fried fish or highly seasoned (e.g. curried fish).

Vegetables

Include all soft vegetables, steamed, boiled or baked (e.g. potato, young carrots or beetroot, marrow, parsnips, cauliflower florets, and petit pois or tinned peas).
Avoid cabbage, onions (except grated for flavouring), cauliflower stalks, fresh or dried peas, beans or lentils, raw salads (e.g. cucumber, celery and tomatoes).

Fruit

Include peeled raw or stewed fruits with limited fibre (e.g. ripe apples, pears, bananas, ripe peaches, avocado pears), also fruit juices and sieved cooked fruits.

Avoid fibrous fruits such as pineapple, plums, guavas, grapes, oranges and figs.

Sweets, jams and sugars

Include jelly, stoned fruit jam, shredded marmalade, honey, syrup, sugar, plain sweets and chocolate.

Avoid whole fruit and berry jams, sweets containing nuts and coarse ingredients.

Miscellaneous

Include strained and puréed soups, herbs for flavouring, and finely grated onion.

Avoid nuts, strong condiments such as pepper, chillis, horseradish and highly seasoned sauces, pickles and chutney.

Appendix B: The high-residue diet

Basic principles

1. The most important foods to include are those high in wheat bran. Two or three tablespoons of wheat bran can be sprinkled on cereal, mixed with salad or used for coating fish prior to baking. Wholewheat bread, biscuits and breakfast cereals should be included daily.
2. Other sources of *cellulose* such as fruit and vegetables should also play a major role in the diet. Tomatoes, cucumber, lettuce, cauliflower, cabbage, Brussels sprouts and beans all have a high fibre content. High-fibre fruit include oranges, grapefruit, grapes, apricots, berries and unpeeled apples and pears.
3. Adequate *fluid* is required, to combine with fibre and increase the bulk in the digestive tract. Eight to ten glasses of water or juice or cups of tea or coffee or other beverages are necessary each day.
4. A small amount of *fat* is helpful for lubricating purposes.

Sample menu

Breakfast
    stewed dried fruit
    rolled oats porridge with milk
    sweetcorn on wholewheat toast
    tea or coffee
Lunch
    wholewheat bread sandwiches spread with butter or margarine
        and meat, cheese, etc
    salad (carrot sticks, tomato, celery, cucumber)
    a high-fibre fruit
    tea or coffee

Dinner
vegetable soup
fried fish, chips, stewed onion and tomato
fruit salad and custard
tea or coffee

Appendix C: Potassium content of common foods

The potassium content of fruit and vegetables is largely dependent on the method of cookery. Raw and fried products have considerably higher potassium content than those diced and cooked in a lot of water which is then discarded.

High-potassium foods (over 300 mg/100 g)

Fruit — all dried fruit, plus apricots, avocado pears, bananas, blackcurrants, dates, greengages, passion fruit, prunes, rhubarb

Vegetables — Jerusalem artichokes, beetroot, mushrooms, parsley, potatoes, tomato paste and sauce

Nuts

Soya

Full-grain breakfast wheat and oats products — Weetabix, grapenuts, wheat flakes

Molasses

Milk chocolate

Some meat (liver, turkey), *fish* (haddock, salmon, sardines)

Moderate-potassium foods (150–300 mg/100 g)

Fruit — apricots (fresh or canned), blackberries, cherries, red- or whitecurrants (fresh or stewed), damsons, figs, grapes, grapefruit, loganberries, yellow melons, mulberries, nectarines, oranges, peaches, pineapples, plums, quinces, raspberries, strawberries

Vegetables — asparagus, broadbeans, Brussels sprouts, cabbage, cucumber, raw celery, pumpkin, sweet potatoes, tomatoes, turnips

Wholewheat bread

Milk (high in protein)

Some meat (beef, pork), *fish* (plaice, skate)

Chocolate

Low-potassium foods (less than 150 mg/100 g)

Fruit — fresh apples, cranberries, lemons, pears, tangerines, watermelon; *canned, drained* cherries, fruit salad, gooseberries, loganberries, mandarins, peaches, pears, plums

Vegetables — globe artichokes, green beans, broccoli, carrots, cauliflower, cooked celery (root), marrow, olives, onion, spinach

All vegetables diced and cooked in large amounts of water which is then discarded

White bread and *biscuits*

Jam

Jellies

Eggs, many cheeses (e.g. cheddar, parmesan, ricotta)

Butter

Oil

Appendix D: Gluten-free products obtainable in Britain

Supplier's name and address

A Montedison Pharmaceuticals Ltd.
   Kingmaker House
   Station Road
   Barnet
   Hertfordshire EN5 1NU

B Farley Health Products Ltd.
   Torr Lane
   Plymouth PL3 5UA

C Cow and Gate Ltd.
   Trowbridge
   Wiltshire BA14 8HZ

D Welfare Foods (Stockport) Ltd.
   63 London Road South
   Poynton
   Stockport
   Cheshire SK12 1LA

E G F Dietary Supplies Ltd.
   7 Queensbury Station Parade
   Queensbury, Edgware
   Middlesex HA8 5NP

Reprinted, with kind permission, from *The Crossed Grain*, April 1979.

Index

Page numbers in *italics* indicate tables or diagrams.